unsettling welfare:
the reconstruction of social policy

social policy: welfare, power and diversity

series editor: john clarke

This book is part of a series produced in association with The Open University. The complete list of books in the series is as follows:

Embodying the Social: Constructions of Difference, edited by Esther Saraga

Forming Nation, Framing Welfare, edited by Gail Lewis

Welfare: Needs, Rights and Risks, edited by Mary Langan

Unsettling Welfare: The Reconstruction of Social Policy, edited by Gordon Hughes and Gail Lewis

Imagining Welfare Futures, edited by Gordon Hughes

The books form part of the Open University course D218 *Social Policy: Welfare, Power and Diversity*. Details of this and other Open University courses can be obtained from the Course Reservations Centre, PO Box 724, The Open University, Milton Keynes MK7 6ZS, United Kingdom: tel. (00 44) (0)1908 653231.

For availability of other course components, contact Open University Worldwide Ltd, The Berrill Building, Walton Hall, Milton Keynes MK7 6AA, United Kingdom: tel. (00 44) (0)1908 858585, fax (00 44) (0)1908 858787, e-mail ouwenq@open.ac.uk.

Alternatively, much useful course information can be obtained from the Open University's website http://www.open.ac.uk.

unsettling welfare: the reconstruction of social policy

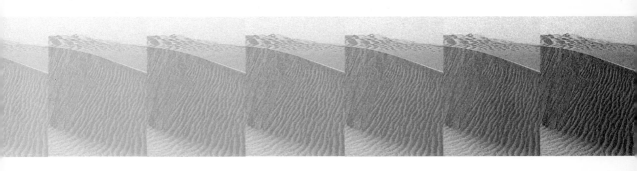

edited
by
gordon
hughes
and
gail
lewis

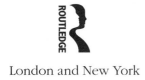

London and New York

in association with

The Open
University

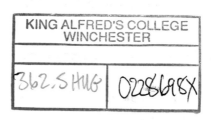
First published 1998 by Routledge
11 New Fetter Lane, London EC4P 4EE

Simultaneously published in the USA and Canada
by Routledge
29 West 35th Street, New York, NY 10001

Edited, designed and typeset by The Open University
Printed and bound by Scotprint Ltd, Musselburgh, Scotland

British Library Cataloguing in Publication Data
A catalogue record for this book is available from The British Library

Library of Congress Cataloging in Publication Data
Unsettling welfare: the reconstruction of social policy / Gordon Hughes and Gail Lewis, eds.
p. cm. – (Social policy – welfare, power and diversity: 4)
Includes bibliographical references and index.
1. Public welfare – Great Britain. 2. Great Britain – Social policy – 1979 – . 3. Great Britain – Social policy. I. Hughes, Gordon, 1952. II. Lewis, Gail. III. Series.
HV248.U57 1998
362.5'0941 – DC21   97–48928
                                                                                       CIP.

ISBN 0-415-18133-X (hbk)
ISBN 0-415-18134-8 (pbk)

1.1

Contents

Preface

Unsettling Welfare: The Reconstruction of Social Policy is the fourth of five books in a new series of introductory social policy texts published by Routledge in association with The Open University. The series, called *Social Policy: Welfare, Power and Diversity*, examines central issues in the study of how social welfare is organized in the UK today. The series is designed to provide a social scientific understanding of the complex and fascinating issues of social welfare in contemporary society. It specifically examines the key issues arising from questions concerning the changing nature of the welfare state and social policy in the UK, giving particular emphasis to the processes of social differentiation and their implications for social welfare. The series also emphasizes the ways in which social problems and solutions to them have been socially constructed and are subject to historical change. More generally, the books use social scientific theories and research studies together with, and in contrast to, other forms of 'knowing' about social welfare and social issues (such as common sense). This is done in order to raise key questions about how society 'works', how social change occurs, and how social order is maintained.

The five books form the core components of an Open University course which shares the title of this series. The first book, *Embodying the Social*, examines the central issue of how patterns of social difference are socially constructed. It traces the implications of such constructions for social policy – for example, the effects of shifting conceptions of disability – and examines their contested character. In exploring these concerns, this first book begins to establish the central focus of the course and series on *diversity*, the formations of *social difference*, and *power*, in particular the power to define our understanding of such differences.

The second book, *Forming Nation, Framing Welfare*, addresses the relationships between nation, state and social welfare by tracing the historical conflicts and constructions that have shaped our modern conceptions of national belonging and welfare rights and duties. The book explores the making of the nation – the inclusions and exclusions of different social groups – and the role of social policy in that process.

The third book, *Welfare: Needs, Rights and Risks*, focuses on a rather different issue, namely the questions of who gets welfare and under what conditions. This book examines how categories of need, desert, risk and rights play a central role in constructing access to welfare, particularly in circumstances where arguments over rationing, priority setting and limited resources are central to the forming of social policies.

This fourth book, *Unsettling Welfare*, deals with the rise and fall of the welfare state in the UK, and traces the ways in which the relationship between social welfare and the state has been reconstructed at the turn of the twentieth century. In particular, it focuses on the consequences of the break-up of the political, economic and social settlements that had sustained the 'old' welfare state in the thirty years after the Second World War.

The fifth and final book, *Imagining Welfare Futures*, looks at the prospects for the further remaking of social welfare around the focal points of citizenship, community and consumerism.

Because these books are integral elements of an Open University course, they are designed in distinctive ways in order to contribute to the process of student learning. Each book is constructed as an interactive teaching text, and this has implications for how the book can be read. The chapters form a planned sequence, so that each chapter builds on its predecessors and each concludes with a set of suggestions for further reading in relation to its core topics. The books are also organized around a series of learning processes:

- *Activities*: highlighted in colour, these are exercises which invite you to take an active part in working on the text and are intended to test your understanding and develop reflective analysis.

- *Comments*: these provide feedback from the chapter's author(s) on the activities and enable you to compare your responses with the thoughts of the author(s).

- *Shorter questions*: again highlighted in colour, these are designed to encourage you to pause and reflect on what you have just read.

- *Key words*: these are concepts or terms that play a central role in each chapter and in the course's approach to studying social policy; they are highlighted in colour in the text and in the margins.

While each book in the series is self-contained, there are also references backwards and forwards to the other books. Readers who wish to use the series as the basis for a systematic introduction to studying social policy should note that the references to chapters in other books of the series appear in bold type. The objective of this approach to presenting the material is to enable readers to grasp and reflect on the central themes, issues and arguments not only of each chapter, but also of each book and the series as a whole.

The production of this book and the others that make up the series draws on the expertise of a whole range of people beyond its editors and authors. Each book reflects the combined efforts of an Open University course team: the 'collective teacher' at the heart of the Open University's educational system. Each chapter in these books has been through a process of drafts and comments to refine both its content and its approach to teaching. This process of development leaves us indebted to our consultant authors, our panel of tutor advisers and our course assessor. It also brings together and benefits from a range of other skills – of our secretarial staff, editors, designers, librarians – to translate the ideas into the finished product. All of these activities are held together by the course manager, who ensures that all these component parts and people fit together successfully. Our thanks to them all.

John Clarke

Introduction

by Gordon Hughes and Gail Lewis

This book explores the reconstruction of social welfare in the UK in the last decades of the twentieth century. In the 1970s there was a consensus among academics, political commentators and much of the public that there was something called 'the British Welfare State'. A collection such as this would therefore have been assumed to be about this 'thing' called 'the Welfare State'. Changes since the 1970s now mean that we cannot write about the welfare state as an obvious and unproblematic reference point for studying how social welfare 'works' in the contemporary UK. Social welfare has been subject in the last decades of the twentieth century to a profound, though uneven, process of deconstruction and reconstruction which together we have called 'unsettling'.

The implications of these changes for the study of welfare have been two-fold. First, it has meant that attention must be paid to the shifts in the production and distribution of welfare services. This involves analysis of the economic, political, social and organizational contexts in which such production and distribution take place. Second, it has required a consideration of the very *meanings* attached to state-organized and state-legitimated welfare services. These two aspects form the central threads of this collection.

The book begins with two introductory chapters which offer the reader a broad mapping of what we term the 'old' and 'new' welfare settlements in the UK since the Second World War. Chapter 1 focuses on the nature of the 'old' social democratic welfare state of the immediate post-war period; in particular, we explore the myths and contradictions of this complex project of social reconstruction. Four types of welfare settlement – 'political', 'economic', 'social' and 'organizational' – are introduced as an analytical means for understanding both the consolidation of the 'old' welfare state and its subsequent demise. Chapter 2 examines the main criticisms and crises of the social democratic welfare state. This chapter also offers an overview of the major processes of welfare reconstruction since the 1970s and not least how the public sphere has been reconstituted.

In Chapters 3 to 8 we focus on six specific areas of social policy – health, housing, probation, education, social care and income maintenance – in the light of the broad processes of change and 'unsettlement' mapped in Chapters 1 and 2. These chapters thus provide the reader with the opportunity to concentrate on how the reconstruction of social welfare in the UK has impacted, often unevenly, in particular areas of social welfare and social policy. In reading these specific 'case studies', the reader will encounter rich and detailed material illustrating both the common cross-sector and sector-specific changes. It will become evident that the reconstructions around social welfare cannot easily be explained in terms of any simple break between the 'old' and the 'new'. The chapters highlight important points of continuity as well as of discontinuity with the past, and our focus on the four 'settlements' provides the analytical framework for thinking about such continuities and discontinuities. These chapters are necessarily selective in their focus, concentrating on welfare reconstruction and policy shifts in each field within the framework established in the first two chapters. Changes in welfare policies, criteria of entitlement, and systems of delivery continue at a rapid pace and in this sense some of the detail outlined in this collection will be quickly superseded. The unique contribution of this book lies in its demonstration of a framework for analysing welfare policy and practice which retains its strength despite the speed with which further shifts in welfare policy are occurring.

Chapter 9 turns its attention to the discourse and practice of managerialism, analysing its content, contradictions and status as a mode of co-ordinating relations within and between welfare organizations. This allows us to revisit the wider processes of welfare restructuring which Chapters 1 and 2 analysed in terms of four 'settlements' and to consider the more specific welfare policies, explored in Chapters 3 to 8, through the lens of managerialism.

Finally, Chapter 10 offers a conceptual review of the whole book. It focuses on the following questions:

- Is it possible to discern 'new welfare settlements' in the 1990s in contrast to those of the 'Beveridgean' welfare state?
- Have new 'welfare subjects' been created as a result of the post-1970s processes of welfare restructuring?
- And, finally, is there now a new welfare order, built around a repositioning and reconstitution of the public, the state and social welfare in the UK at the end of the twentieth century?

This book emphasizes that social welfare in the contemporary UK has been subject to a profound 'unsettling' during the 1980s and 1990s. What is less clear is what new welfare order may emerge in future years. Our concern here is to illustrate the social and political conflicts that played a part in the making, dismantling and reconstruction of social policy during the second half of the twentieth century. By the end of this book the reader will nonetheless be clear that it is vital to understand that social welfare has always been an object of both political and theoretical controversy. This situation is unlikely to change in the twenty-first century.

CHAPTER I

'Picking over the Remains': the Welfare State Settlements of the Post-Second World War UK

by Gordon Hughes

Contents

1 Introduction

There have been major changes in welfare policies across many different countries over the last decades of the twentieth century, so much so that the term 'welfare state' is no longer taken for granted as a point of reference for understanding social policy in the contemporary UK. Indeed, the changes since the 1970s mean that it is now arguable as to whether we any longer live in a welfare state. The nature of these changes and the questions they raise for the nature of UK society are the key concerns of this book. For the most part, this book is focused on the developments in social welfare in the UK during the last decades of the twentieth century. However, we also place great emphasis on understanding social issues, events and processes in terms of their historical context and thus their historical antecedents. Any investigation of the changing character and context of social welfare in the late twentieth and early twenty-first centuries therefore needs to be aware of the structures, conditions and discourses which prevailed in the era of the supposedly fully-fledged welfare state in the UK in the period after the Second World War.

This chapter's aim is therefore to provide a thorough and critical understanding of the 'old' welfare state as a starting-point for this book. However, our discussion is not of the descriptive 'nuts and bolts' variety – until recently the common content of UK social policy literature. We will, of course, attempt to clarify the nature of this social construction termed the welfare state, but you will also discover that it never was a homogeneous or unified entity. Rather, the welfare state may be more productively understood as the result of a complex, contested and fragile set of arrangements which in this book we term 'settlements'. Furthermore, you will examine the ways in which the welfare state itself became, and remains, a powerful metaphor in its own right for, alternatively, images of the 'good' or 'bad' society, according to the perspective of different commentators. The study of the 'thing' we call the welfare state, and indeed the 'post-welfare state' discussed in Chapter 2, is central to the book-wide theme of seeing phenomena as the product of contested constructions through competing discourses, political struggles and ideologies.

settlement The concept of settlement is central to the whole project of this book. It is therefore important to clarify in concrete terms what the concept of settlement means. By 'settlement', we do not want to imply that the frameworks through which state-regulated welfare is delivered are fully fixed and agreed upon by everybody. Rather, a kind of framing consensus becomes established which sets the limits within which compromises over what and how, and by whom and for whom, welfare services and benefits are delivered. In this sense, then, a 'settlement' is a set of positions negotiated by the key or most powerful groups in society. The concept of 'settlement' as used here refers to a set of arrangements that create a temporary period of stability or equilibrium, even while they remain complex, contested and fragile. As such, there will always be some groups who are marginalized or subject to conditional inclusion in the process of negotiation. Such groups either have their welfare needs ignored by the state-organized institutions or have them met to some extent, but in a stigmatized or 'residual' way. There is thus a hierarchy of inclusions in the welfare state.

This chapter suggests that what we call the 'welfare state' was a complex and contradictory project. Its social effects have been evaluated in different ways: some have emphasized how the welfare state provided collective security and promoted social cohesion; others, however, have argued that it created dependency and excluded or oppressed some social groups in the process of providing social welfare. It is important to recognize that the concern with collective provision and social security grew out of pre-war experiences of, and popular struggles against, insecurity, gross inequality and lack of social justice. The welfare state emerged from varieties of political and social struggles against inequality, vulnerability and oppression. However, the post-war welfare state project was also tied to the keen interest among economic and political elites in managing and regulating the disorderliness of markets and labour forces as ways of making UK capitalism work more efficiently.

The idea of a 'settlement', then, points us to two issues. First, it directs our attention to the terms of reference of the compromise: the frameworks of ideas, principles and commitments within which (most) thinking about social welfare takes place. Secondly, it points to the different special interests, groups or demands that are (temporarily) reconciled in this compromise – and reminds us that there may be other groups who are excluded, marginalized or subordinated in this process. Settlements, then, are central to how social welfare is defined, constructed and organized.

You may feel this definition is very vague and abstract. Let us try to make it more tangible by looking at a specific illustrative example from welfare policy during the post-war period in the UK. There was, for example, a 'settlement' between the organized labour movement, capital and government structured in part around the notion of the 'social wage' for the male 'breadwinner' and a commitment to full male employment throughout the period of 1945 through to the 1960s. This settlement involved key competing interest groups or power blocs (the Labour and Conservative parties, the trade union movement, big business or corporate capital) arriving at a negotiated ideological consensus in which conflicts and differences existed between the key players, but all within a constraining and bounded framework of compromise. Thus, despite important differences between the Attlee Labour government of 1946–51 and the Conservative governments of 1951–64 (Whiteside, 1996), a commitment was maintained towards the principle of full (male) employment and the 'family wage'. The organization of welfare and the categories of people (whom we term welfare subjects) and types of need to which it was directed, thus establish the shape of the social relations of welfare. Apart from reflecting the patriarchal nature of the powerful blocs involved in the compromise, it is important also to note that the settlement over the 'family wage' and full (male) employment also reflected the colonial/imperialist assumptions and institutional practices of the time in the increasingly post-imperial UK state. It was assumed, for example, that migrant workers from New Commonwealth countries would not be beneficiaries of this 'racialized' settlement, positioning them as an excluded category of people (excluded welfare subjects). This example also reminds us it is important to remember that the welfare state in the UK was (profoundly) influenced by processes beyond the boundaries of the nation-state. Sections 3, 4 and 5 of this chapter in particular offer an analysis of the post-war processes of social policy and social welfare in terms of the international context in which the society was structurally located. Arising out of this discussion, we argue that a complex set of settlements (separated out for analytical purposes only and distinguished in terms of being *political, economic, social* and *organizational* in character) emerged and merged to make up what we may term for short-

consensus

welfare subject
social relations
of welfare

5

hand purposes the 'old' welfare state. Having established the complex realities of this welfare state formation, we will then be in a better position to explore and explain its demise in Chapter 2 and later chapters of this book.

2   Myths and 'realities' about the UK welfare state

The welfare state in the post-war UK has had an existence which is more than simply a collection of institutions and practices aimed at the delivery of social welfare. Indeed the UK welfare state has also been surrounded by myths and symbolic imagery of what it is to be a 'UK citizen'.

ACTIVITY 1.1

Let us begin with a seemingly simple question: when did the welfare state come into existence and what was its duration? In answering this question you should try to put a date to or to specify a period of time when you would estimate the welfare state in the UK emerged historically and how long it lasted.

COMMENT

Like me, you may well have struggled to have come up with an entirely satisfactory or conclusive answer to the question. However, some of you, perhaps drawing on your own experiences and memories, may have come up with a specific date such as 1948 when the National Health Service (NHS) Act was passed in Parliament. For others, it may have been dated in terms of the end of the Second World War and the Labour electoral victory in 1945. There is therefore no right or wrong answer to this question. For some very influential commentators in the academic discipline of British social policy, it was a distinct era in social policy in the mid twentieth century when there was a widespread consensus in society about the need for state intervention of a positive nature in the lives of the citizenry to guarantee a secure and decent life for all (Marshall, 1950). In a more chronologically exact and perhaps intellectually foolhardy fashion, Moran (1995) has dated the emergence of the welfare state in the UK fairly precisely in terms of the entry of Labour politicians into Churchill's war-time Coalition government in 1940 and suggested that the era of consensus ended with the changes in economic policy forced on the Labour government by the economic crisis of 1976. And yet for some commentators the welfare state never existed as a distinct post-war creation but was instead a messy mishmash of policies drawing on long-term trends in the state–society interface (or boundary) in modern societies, with severe limitations to any notion of a cross-party political consensus on welfare (Glennester, 1995). For others, such as Ginsburg (1992), the post-war welfare state is seen as a distinct formation, whose roots can be traced to the late nineteenth century, in which the state takes on substantial and complex welfare functions within capitalist, patriarchal and racialized societies. In turn, historians such as Evans (1994) point to the period between the First World War and the 1970s as an age of collectivism, and the inevitable development of the social policy reforms of the Liberal government of 1906–14. There is therefore no settled view as to the precise origins and periodization of the 'welfare state'.

■ ■ ■

Can you think of different ways in which the idea of the welfare state has been used?

There are several possible answers to this question which come to mind.

1   The welfare state describes a distinct set of institutional arrangements.
Arguably, the welfare state has most commonly been viewed and understood as a supposedly distinct set of institutional arrangements for the state delivery of social welfare. Thus, for example, Bryson defines the welfare state as follows: 'The term *welfare state* is used when a nation has at least a minimum level of institutionalized provisions for meeting the basic economic and social requirements of its citizens' (Bryson, 1992, p.36). Key components among such provisions would be a system of social security/income maintenance, education, health, social services and the near universal provision of basic needs (for a fuller outline, see **Langan, 1998**).

2   The welfare state can be seen as an ideological representation.
In contrast to the first answer above, another answer would be that the welfare state has really only existed as a powerful image within a discourse about 'the British nation', both after the Second World War and in the throes of imperial decline. The image of the welfare state may thus be viewed as an ideological and imaginary representation of the 'state of the nation' in the post-war UK and   **representation**
beyond. If you are old enough, you may have memories of how the 'coming' of a free and comprehensive health service, perhaps tangibly embodied in a figure such as the school nurse (the 'nit nurse' in the common parlance of the 1950s), appeared to usher in a new, more collectivist, 'deal' for 'ordinary' British people. Furthermore, protection from 'the cradle to the grave', celebrated in the arrival of the NHS in 1948, retains a powerful appeal decades later. Indeed, following

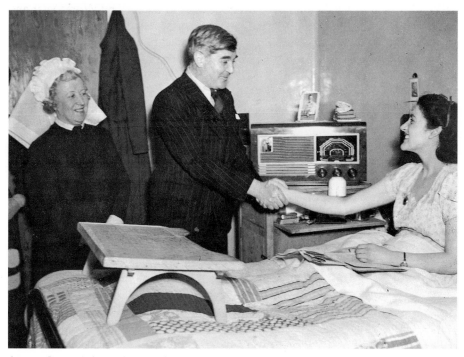

Aneurin Bevan, Labour Minister of Health, visiting Papworth hospital, a centre for tubercular diseases, in May 1948, just before the National Health Service came into operation

the hardship of the 1930s and the grim struggles of the Second World War, the arrival of state-run welfare schemes in the post-1945 UK was accorded a utopian potential for an altruistic and more collectivist (as against individualist) society by some social science commentators (for example, Titmuss, 1958). With the powerful rallying calls of social security, social justice, collectivism and altruism, it is perhaps easy to see why the post-war programme of reconstruction appeared to offer a 'social democratic vision of the welfare state as the mechanism for taming capitalism through redistributive social policy' (Pierson, 1991, p.177). Such altruistic tendencies in post-war collectivism continue to be celebrated by defenders of the 'old regime' (Page, 1995).

3   The welfare state has been a key concept in the discipline of social policy. Apart from its status as a powerful ideological icon or image in the post-war UK, the welfare state has also been the key concept in the academic study of social problems and social welfare, in other words in the discipline of social policy. Indeed, we may note that the academic study of social policy itself has been built up around the conceptualization of social welfare as the province of the state. Thus social policy as a discipline has been dominated by the notion of the state as the embodiment of social reform which through the application of expertise will promote universal social citizenship. Similarly, Sullivan has observed that the dominant notion of the welfare state in both popular and academic representations has been constructed on the assumption of state control and state provision (Sullivan, 1992, p.216).

<hr>

ACTIVITY 1.2

This assumption of social welfare as being the almost exclusive province of the state has been a dominant notion in the discipline of social policy. In the light of this, consider the following question:

What limitations does this view of the central role of the state in the organization and delivery of welfare impose on the study of social welfare, past, present and future?

<hr>

COMMENT

This assumption about the central importance of the state to any understanding of social welfare in much of the academic literature in part reflects the powerful effects of the post-war welfare state settlements on supposedly detached academic commentators. A major limitation of this view of social welfare as the almost exclusive province of the state is its conceptual tunnel vision towards non-state forms of social welfare provision. In particular, we may point to such activities as 'informal care' in the domestic sphere (performed largely by women) which have, arguably, always been more significant in meeting human needs than the state-organized delivery of welfare. But we might also mention welfare purchased from private sources (such as personal pensions) or welfare services provided by voluntary or charitable organizations.

■ ■ ■

Thinking further on the problem of defining the welfare state as an integral institutional entity, it may be argued that there has never been a coherent and tightly organized institutional entity that forms the welfare state. In the post-war

UK, the welfare state has been loosely made up of a combination of government departments and both central and local arrangements through which the state has pursued social policies or performed its welfare functions. Once again, such questioning of the idea of the welfare state as a coherent and homogeneous institutional entity is not intended to detract from its crucial importance in promoting social welfare or creating tangible improvements in the quality of the lives and life-chances of many people during this period. We should not lose sight of the effects of different welfare policies and practices on real human beings, but this is not the same as treating these in an undifferentiated way as 'the welfare state'.

Alongside these social effects, the welfare state has also served a profound symbolic function in political and ideological formations since the reforms of the 1940s in the UK. It may be suggested, then, that the welfare state represented a particular but powerful symbolic conception of the relationship of the 'British people' to the state, as we will explore in some depth in section 3 below. In much British social policy literature the welfare state has also been given a peculiarly British meaning, epitomizing something akin to the national spirit, as the following quotations from two influential textbooks illustrate:

> ... the term 'Welfare State' is a useful description of that synthesis of past pragmatism and future aspirations which was the achievement of social policy in 1948. The Welfare State represented the social consensus of the British people in the middle of the twentieth century.
>
> (Fraser, 1973, p.222)

> ... the Welfare State is the practical British answer to the practical problems of industrial development and mass society which, though Britain was the pioneer, every people in the world has to face.
>
> (Bruce, 1968, p.30)

You may already be well aware that much of the work of the social scientist is concerned both with the deconstruction of popular myths and also with unveiling the story of particular social constructions (see **Saraga, ed., 1998**). Much of what follows in this chapter will develop Jordan's remark that the post-war welfare state consensus in the UK was 'a very complex social construct' (Jordan, 1987, p.8).

This section has introduced you to the complex and contested idea of the welfare state in the UK. We have suggested that it is difficult to try and say when the welfare state emerged historically. Furthermore, it was argued that we may wish to be sceptical about seeing the welfare state as a unified, homogeneous institutional entity. Instead, this chapter and Chapter 2 will attempt to offer an alternative framework to that of traditional social policy explanations for the understanding of the changing strategies of organizing social welfare in the post-war UK state.

3   Traditional explanations of the rise and consolidation of the welfare state in British social policy

In this section we will focus on three of the most influential theses on the 'British' welfare state associated with the work of three social scientists – Tom Marshall, Richard Titmuss and John Saville. By analysing these three competing but comparable explanations, you will gain important insights into how both the birth and consolidation of the UK welfare state have been traditionally understood in the discipline of social policy and how we may need to move beyond this traditional paradigm or conceptual framework.

Let us begin by outlining in brief these important traditional explanations of the UK welfare state. We shall first examine Marshall's social reformist and evolutionary thesis on citizenship, followed by Titmuss's sociological analysis in terms of post-war altruism and social solidarity. Finally, we shall focus on Saville's class struggle explanation.

Marshall's interpretation of the rise and subsequent consolidation of a social democratic welfare state in the post-war UK was optimistic about the possibilities of social inclusion and the avoidance of class conflict through the rise of a third form of citizenship, namely social citizenship, following the earlier historical evolution of two other crucial forms of citizenship (legal and political). It is important to note that citizenship in Marshall's formulation is about the possession of formal, equal rights (for example, to vote and equality before the law). There seemed to be a hope expressed by Marshall that equality of status would become more important than equality of income. Let us explore briefly what this distinction implies.

Marshall's work was part of a reforming liberal tradition that saw a line of development towards a state in which injustices of inequality are overcome without fundamental change in economic or social institutions. Marshall (1950) thus envisaged a future in terms of 'a decent and secure life irrespective of the amount earned'. This thesis appears to celebrate a peculiarly British compromise in which the worst excesses of capitalism were tamed and yet the 'extremes' of socialism were also avoided. Thus the capitalist system was profoundly reformed: 'Social policy had not only done so much to humanize conditions of life and work; it had altered the structure of society by admitting the working class to full membership of the community and giving its members the full status of citizenship' (Marshall, 1965, p.96). This British social policy tradition, emphasizing steady or evolutionary progress, has been institutionalized in basic teaching texts (see, for example, the statements by Fraser (1973) and Bruce (1968) above on the gradual but inexorable growth of welfare legislation). In some ways this tradition has read like a story of the triumph of rational social administration and policy over the forces of darkness and ignorance.

Apart from Marshall, the other major mainstream analyst of the welfare state in the discipline of British social policy in the immediate post-war years was Richard Titmuss (1958, 1970). Titmuss emphasized the crucial importance of war-time experiences for the development of the welfare state in the UK. For Titmuss, the significance of the Second World War lay in its effect of generating a national sense of collective solidarity and shared hopes for a better society in the immediate post-war period. This emphasis on *collective solidarity* links

inclusion
citizenship

Titmuss back to the influential work of the nineteenth-century sociologist, Emile Durkheim, and the body of work called 'communitarianism' which emphasizes the crucial function of informal communal bonds in both the maintenance of social order in general and the realization of social welfare in particular (on appeals to community and communitarianism, see **Hughes and Mooney, 1998**). In the context of Titmuss's emphasis on national unity, it is important to recall that the Beveridge Report of 1942 (and thus written during the war) wrote of five giants which the nation needed to vanquish once the war was over. In its portrayal of the five giants of Want, Disease, Ignorance, Squalor and Idleness, the Beveridge Report deliberately endowed these social problems with monstrous personae and made explicit patriotic comparisons between this struggle and the fight against the fascist enemy abroad (Jordan, 1987, p.79). The specific context of the UK's costly victory in the Second World War is thus crucial to Titmuss's (1958) interpretation of the post-war project of social as well as economic reconstruction. According to Glennester, 'The [war-time] experience convinced Titmuss that universal social institutions that met the needs of the whole population were the only way in which a modern state could be held together as an organic whole' (Glennester, 1995, p.100).

Both Marshall and Titmuss contrast in many ways to Saville's influential Marxist interpretation of the welfare state as the result of class conflict and struggle. Put briefly, Saville (1957) emphasized that the basis for welfare reforms lay in large part in the class struggles of the British working class since the nineteenth century to gain some basic rights and protection from the capitalist

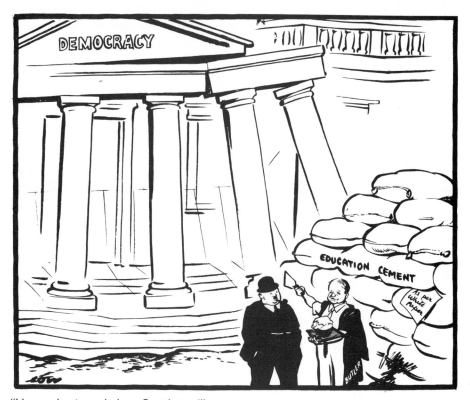

"I know what it needs, boss. Foundations!"
(Butler's Education Act 1944 aiming to create good citizens)

Right turn

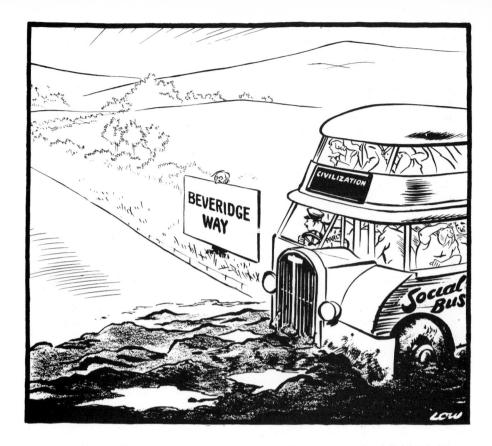

system. At the same time such struggles led to compromises from the ruling capitalist class, such as providing greater security for the working class, albeit a security paid for by the contributions of the workers themselves. Saville thus questions whether the welfare state in the UK was a 'half-way house to socialism' and instead contends that it was an example of a capitalist society adapting to internal pressures from below without leading to any significant redistribution in wealth, property or power.

ACTIVITY 1.3

Drawing on the introductory comments on each theorist above, you should now read the brief extracts from Marshall, Titmuss and Saville given in Extracts 1.1, 1.2 and 1.3. In particular, you should try to identify and unpack the major assumptions implied in the three accounts presented about the nature of the welfare state in UK society. When reading these accounts remember that they represent competing perspectives on the welfare state rather than necessarily being the 'truth'.

Extract 1.1 Marshall: 'Citizenship and welfare'

The basic human equality of membership has been clearly identified with the status of citizenship. (p.9)

… the modern drive towards social equality is, I believe, the latest phase of an evolution of citizenship which has been in continuous progress for some 250 years. (p.10)

I propose to divide citizenship into three parts. I call these three parts or elements, civil, political and social. (p.10)

... By the social elements I mean the whole range from the right to a modicum of economic welfare and security to the right to share to the full in the social heritage and to live the life of a civilised being according to the standards prevailing in the society. The institutions most closely connected with it are the educational system and the social services. (p.11)

Citizenship requires ... a direct sense of community membership based on loyalty to a civilisation which is a common possession. It is a loyalty of free men [sic] endowed with rights and protected by a common law. Its growth is stimulated both by the struggle to win those rights and by their enjoyment when won. (pp.40–1)

The extension of the social services is not primarily a means of equalising incomes. In some cases it may, in others it may not. The question is relatively unimportant; it belongs to a different department of social policy. What matters is that there is a general enrichment of the concrete substance of civilised life, a general reduction of risk and insecurity, an equalisation between the more and the less fortunate at all levels – between the healthy and the sick, the employed and the unemployed, the old and the active, the bachelor and the father of a large family. Equalisation is not so much between classes as between individuals within a population which is now treated for this purpose as though it were one class. Equality of status is more important than equality of income. (p.56)

(Marshall, 1950, pp.9–11, 40–1, 56)

Extract 1.2 Titmuss: 'War and the welfare state'

Not only was it necessary for the State to take positive steps in all spheres of the national economy to safeguard the physical health of the people; it was also an imperative for war strategy for the authorities to concern themselves with that elusive concept 'civilian morale'; with what Professor Cyril Falls called, in his Lees Knowles lectures in 1941, 'demostrategy'. By this he meant, in military terms, that the war could not be won unless millions of ordinary people, in Britain and overseas, were convinced that we had something better to offer than had our enemies – not only during but after the war. This requirement of war strategy was stated, more explicitly, in a memorable leader in *The Times* soon after the last British troops had left the Dunkirk beaches. It was a call for social justice; for the abolition of privilege; for a more equitable distribution of income and wealth; for drastic changes in the economic and social life of the country.

...

The social measures that were developed during the war centred round the primary needs of the whole population irrespective of class, creed or military category. The distinctions and privileges, accorded to those in uniform in previous wars, were greatly diminished. Comprehensive systems of medical care and rehabilitation, for example, had to be organized by the State for those who were injured and disabled. They could not be exclusively reserved for soldiers and sailors, as in the past, but had to be extended to include civilians as well – to those injured in the factories as well as the victims of bombing.

(Titmuss, 1958, pp.82–3)

Extract 1.3 Saville: 'Welfare in capitalist society'

The Welfare state, it will be suggested, has come about as a result of the interaction of three main factors: (1) the struggle of the working class against their exploitation; (2) the requirements of industrial capitalism (a convenient abstraction) for a more efficient environment in which to operate and in particular the need for a highly productive labour force; (3) recognition by the property owners of the price that has to be paid for political security. In the last analysis, as the Labour movement has always recognised, the pace and tempo of social reform have been determined by the struggle of working class groups and organisations; but it would be historically incorrect and politically an error to underestimate the importance of either of the other factors in the situation. To do so would be to accept the illusion that the changes are of greater significance than in fact they are, as well as to misread the essential character of contemporary capitalism.

...

... There are three points to be made in this connection. The first is that at least part of the additional share of the national income accruing to the working class in the post-war years has been absorbed by higher indirect taxation to pay for the increased social services. Secondly, the major redistribution occurred during the war years: and since then, the official calculations show a slow but persistent trend towards greater inequality. This is, of course, what must always be expected of capitalism, for it continuously generates inequality. Thirdly, the official calculations of income distribution, the basis for many sweeping generalisations made by those who are convinced they have been living through major historical changes in Britain since 1945, omit three factors whose individual and collective effect is to increase sharply the inequality of incomes. These are (i) capital gains, (ii) expense allowances, and (iii) tax evasion; and only the politically innocent really believe that the official figures of taxable income for the upper income brackets represent the true position.

Concerning the distribution of property in the country there is no dispute. The Welfare state, with its higher death duties and its supposedly crippling and burdensome taxation upon the rich, has effected practically no change in the distribution of private capital ...

The Welfare state is the twentieth-century version of the Victorian ideal of self-help: and since this involves, in addition to benefits, high taxation on alcohol and tobacco, it must be said that these aspects of the Welfare state, taken by themselves, cannot be objected to by Socialists. The state now 'saves' for the working class and translates the savings into social services. As the *Economist* remarked in 1950 of the social services: 'It is still true that nobody – or practically nobody – gets anything for nothing.' Since the Welfare state in Britain developed within a mature capitalist society, with a ruling class long experienced and much skilled in the handling of public affairs, its growth and development has been slow and controlled: and the central interests of private property have never seriously been challenged. Britain remains a society in which the distribution of capital wealth is no more equal than it was half a century ago: and although income distribution has proved more amenable to political pressure from the Labour movement, there exists within any capitalist society strong and powerful tendencies offsetting egalitarian measures.

(Saville, 1957, pp.5–6, 23–4)

COMMENT

There are clearly important differences of viewpoint between the three accounts. Marshall offers an evolutionary theory of the rise of the third form of citizenship, namely social rights, implying equality as a member of the community rather than economic equality per se. The evolution of social citizenship thus appears to be the result of processes going deep back into British history. Titmuss, on the other hand, places great emphasis on the specific conditions and challenges resulting from the war whereby altruism and collectivism came to the fore. Titmuss also holds what we have termed a 'communitarian' view of welfare which means that he saw welfare as an expression of common values that bind otherwise disparate individuals together. By way of contrast with both Marshall and Titmuss who in their different ways 'celebrate' the rise of the welfare state in the UK, Saville offers a much more sceptical explanation of the phenomenon. In particular, Saville views the welfare state as a crucial means of 'saving' capitalism in the long run from the threat of class revolution.

■ ■ ■

There are important differences in their accounts of the nature of UK society and how the rise of the welfare state is to be understood in this context. However, the authors may also be said to share certain assumptions in their diagnosis of the crucial 'subject' in the story of welfare in the UK. All three commentators appear to carry assumptions about the gendered and racialized nature of their respective subject, namely the central social groups involved in the formation of the welfare state. For Titmuss, it is the returning soldier; for Marshall, the new, white, heterosexual, male and working 'social citizen'; while Saville gives the central role to the British, white, male working class. The highly gendered nature of assumptions in traditional social policy literature about citizenship (equated with being a male worker with dependent wife and children) has been clearly noted by feminist work (Williams, 1989). We will explore in section 4 below how such assumptions may have structured the dominant demographic picture of the post-war UK. Furthermore, the body of traditional social policy analysis associated with key writers such as Marshall, Saville and Titmuss was arguably marked by profound absences with regard to the complex international dimension to the post-war welfare state in the UK and to the UK's place in the new world order of the post-war years. With the benefit of hindsight, it is noticeable that no mention is made in the three accounts of the global context within which the UK had been a privileged and powerful player in the pre-war period and how the post-war period saw a serious erosion of this privileged and powerful role.

More recent scholarship on the UK's colonial and imperialist legacy has begun to challenge the neglect by the discipline of social policy of the 'outside' world (which also had a largely hidden internal presence in the UK in the 1940s and 1950s) (Williams, 1991). It may be argued that the powerful symbolic function played by the notion of the 'British' welfare state is only explicable in the context of international processes such as the loss of empire and the UK's more subordinate economic and political role in a world dominated by the rise of the USA to 'super-power' status and the perceived threat of the Soviet Union during the Cold War. You will note that this chapter does not attempt to be comparative in the sense of comparing the similarities and differences between countries with regard to their specific welfare states (see Esping-Andersen, 1990; Cochrane and Clarke, eds, 1993). However, it does see the international context as relevant to the discussion of the origins and development of the UK welfare state.

In the sections which follow we build on the knowledge gained here about the limitations in the traditional social policy literature to develop an alternative framework for understanding the post-war state and its particular 'settlements' in the UK.

4 'Picture the nation': demographics and the post-war UK

Every social policy pursued by a nation-state presumes a certain general population profile or knowledge of particular categories of people within the general population. Any mass vaccination programme of young children, for example, requires a fairly accurate notion of how many needles, number of doses and nurses may be required to carry out such a project. Statistical profiles are thus a vital tool of the modern state. The experts who undertake the study and compilation of population profiles are termed demographers and these **demographics** (sub-)population profiles are generally termed demographics. Demographics may be most easily understood as being about the characteristics associated with a given national population at a particular time. It is argued in this section and in Chapter 2 that a critical understanding of demographics at particular times in the history of the welfare state is crucial to an understanding of the changing ideology and practices of social welfare provision. We also contend that demographics are themselves socially constructed.

Having described demographics as the characteristics associated with a given national (sub-)population at any one time, it may appear at first sight that the demographics of a nation are nothing more than the numbers of people who live within the borders of the nation-state. In other words, demographics may seem to be merely a descriptive and technical picture or 'snapshot' of the nation at a specific point in history. This simple understanding is one aspect of a national demographics but it is only the starting-point for the social scientist. This statistical picture of the nation at any one historical moment may be broken down into a whole range of smaller groupings according to criteria such as age, sex, 'race' and ethnicity, region, health, sectoral and occupational grouping, patterns of employment, type and place of residence, marital status. Apart from being interesting in themselves, such demographic profiles are also important for welfare states because they have implications for estimates about the level of need, the types of needs, their geographical and social distribution, and the ways in which they may shift over time.

In the rest of this section we briefly consider the demographic profile of the United Kingdom in the immediate post-war period and by implication the population profiles which were assumed by the architects of the welfare state. It is important to do this for three interrelated reasons.

- Firstly, a particular demographic profile forms part of the basis upon which the policies of a welfare state are both conceptualized and made.

- Secondly, it is necessary to consider the demographic profile when thinking about the changes to welfare which were implemented in the immediate post-war period. As you will see in greater depth in Chapter 2, it is on the basis of changes in the demographic profile of the national population that political debate about the need for and forms of a restructured welfare state were in part played out in the last decades of the twentieth century. Demographics are thus not uncontested constructs of the population but are particular portraits that are invoked politically at different times, whether it be the 'idle poor' in the nineteenth century or 'single mothers' in the late twentieth century. It is important to hold on to this point as it reminds us that the national population is also a category constructed out of demographic diversity.

■ The third reason why it is important to consider changes in the demographic profile is because it is from these sites of diversity that particular welfare needs and demands emerge.

In the 1940s and 1950s demographers pointed out that the population trend for the UK was one of declining numbers compared to earlier decades. It was noted, for example, that the mean household size in England and Wales had fallen from 4.6 members in 1891 to 3.7 in 1931 to 3.2 in 1951 (Stevenson, 1984). Table 1.1 illustrates how the birth and death rates in Great Britain had also changed between 1901 and 1945.

Table 1.1 Birth and death rates in Great Britain, 1901–45

	Births per thousand population		*Deaths per thousand population*	
	England and Wales	*Scotland*	*England and Wales*	*Scotland*
1901–05	28.2	29.2	16.0	17.0
1906–10	26.3	27.6	14.7	16.1
1911–15	23.6	25.4	14.3	15.7
1916–20	20.0	22.8	14.4	15.0
1921–25	19.9	23.0	12.1	13.9
1926–30	16.7	20.0	12.1	13.6
1931–35	15.0	18.2	12.0	13.2
1936–40	14.7	17.6	12.2	13.6
1941–45	15.9	17.8	12.8	14.1

Note: Data from Registrar-General's *Statistical Review of England and Wales*, and Registrar-General, Scotland, *Annual Reports*.

Source: Stevenson, 1984, Table 11, p. 148

The major concern of demographers and policy-makers was 'the question of replacement', namely the decreasing numbers of young people relative to older age cohorts such that the population overall was in decline. As a result of such scientific analyses and the public disquiet generated in political and policy circles, a Royal Commission on Population was established in 1944 which reported its findings and recommendations in 1949. According to the Royal Commission, the chief factors identified as lying behind this trend were emigration, mortality and the size of the family (resulting particularly from the use of birth control). Apart from examining the facts relating to the population trends in the UK, their causes and consequences, the remit of the Commission was to consider what measures should be taken 'in the national interest' to influence the future trend of population. In particular, the Commission was specifically concerned about the loss of the UK's competitive edge internationally versus other countries if the UK's population were to decrease. The greatest problem identified from the demographic trends was the low level of family size. However, the Commission also addressed the difficulties caused by trends in both emigration and immigration.

ACTIVITY 1.4

You should now read Extract 1.4 which outlines the Royal Commission's view on the problem caused by the small average family size of (white) British citizens in the immediate post-war period. In particular you should think about the ideological assumptions carried in the extract with regard to the role of (white) British citizens in the world and that of (black) Commonwealth citizens in the UK. What policy implications might result from such an analysis of the 'nature' of the immigrant population entering the UK?

Extract 1.4 Royal Commission on Population: 'Immigration and emigration'

Problems of immigration

Immigration on a large scale into a fully established society like ours could only be welcomed without reserve if the immigrants were of good human stock and were not prevented by their religion or race from intermarrying with the host population and becoming merged in it. These conditions were fulfilled by intermittent large scale immigration in the past, notably by the Flemish and French Protestant refugees who settled in Great Britain at different times. There is little or no prospect that we should be able to apply these conditions to large scale immigration in the future, and every increase of our needs, e.g., by more emigration from Great Britain or by a further fall in fertility, would tend to lower the standards of selection.

All these considerations point to the conclusion that continuous large scale immigration would probably be impracticable and would certainly be undesirable, and the possibility – it can be regarded as no more than a possibility – that circumstances might compel us to consider or attempt it is among the undesirable consequences of the maintenance of family size below replacement level.

…

The trend of population and the national interest, 1949

Migration

A low level of average family size discourages emigration and encourages immigration; and it seems on the whole likely that the present boom in emigration will be short, emigration will tend to diminish, and there may be continuing pressure to bring in immigrants to make good shortages in particular occupations. This prospect we regard as among the undesirable consequences of a sub-replacement family size because (*a*) the sources of supply of suitable immigrants are meagre and the capacity of a fully established society like ours to absorb immigrants of alien race and religion is limited and (*b*) a diminishing flow of British emigrants to other parts of the Commonwealth may have serious consequences for the economic and political future of Great Britain and the Commonwealth as a whole.

Even if average family size in Great Britain were maintained at replacement level or a little over, which is the most that seems probable, it is unlikely, given good economic conditions here, that emigrants from Great Britain would amount to more than a third or a quarter of the immigrants which the Dominions would need if they wanted to maintain their pre-1930 rates of growth. It is likely therefore on present trends that the British element in the Commonwealth will tend to diminish. This fact presents a problem of vital concern to the whole Commonwealth, and we urge that it should be studied jointly by the Governments of Great Britain and the other Commonwealth countries. This study would of course bring under review Great Britain's economic prospects and the political and strategic implications of the use of atomic energy and other developments that affect national defence.

Imponderables and conclusions

Among the many imponderable considerations that must enter into the question of the desirable trend of population are the effects on the security and influence of Great Britain. The population of the USA is now nearly three times, and that of Soviet Russia, nearly four times, that of Great Britain, and no change in future numbers that is at all likely would reduce these proportions; indeed they must be expected to increase. Great Britain however, is the centre of a Commonwealth spread throughout the world. Even this is an unduly narrow approach to modern problems of power and influence. Not only in the eventuality of war but in maintaining a balance of strength by which war may be averted, it is in association or alliance with other States that the British Commonwealth is likely to be important. The drift of world affairs is giving a new emphasis to the conception of Western civilisation as an entity possessing reality and value. This lends significance to the fact that the modern fall in the size of the family towards and often below replacement level is a phenomenon common to most of the peoples of Western civilisation and virtually confined to them. Their rate of increase has markedly declined while that of Oriental peoples has markedly accelerated. The establishment or continuance of size of family below replacement level might accentuate a change in relative numbers as radical as that which occurred between France and Germany in the 19th century and might be as decisive in its effects on the prestige and influence of the West.

This question is not merely one of military strength and security; it merges into more fundamental issues of the maintenance and extension of Western values and culture. The effective force of this wider commonalty depends on the vitality of its constituent parts, which in turn is affected by their trends of population.

(Royal Commission, 1949, pp.124–5, 225–6)

COMMENT

The Royal Commission on Population (1949) gives us a clear illustration of the profoundly racialized nature of debates on the population and welfare during this period and beyond. In particular, the Commission was part of a wider debate on the need for new sources of labour for the UK economy. The diminishing flow of British emigrants to parts of the Commonwealth was viewed as a threat to the post-imperial success of both the UK and the Commonwealth. The colonialist and racist notion of 'the white man's burden' as civilizing agency had clearly not disappeared from mainstream political discourse. In terms of the policy implications arising out of its analysis of the 'nature' of the immigrant population entering the

UK, the Commission discussed the problem of how to dispose of migrant labour when surplus to requirement and who should be eligible to stay. Explicit in the categorization of the new immigrants from the 'New Commonwealth' countries (for which, read 'black' people) was a concern that the nation's 'stock' would be diminished in quality as a result of 'continuous large-scale immigration'. The Commission emphasized that those who stayed should be 'of good human stock' and were not prevented by their religion from intermarrying with the 'host' population and becoming merged in to it. This racialized discourse was to continue to re-surface and influence subsequent immigration and race relations policies throughout the post-war period in the UK (Ginsburg, 1992).

■ ■ ■

The demographics of this immediate post-war period suggested a specific picture of the UK population. It was assumed that there was a clear (and natural) division of labour between men and women based on the role of women as 'homemaker', in other words wife and mother. Men, on the other hand, were primarily understood as the 'breadwinner', that is the head of household as husband and father. In turn, full-time paid employment was the norm for men. Heterosexual monogamy institutionalized in marriage was the normal, 'natural' framework for adults living together. It is important to note again that such normative assumptions became institutionally embedded in the laws regarding, and everyday practices of, state-provided welfare.

'Ah ... Bisto!' The 'British' family at home?

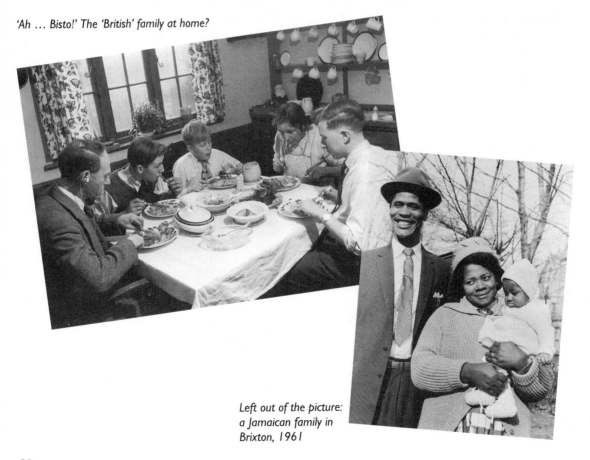

Left out of the picture:
a Jamaican family in
Brixton, 1961

5 Beyond the monolithic welfare state: the post-war welfare settlements in the UK

This final section introduces you to the four analytically distinguished welfare settlements – political, economic, social and organizational – which emerged in the post-war period in the UK. As you will remember, the term 'settlement' in this context is used to capture the complex compromises and negotiated positions reached by competing interest groups and power blocs in specific historical contexts. The concept of settlement does not thus exclude political and ideological differences but instead points to the bounded limits to such differences. A settlement thus establishes the frameworks of reference within which conflict, negotiation and shifting alliances take place. Furthermore, such settlements also served to exclude or marginalize a range of interests (Clarke and Newman, 1997). In particular, we draw on the work of Fiona Williams (1989, 1991, 1996) who has argued that conventional social policy analysts have ignored the highly gendered, racialized and disablist character of the post-war welfare state in the UK.

Whereas most previous social policy literature conventionally treated the development of the UK welfare state as a process resting on a double settlement based on economic and political conditions (see, for example, Mishra, 1984), Williams' work introduced a third crucial settlement, which we may term the social settlement, organized around the ideological triangle of 'nation, family and work'. Williams' analysis thus opened up the study of social policy in general, and of the UK welfare state in particular, to the investigation of the ideological formations and material social relations which were produced and reproduced in the activities of the welfare state. More specifically she also pinpointed the discriminatory racist, sexist and disablist consequences of such activities. In other words, the social settlement involved the production of the types of 'included' people who were the subjects imagined and realized by the 'Beveridgean' welfare state, such as the 'universal citizen' figure of the male breadwinner bringing home the social wage for his dependants (wife and offspring). At the same time, this social settlement also produced those who would be marginalized from full membership of the UK citizenry but conditionally included as 'inferior' or 'dependent' welfare subjects – such as black people, women, 'immigrants', disabled people.

Beveridgean welfare state

Clarke, Cochrane and McLaughlin (eds, 1994) have opened up the study of the welfare state further by means of their conceptualization of a fourth settlement which they term organizational. As we will see shortly, this settlement concerned the specific organizational conditions for the provision and delivery of social welfare in the post-war welfare state in the UK.

We will now introduce you to each of the four settlements. Following this exposition of the complexly constituted construction which was the 'old' Beveridgean welfare state, more recent developments around the 'crisis' of the welfare state, examined in the subsequent chapters of this book, should be better understood. It should also be apparent from what follows that the welfare state was a product of quite specific historical processes and compromises rather than the inevitable and natural evolution of the British 'national spirit' implied in some influential traditional social policy interpretations discussed in section 3 above.

5.1   The political settlement

social
democratic
consensus

Although there is the danger of exaggerating the unity of opinion across political parties with regard to the post-war welfare state project (see Glennester, 1995), most commentators point to the existence of a social democratic consensus during the period from 1945 to 1975.

What do you think is meant by a social democratic consensus?

Let us try to clarify what this notion of a social democratic consensus in post-war Britain implies. A political consensus may be defined as the set of common assumptions and the continuity in the main policies pursued by the chief political parties when in power over a given period of time. In turn, the term 'social democratic' may be understood as implying the ideological commitment to the gradual transformation of capitalism through the agencies of parliamentary democracy and the state. Social democratic consensus thus captures the common ground shared across the main political parties as to the desirability and commitment to reforming capitalism through gradual reform from 'above' (i.e. the state) rather than revolution from 'below'. Furthermore, throughout this period both the Labour and Conservative parties claimed credit for the expansion of the welfare state, improvements in education and housing, and the claimed reductions in inequality and poverty which were often financed by increases in public expenditure and redistributive taxation.

The main planks of this post-war political consensus have been usefully summarized by Kavanagh and Morris (1994) as follows:

- support for the 'mixed economy', epitomized by the nationalization of key public utilities such as coal and steel and a commitment to the government's management of the economy but with the bulk of the economy remaining in private hands and run on capitalist lines;

- commitment to full employment which remained below 3 per cent for most of the period;

- active conciliation of the trade unions;

- support for and expansion of the welfare state following the Beveridge Report of 1942;

- foreign and defence policies which supported the shift from Empire to Commonwealth and the consolidation of close links with the USA and Western Europe against the Soviet threat.

As Kavanagh and Morris (1994, p.6) note, 'These policy goals formed something of a social democratic package. It was a middle way: neither free market capitalism (as in the United States) nor state socialist (as it was to emerge in Eastern Europe).'

The notion of a social democratic consensus does not imply that there were no dissenting voices. As early as 1952, two leading young Conservative MPs, Iain Macleod and Enoch Powell, argued against the redistributive nature of social service delivery and argued for a selective means-testing of claimants to relieve destitution and misfortune. They argued that there would be a decline in individual initiative and family responsibilities with the expansion of social services. High taxes in turn were viewed as a disincentive to work (Macleod and Powell, 1952). However, such voices were to remain marginal until the

1960s when there was a gradual growth of selective benefits and services, in part to save money and in part to target the worse off. This latter period (1960s–1970s) did, then, see a partial shift from the universalist principle of welfare, but there was still cross-party commitment to public provision through the welfare state.

During the immediate post-war period there were also critics on the left who argued that the welfare state had not gone far enough. Thus Aneurin Bevan (1952) defended the original National Health Service as a socialist project in the following manner:

> The National Health Service and the Welfare State have come to be used as interchangeable terms, and in the mouths of some people as terms of reproach. Why this is so it is not difficult to understand, if you view everything from the angle of a strictly individualistic competitive society. A free health service is pure Socialism and as such it is opposed to the hedonism of capitalist society. To call it something for nothing is absurd because everything has to be paid for in some way or another.
> (Bevan, 1952, p.106)

We may note in passing that Bevan resigned from his post as Minister for Health when the Labour government introduced further charges for prescriptions in 1951.

Let us return to a description of the dominant political settlement in this post-war period. Throughout the decades of the 1950s, 1960s and early 1970s, key politicians and policy-makers appeared to share many common assumptions about the need for state intervention, both to regulate the workings of the economy and to deliver public goods. Important differences did exist in the priorities of, for example, the Attlee Labour government of 1945–51 and the Conservative governments of 1951–64, with the former committed to universalism, the planned economy and 'fair shares for all', whilst the latter were committed to a return to 'sound finance' and, if possible, 'targeting' of the needy (Whiteside, 1996). However, all administrations of this period had a shared faith in the state as an agency of social improvement or what has often been called 'big government' in the late twentieth century. In this vein, the Conservative journalist T.E. Utley (1949, p.10) accepted that: 'The central problem of British home policy since the war has been the problem of how to combine full employment with low wages and a production great enough to make the welfare state safe. Everything that any political party says or does in home affairs must be referred back to that.'

In accord with the influential thinking and policy recommendations of both the policy adviser William Beveridge and the economist John Maynard Keynes (both seen as key architects of the post-war reconstruction of the UK), leading political actors in Britain and in other Western capitalist societies 'assumed state power could become the caretaker and moderniser of social existence' (Keane, 1988, p.4). Indeed, as early as 1926, Keynes had predicted that, 'In the future, the government will have to take on many duties which it has avoided in the past' (p.301). Post-war developments appeared to confirm this prediction.

In turn, the Beveridge Report of 1942 put forward a plan for social insurance based on a universal flat rate of insurance contributions and benefits. Beveridge thus offered a plan for social security based on the contributory social insurance principle of 'giving in return for contributions, benefits up to subsistence level, as of right and without means tests' (Beveridge Report, 1942, p.42). The logic of the Report was inclusive, that is, it intended to give people a greater stake in

political settlement

society than had been the case in the pre-war period. However, at the same time the key theme of the Report was that of security for all citizens (paid by their own compulsory contributions) – a 'domain of collective security' (Rose, 1996) – rather than promoting greater equality. This emphasis on creating a more secure society within the 'shell' of a capitalist mode of production reflected the political settlement in this period.

Neither Keynes nor Beveridge were radical critics of either capitalism or indeed of the ethos of self-help and individual responsibility. The notion of a guaranteed minimum to create security was certainly seen as an advance on pre-war welfare provision but it was not meant by Beveridge to usher in dramatic changes in redistribution. Thus the Beveridge Report may be seen as offering a middle way with its mixture of radicalism (universal and comprehensive insurance) and caution (familiar and 'familialist' core values, for example, about the roles of men and women and individual self-reliance). In Beveridge's words: 'The State should offer security for service and contribution', but 'the State in organizing security should not stifle incentive, opportunity and responsibility' (Beveridge Report, 1942, p.92). By 1950 influential Conservative politicians such as R.A. Butler to a great extent shared the same assumptions as those embedded in the Beveridge Report, as shown in the following passage: 'It is the task of the present generation of Conservatives to found our modern faith on the basis of two features of this age, namely the existence of universal adult suffrage and the acceptance by authority of the responsibility for ensuring a certain standard of living, of employment and of security for all' (Butler, 1950, p.3).

It is obvious that the Beveridgean welfare state does not represent the transcendence of capitalism nor a Fabian 'half-way house' to socialism (Saville, 1957). However, the project was important in other ways, in creating the conditions of existence of greater social justice and solidarity in capitalist societies, particularly by means of increased opportunity and mobility for constituencies in the working and lower middle classes. Commenting on comparative trends in the development of welfare states across different countries, Baldwin (1990, p.18) has noted that, 'Protection against risk has been sought more universally than a redistribution of resources.' We should add that only *certain* risks affecting social groups in *specific* ways have been the focus of such protection. Post-war welfare states appeared to be important examples of collective political attempts, not least including middle-class beneficiaries, to protect against risk and develop forms of 'social security' in the generic sense of the word. For example, during the 1940s it was assumed that the state would be able to weld society together through such initiatives as the NHS by advancing goals worthy of collective pursuit. This emphasis on the crucial role of the state in the planning and realization of social development (and thus a more 'open' society based on merit) is generally termed 'statism' as opposed to approaches such as the New Right which emphasize the strictly limited role of the state in the workings of the economy and the key role of the free market in creating progress (see Chapter 2).

There also appeared to be some consensus across political parties over the style of government or 'statecraft' at this time, in contrast to the period covered in Chapter 2. This aspect of the political settlement involved the incorporation of the powerful, patriarchal, white British and able-bodied trade union movement into the process of policy-making. It was symbolized during the war by the entry into Churchill's Coalition government of the most influential trade union leader of the time, Ernest Bevin. In subsequent decades, there was a high level of consultation about policy between the government and bodies like the trade union movement leadership, employers' organizations and business federations, aimed at a consensus across potentially conflicting sides. This system of negotiation and consensus-building is often termed corporatism by social scientists. Such political incorporation may be viewed as an attempt to ensure that the organized (male, white and 'able-bodied') working-class movement would co-operate in the pursuit of reforms needed to ensure that the British economy might regain its edge in international competition.

    The political settlement was closely linked to the economic settlement, which is the focus of the following section.

corporatism

5.2   The economic settlement

The economic settlement was in large measure structured by the Keynesian solution to the world-wide problem of an unmanaged capitalist economy which was prone to crises. Keynesianism represented an immensely influential approach to economic theory and policy in the post-Second World War period. It was highly critical of traditional laissez-faire economics. The latter assumed that the unregulated, 'free' market would tend towards full employment and hence equilibrium by its own 'natural' processes. Keynes questioned this orthodoxy. Instead, he argued that governments wishing to achieve full employment had to intervene actively in the economy by stimulating aggregate or collective demand. Conversely, if full employment resulted in inflation (that is, the rise in the general level of prices which brings about an increase in the money supply), then governments had to act to reduce demand. On both accounts, governments needed to use the interventionist devices of tax policy, government expenditure and monetary policy. This approach formed the basis of most Western societies' economic policies from the 1940s through to the early 1970s. Put simply, the Keynesian solution was that of a (state) managed capitalist economy, based on full (male) employment and economic growth. The oscillations of the capitalist economy (booms and slumps) were to be reduced by the strategy of 'demand management' by the state. Continued economic growth would sustain the increased public spending necessary to fund the welfare state. This settlement in turn implied that the UK's financial and industrial base would be restructured and modernized, not least with the active agreement of both capital and labour.

economic settlement

Keynesianism

    Reflecting the intellectual and practical influence of Keynes on the development of economic policy in the post-war period, the post-war welfare state has been widely referred to as the 'Keynesian welfare state'. According to one commentator, 'This term is meant to denote not only a society characterized by the existence of a welfare state and the manipulation of the economy to retain full employment: it also refers to a way of funding the development and growth in the welfare state' (Sullivan, 1992, p.226).

    In a similar fashion, Beveridge's proposals supported full (male) employment as a means to more consumption, leisure and thus a higher standard of living. Full employment and ambitious welfare schemes were thus seen as going hand in hand with the 'free society' (Beveridge, 1944). The institutional commitment of the state to this approach may be discerned, for example, in the Employment

Policy White Paper of 1944, which committed government to using the resources of the state in a systematic way in order to reduce unemployment.

Apart from the commitment to full (male) employment, the economic settlement involved what we have earlier termed *'corporatist'* decision-making. In a corporatist system, powerful organized groups (i.e. state, organized labour and big business) negotiate between themselves on such issues as incomes, policies and economic planning.

Overall, government responsibility for economic management and the establishment of the 'mixed economy' of private and public industries and utilities seemed the only way to 'civilize' capitalism and further promote economic growth. At the same time, Keynesian economics remained committed to managed markets and thus illustrated the limited role of the state vis-à-vis the capitalist economy in this settlement.

ACTIVITY 1.5

You should now look back over the two subsections on the political and economic settlements. Pay particular attention to the points of convergence and similarity around:

- the process of decision-making in politics and economics;
- the relationship of the state to the economy.

COMMENT

There are clear points of convergence with regard to the preferred process of decision-making at both the political and economic levels. Across both levels, emphasis is placed on consensus and negotiation, as illustrated by the cross-party social democratic consensus and the role accorded to what is often termed corporatist decision-making between the state, organized labour and big business on economic matters. Furthermore, the relationship of the state to the economy is viewed as being that of a 'manager', eager to co-ordinate and intervene in the economic realm when required.

■ ■ ■

At this point, consider how the political and economic settlements can be compared.

It is important to remember that the settlements which we are discussing, such as the political and the economic, are difficult to separate out from each other in practice. There are, in fact, important points of convergence between the political and economic settlements. Thus we have argued that there were two key shared features of the political and economic settlements of the welfare state. The first was the general consensus that the state should intervene to regulate the economy and deliver welfare services and benefits. The second was the incorporation of the two sides of industry in the policy-making process, often termed corporatism. Remember again that we are separating out the settlements chiefly for analytical purposes to help us grasp the complex nature of the processes captured by the term 'the Keynesian welfare state'.

5.3   The social settlement

It should be clear by now that welfare institutions and policies are not separate from the wider patterns of social relations in the UK. The welfare state is thus the product of a society characterized by particular social patterns of, for example, class, 'race', gender, regional and disability differences and inequalities. Furthermore the welfare state in turn impacts on these patterns. This brings us to the notion of the social settlement of the Beveridgean welfare state. We have already referred to Williams' (1989) notion of a social settlement around the ideological triangle of nation, family and work. To explore its importance to the post-war social settlement further, it would appear that this triangle organized welfare practices around:

social settlement

- formations of national identity around 'race';
- familial divisions of labour around gender;
- work–welfare linkages around class.

In turn, such formations were articulated as an imaginary field of 'naturalized' social relations that constructed 'the British people' as particular types of citizens and beneficiaries of social welfare. In other words, it constituted them as 'welfare subjects'.

Let us now try to unpack this complex argument through the use of some illustrative examples of how this dominant 'naturalizing' ideological triangle operated (on 'naturalization', see **Saraga, ed., 1998**). Put differently, who were the 'subjects' and what was the nature of the population envisaged in the Beveridgean social welfare settlement? In this ideological triangle of nation, family and work, there is an unambivalent conception of the normal (British, white, non-'alien', 'able-bodied') family as the cornerstone of society (as literally 'pictured' in contemporary imagery of the family). In turn, the notion of the normal and natural family is predicated upon the desirability and importance of 'successful' monogamous heterosexuality within marriage: successful because enduring, productive of legitimate children and the socialization of the 'normal' future citizens. This assumption about the normal composition of the household as that of the nuclear family is not least reflected in the size of the typical post-war council house as three to four bedrooms. As you will see in Chapter 4, in the immediate post-war period council housing was viewed as modern, high-quality tenure, occupied mostly by the better-off working class. In turn, within this social settlement of the British welfare state, motherhood came to be defined in terms of full-time childcare and homemaking. This highly gendered notion of childcare responsibilities was, for instance, concretely reinforced and reflected by the Family Allowance Act 1946 as a result of which married mothers were granted non-contributory allowances to be paid to the mother for each child other than the first. The norm of secure and permanent employment for the majority of household heads – for which read predominantly white, heterosexual, able-bodied males – was also built into the structures of the social insurance scheme (national insurance, pensions, family allowance and so on) and, of course, presupposed a key role for the 'link worker' (i.e. women) in supporting the male head of household (Penna and O'Brien, 1996, p.44).

Of course, the socialization and training of children were not left solely to the family in this social democratic settlement. There was a whole range of public mass projects (such as schools, public housing, public broadcasting, social

'My baby works from nine to five ...' 1957 John Bull cover illustration

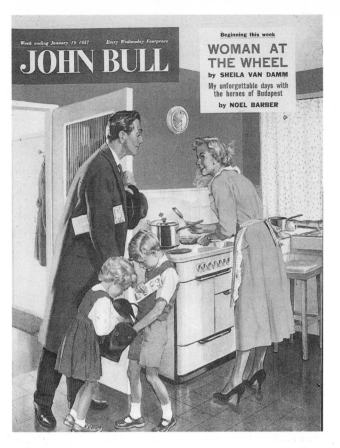

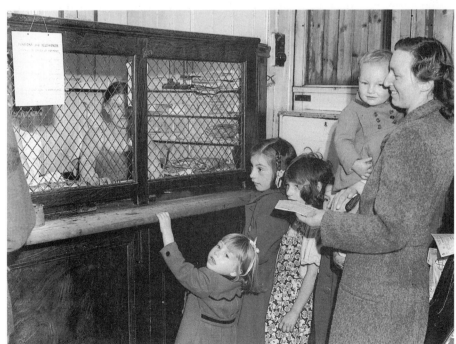

Collecting the 'family allowance': the implementation of the National Insurance Act 1946

insurance) whose ideological goal was to create and reproduce new forms of identity among the citizenry. In the field of schooling, for example, the state provided for the first time compulsory and free secondary education for all as a result of the Education Act 1944 (Chapter 6 covers this in more detail). As one instance of the positive drive towards change, by 1950 expenditure on education was four times greater than in 1940. It was an era of opportunity and mobility for some sections of the population, involving the selective promotion of social efficiency, meritocracy, social justice and the means of self-realization. As Evans notes, the new educational system provided an institutional highway to social and political advancement for a generation of 'able' working-class and lower middle-class children and this acted as a powerful piece of social engineering (Evans, 1994, p.21).

The 'normal' majority of the population was thus made up of the insured population of patriarchal, 'British'/white families supported by the family wage. However, a new space was also opened up for what we may term the 'safety-net' people who were no longer pauperized as in the pre-welfare state days (for further discussion, see Chapter 8). In Marshall's optimistic and influential account, welfare services for the first time were 'offered to all who needed them and free from any flavour of charity or taint of pauperism' (Marshall, 1965, p.84). However, the changes and resultant settlement would seem to be more complex and contradictory than Marshall allowed for. It would appear that a taint did cling tenaciously to those receiving means-tested assistance from the National Assistance Board and later from Social Security. In Beveridge's own words, assistance was cast as of lower moral standing than of insured ('earned') benefits. It was thus the recourse of 'cripples, the deformed ... and moral weaklings' (Glennester, 1995, p.41). With the exception of the minority of 'deviants', the population (both imagined and enshrined in the policies) of the Beveridgean welfare state was thus homogeneous, though class-divided, made up of a vast majority of solidly British/white nuclear families. As **Langan (1998)** notes, the welfare state arguably was founded on the projection of the particular interests of the adult male, white and able-bodied worker as the universal interests of society. And as Chapter 2 will show, this settlement was based on a highly circumscribed form of welfare universalism based on a hierarchy of dependencies.

What we may term the 'Beveridgean citizen' was thus effectively constructed as the fully employed, married, male worker who, through his taxes, supported the state, and the state in turn supported him through the provision of social welfare. Although this figure of the citizen emerges out of a quite specific politics of class compromise (between organized labour and capital), it is a profoundly gendered and ethnicized one. It is important to note that the British Nationality Act 1948 did confirm the rights of Commonwealth and colonial citizens to enter and settle in the UK (although these rights were consistently and increasingly undermined in subsequent decades). However, radical social policy analysts such as Norman Ginsburg (1992) have also noted that racism was institutionalized in several ways in the administration of social welfare during this period. There was thus a denial of access to 'persons from abroad' and the requirement of sponsorship for incoming settlers who should have no claim on public funds. Council house allocation policies similarly discriminated against recent immigrants through the residency qualification period and 'waiting-list' policy (Ginsburg, 1992, p.153). At a more general level, throughout the 1950s and

The Furnace: *painting by
Stanley Spencer celebrating
male physical labour*

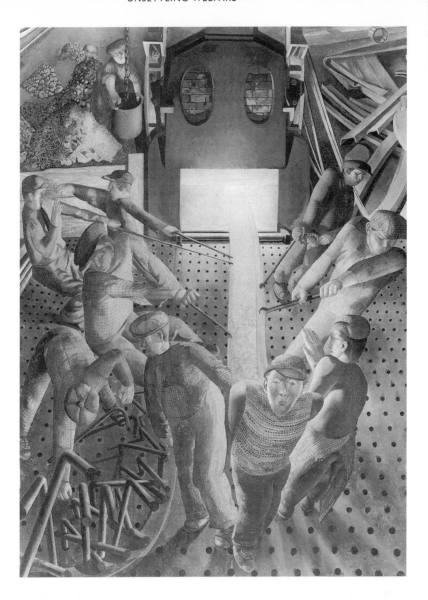

1960s black workers were recruited from the Caribbean by both private and
public sector employers as a cheap labour reserve. To give a concrete example,
Enoch Powell as Minister for Health in the late 1950s actively recruited 'cheap'
Caribbean workers to overcome labour shortages in the health and transport
industries and other public services.

Such examples from the immediate post-war period begin to show that the
social settlement in Britain was clearly racialized and affected by the colonial/
post-colonial context of the UK state. As the decades progressed, the racialization
of British politics in general was manifested in such apocalyptic speeches as
that of Enoch Powell in the 1960s – the same politician who had recruited
Caribbean workers into Britain in the 1950s – when in 1969 he forecast that
further immigration of black people into Britain would result in blood on the
streets and thus fanned the flames of white racism across the country: 'Like the
Roman I seem to see "the River Tiber foaming with blood".'

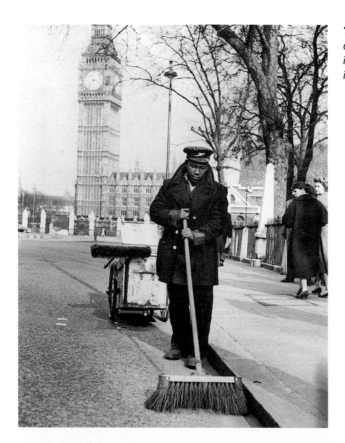

'A useful job and no-one objects': the conditional inclusion of black people in the post-war UK

ACTIVITY 1.6

You should now try to answer the following questions:

1 What were the central features of the new figure of the 'Beveridgean citizen'?
2 Which categories of people were excluded from this image of the archetypal citizen subject?

COMMENT

We saw that the quintessential new 'Beveridgean citizen' was the fully employed (and insured) married, white, able-bodied, male worker. Other categories of people included women, ethnic minorities, disabled people, children and the elderly, who, although not excluded from the welfare state, were subject to hierarchically organized forms of state welfare. In turn, such categories as minority ethnic groups and women were recipients of highly conditional forms of welfare inclusion and tended to occupy more dependent statuses in the welfare state compared to the 'Beveridgean citizen' of the mythical one-dimensional British nation.

■ ■ ■

Overall, then, the ideological triangle of nation, family and work established the mythology of this one-dimensional nation. In our discussion of this third, 'social', settlement, it has been argued that the key organizing principles of welfare state development in the UK should not be simply identified with paid work and thus class but must also recognize the crucial importance of the themes

31

of family and 'race'/nation. Any adequate analysis of the development of the welfare state needs to pay particular attention to the shifting relations of the massive historical forces of imperialism, patriarchy and capitalism (Williams, 1989, p.150).

5.4   The organizational settlement

The period under review witnessed an expanded role for the state and its organizational forms, both nationally and locally. Responsibilities for the organization and delivery of welfare provision were divided between different ministries at the national level and between central and local government in such areas as the administration of primary and secondary education and the provision of public housing. The organizational form of the welfare state was thus never monolithic but rather was made up of different departments, agencies and tiers of government which themselves were differently organized and constituted in England and Wales, Northern Ireland and Scotland. The welfare state was therefore a complex organizational structure.

organizational settlement

At the risk of over-simplifying the complexity of the organizational settlement in the Beveridgean welfare state, both professional and bureaucratic modes of co-ordination appear to have played a crucial role in this organizational settlement. Although different in important respects as modes of institutional organization, bureaucracy and professionalism were fused together as relatively compatible ideological components in this fourth settlement. Common to both components was an emphasis on *public service*, made up of distinct set of values, code of behaviours and forms of practice. Indeed Clarke and Newman (1997) have pointed out that both professionalism and bureaucracy, often as uneasy allies, became the characteristic mode of organizational co-ordination within the institutional arrangements of the 'old' welfare state. Despite critiques of bureaucracy and professionalism from both the right and the left (see, for example, Niskanen, 1971, and Wilding, 1982), it is important to remember the public service ethos in the past associated with both the bureaucrat, who was able to separate personal interest from the performance of organizational duty, and the professional driven by the vocation of expert service.

Neither bureaucracy nor professionalism were new modes of co-ordination specific to the post-1945 situation. As the sociologist Max Weber first noted, the notion of bureaucracy emergent in the nineteenth century aimed at the exclusion of partiality, patronage and corruption through the institutionalization of rule-bound procedures (Bendix, 1966). As a consequence, bureaucracy offered the promise of social impartiality and predictable outputs from trained staff. Similarly, professionalism was not new to the post-1945 situation given its nineteenth-century roots, but it was in the post-war period that it became nationalized and generalized, offering to all the promise of the application of valued, expert knowledge in the service of the public and embodied in the person of the professional. The merger of these principles of bureaucratic and professional

bureau-professionalism

co-ordination is sometimes described in the social sciences by the term bureau-professionalism. Bureau-professionalism played a distinctive ideological role in the routine operation of the Beveridgean welfare state in the UK.

Again, as we noted with regard to the very idea of the welfare state, bureau-professionalism was not just a set of technical, organizational practices. It carried clear implications for the social relations of welfare, particularly between the lay client and the professional expert. Bureau-professionalism thus also functioned at the level of what we term the *representational* dimension, depicting and symbolizing a quite specific people/state relationship of trust and deference from one actor (the lay person) to the other (the state expert). It also carried a very limited view of the role of the citizen with regard to the state (and its experts established as the all-knowing providers). This was confirmed by the general ascendancy of the objective determination of need over the subjective demand for services in the post-war welfare state. Such ascendancy in turn lay with the old professionals like doctors but also, to a lesser extent, with the new bureau-professionals such as social workers in the early 1970s (see Chapters 4 and 7).

The creation of a 'passive' and 'dependent' role for citizens with 'special' welfare needs was nowhere more apparent than in terms of what happened to disabled people in the welfare state. Although the Disabled Persons (Employment) Act 1944 represented an important 'advance' in treating disabled people as a single group for the first time, it remained focused on employers' attitudes rather than on the rights of disabled employees (Oliver, 1995, p.68). In a similar manner, Section 26 of the National Assistance Act 1948 placed a duty on local authorities to 'arrange' services for disabled people. Such policies, and the manner in which they were organized, established the professional and bureaucratic domination of welfare provision for disabled people throughout the post-war period, with concomitant disablist consequences (see **Hughes, 1998**).

The organizational settlement of the welfare state was predicated upon a paternalistic view of the role of the state and its technocrats in relationship to that of welfare recipients who were themselves often seen as 'inadequate' or problem people. Such paternalism was no doubt at times of positive value in enabling the power of the state to be used to protect people who needed special care. There was in Titmuss's (1970) terms a special moral quality in meeting the needs of strangers which was best effected through the anonymity of the state. However, what Bill Jordan terms 'the imperious certainties of bureau-professionalism' could also, in its well-meaning but patronizing delivery of assistance, 'crush or distort the lives of those who receive it' (Jordan, 1976, p.213).

In the old welfare state, then, the provision of services was delivered by state agencies and based on strategic planning within a unified service (rather than for example, by today's 'multiple providers'). For example, the Beveridge Report aimed at, and succeeded in, unifying the provision of unemployment and sickness insurance from being a system administered by both civil servants in the Ministry of Labour and 800 approved societies, each of which had thousands of local branches, to one scheme administered by central government (Glennester, 1995, pp.35–6). Thus the Beveridge Report (1942, pp.20–22) recommended: 'Change 1: Unification of social insurance … enabling each insured person to obtain all benefits by a single weekly contribution on a single document … Change 2: Unification of social insurance and assistance … in a ministry of Social Security with local security offices within reach of all insured persons.'

The organization of much of the old welfare state's services was thus based on the virtues of central planning and monopoly provision. However, these principles were tempered by the continuing importance of countervailing principles of co-ordination such as professional autonomy in health care.

The bureau-professionalism of state-run services has been presented as the dominant means of co-ordination in the old welfare state in the post-war UK. What were the major implications of this organizational settlement for the recipients of welfare services?

In this organizational settlement, the recipient of welfare services was viewed, and socially constructed, as a passive, deferential and dependent 'client'. In turn, this welfare client had no choice in terms of their preferred method of treatment or type of service (unlike that of an active consumer). The expertise of the monopolistic state service was not to be challenged in the organizational settlement of the old welfare state.

■ ■ ■

This section has introduced you to a more complex analysis of the so-called Beveridgean welfare state than that traditionally associated with both orthodox social policy accounts and popular commonsensical notions about the UK welfare state. Indeed, instead of assuming any simple homogeneity and consensus, it has examined how four major settlements – political, economic, social and organizational – may be distinguished analytically. Even these four settlements, used as analytical frames, cannot fully capture the complexity and interplay of social forces at work on the welfare state. However, they are valuable in alerting us to the complex processes of construction involved in the 'story' of the post-war welfare state. Awareness of these never truly 'settled' settlements will provide you with a useful basis for understanding the concerns of the following chapters in this book. Furthermore, understanding the complex nature of these settlements will, for example, help you to answer both the broad question of 'what has happened to the welfare state in Britain since the 1970s?' and the question of how the settlements were manifested and realized in the specific sites of welfare covered in Chapters 3–8 below.

6   Conclusion

This chapter has focused on the study of the welfare state as a complex product of specific historical conditions and compromises. It has been argued that the welfare state was never a unitary entity but rather was a complex pattern of relationships between the state, the market, and families and communities. As such, our narrative almost has the status of telling the story of something that never existed in the form in which it is usually understood! In this sense much of our discussion has dealt with the realm of what we have called the 'representational'. In simpler language this chapter is more about how one approaches and analyses the welfare state than it is about the welfare state 'in action'. Despite this, there are some key features to the Beveridgean welfare state which mark it off from more recent shifts in welfare organization and provision. Its distinctiveness lay in the general agreement that the state had a responsibility for ensuring a minimum standard of welfare for all its citizens and the *welfare state* was the form which emerged as being the most appropriate for implementing this responsibility.

To reiterate, the key features of the Beveridgean welfare state were:

- a systematic structure to organize and deliver social welfare;
- a degree of political consensus around the ideology of social democracy;
- a wide acceptance of the need for the state to manage the economy and maintain a high level of (male) employment together with economic growth;
- the establishment of a dominant norm around the patriarchal, white nuclear family and the social wage;
- in organizational terms, a bureau-professional mode of co-ordination together with a high degree of centralized provision of welfare;
- through the icon of the welfare state, the relationship of the state to 'the people' ideologically represented as one of unity.

By the mid to late 1970s these distinctive features were being seriously questioned and undermined. This was accompanied by an erosion of the economic growth which had underpinned the Beveridge reforms. Together these two factors established the pre-conditions for a radical attack on the welfare state which is the subject of Chapter 2.

Further reading

For useful historical overviews of the post-war history of welfare in the UK, see Glennester's *British Social Policy since 1945* (1995) and Timmins' *The Five Giants: A Biography of the Welfare State* (1996). On the life and work of Beveridge, see José Harris's biography (1977). On the post-war social democratic consensus, Kavanagh and Morris (1994) provide a lively and user-friendly overview. For a provocative contemporary defence of Keynesianism and the welfare state, see Will Hutton's *The State We're In* (1996). On the gendered and racialized welfare settlement, both Williams (1989) and Ginsburg (1992) offer important analyses, while on the Beveridgean organizational settlement, Clarke and Newman (1997) offer the clearest overview.

References

Baldwin, P. (1990) *The Politics of Social Solidarity: Class Bases of the European Welfare State, 1875–1975*, Cambridge, Cambridge University Press.

Bendix, R. (1966) *Max Weber: An Intellectual Portrait,* London, Methuen.

Bevan, A. (1952) *In Place of Fear* (London, Quartet Books, 1979).

Beveridge, W. (1944) *Full Employment in a Free Society: A Report*, London, George Allen and Unwin.

Beveridge Report (1942) *Social Insurance and Allied Services*, Cmnd 6404, London, HMSO.

Bruce, M. (1968) *The Coming of the Welfare State*, (4th edn; first pub. 1961), London, Batsford.

Bryson, L. (1992) *Welfare and the State: Who Benefits?*, London, Macmillan.

Butler, R.A. (1950) *Conservatism 1945–50*, London, Conservative Political Centre.

Clarke, J., Cochrane, A. and McLaughlin, E. (eds) (1994) *Managing Social Policy*, London, Sage.

Clarke, J. and Newman, J. (1997) *The Managerial State: Power, Politics and Ideology in the Remaking of Social Welfare*, London, Sage.

Cochrane, A. and Clarke, J. (eds) (1993) *Comparing Welfare States*, London, Sage/The Open University.

Esping-Andersen, G. (1990) *The Three Worlds of Welfare Capitalism*, Cambridge, Polity.

Evans, E. (1994) 'The enabling state: welfare and industrial society', *History Today*, June, pp.17–23.

Fraser, D. (1973) *The Evolution of the Welfare State: A History of Social policy since the Industrial Revolution*, London, Macmillan.

Ginsburg, N. (1992) *States of Welfare*, London, Sage.

Glennester, H. (1995) *British Social Policy since 1945*, Oxford, Blackwell.

Harris, J. (1977) *William Beveridge: A Biography*, Oxford, Clarendon.

Hughes, G. (1998) 'A suitable case for treatment? Constructions of disability' in Saraga (ed.).

Hughes, G. and Mooney, G. (1998) 'Community' in Hughes, G. (ed.) *Imagining Welfare Futures*, London, Routledge in association with The Open University.

Hutton, W. (1996) *The State We're In*, London, Vintage.

Jordan, B. (1976) *Freedom and the Welfare State*, London, Routledge and Kegan Paul.

Jordan, B. (1987) *Rethinking Welfare*, Oxford, Blackwell.

Kavanagh, D. and Morris, P. (1994) *Consensus Politics from Attlee to Major*, (2nd edn) Oxford, Blackwell.

Keane, J. (1988) *Democracy and Civil Society*, London, Verso.

Keynes, J.M. (1925) 'Am I a Liberal?', *The Collected Writings of John Maynard Keynes* (1972), vol.IX, *Essays in Persuasion*, London, Macmillan for The Royal Economic Society.

Langan, M. (1998) 'The contested concept of need' in Langan, M. (ed.) *Welfare: Needs, Rights and Risks*, London, Routledge in association with The Open University.

Macleod, I. and Powell, E. (1952) *The Social Services: Needs and Means*, London, Conserative Political Centre.

Marshall, T.H. (1950) *Citizenship and Social Class and Other Essays*, Cambridge, Cambridge University Press.

Marshall, T.H. (1965) *Social Policy in the Twentieth Century*, London, Hutchinson.

Mishra, R. (1984) *The Welfare State in Crisis*, London, Macmillan.

Moran, M. (1995) 'Reshaping the British State', *Talking Politics*, vol.7, no.3, pp.174–7.

Niskanen, W.A. (1971) *Bureaucracy and Representative Government*, Chicago, Aldine Atherton.

Oliver, M. (1995) *Disability: From Theory to Practice*, Basingstoke, Macmillan.

Page, R. (1995) 'The attack on the welfare state – more real than imagined? A leveller's tale', *Critical Social Policy*, issue 44/45, pp.220–28.

Penna, S. and O'Brien, M. (1996) 'Postmodernism and social policy: a small step forwards?', *Journal of Social Policy*, vol.25, pt.1, pp.39–61.

Pierson, C. (1991) *Beyond the Welfare State? The New Political Economy of Welfare*, Cambridge, Polity.

Powell, E. (1969) *Freedom and Reality*, London, Batsford.

Rose, N. (1996) 'The death of the social', *Economy and Society*, vol.25, no.2, pp.327–56.

Royal Commission on Population (1949) *Report of the Royal Commission on Population*, Viscount Simon (Chair), Cmnd 7695 (Simon Report), London, HMSO.

Saraga, E. (ed.) (1998) *Embodying the Social: Constructions of Difference*, London, Routledge in association with The Open University.

Saville, J. (1957) 'The welfare state: an historical approach', *The New Reasoner*, vol.1, no.3, pp.5–25.

Stevenson, J. (1984) *British Society 1914–45*, Harmondsworth, Penguin.

Sullivan, M. (1992) *The Politics of Social Policy*, London, Harvester Wheatsheaf.

Timmins, N. (1996) *The Five Giants: A Biography of the Welfare State*, London, HarperCollins.

Titmuss, R. (1958) *Essays on the Welfare State*, London, Allen and Unwin.

Titmuss, R. (1970) *The Gift Relationship*, Harmondsworth, Penguin.

Utley, T.E. (1949) *Essays in Conservatism*, London, Conservative Political Centre.

Whiteside, N. (1996) 'Creating the welfare state in Britain, 1945–1960', *Journal of Social Policy*, vol.25, pt.1, pp.83–103.

Wilding, P. (1982) *Professional Power and Social Welfare*, London, Routledge.

Williams, F. (1989) *Social Policy: A Critical Introduction – Issues of Race, Gender and Class*, Cambridge, Polity.

Williams, F. (1991) 'The welfare state as part of a racially structured and patriarchal capitalism' in Loney, M. *et al.* (eds) *The State or the Market: Politics and Welfare in Contemporary Britain*, London, Sage.

Williams, F. (1996) 'Postmodernism, feminism and the question of difference' in Parton, N. (ed.) *Social Theory, Social Change and Social Work*, London, Routledge.

CHAPTER 2

'Coming Apart at the Seams': The Crises of the Welfare State

by Gail Lewis

Contents

1   Introduction

In the previous chapter we saw how the welfare state comprised a number of 'settlements' and sets of institutional arrangements for the production and distribution of state-delivered and state-controlled welfare benefits and services. A further three points were stressed as necessary to an understanding of the overlapping settlements. First, it was noted that the 'old' welfare state was not a single, monolithic and homogeneous entity, but rather a complex series of overlapping and negotiated positions through which relations between a number of social actors were both structured and represented. Among these relations were those between the state and the citizen – especially in terms of the gendered positions within 'the family'; between the professional and the client; and between local and central government. In this way, it was argued, the welfare state was also an ideological construct through which the structural relations among the nation's people were imagined. Second, this 'old' welfare state was said to have emerged in the context of a particular set of international economic and political relations which followed on from the end of the Second World War. This economic and political context was exemplified in the declining position of the UK in the world economy; the anti-colonial struggles; the Bretton Woods agreements which set up the International Monetary Fund and the World Bank and established the terms in which financial relationships among nation-states were organized; and the particular mode adopted by the UK in the attempt to restore its economic competitiveness. Finally, the 'old' welfare state was contextualized within a specific national demographic profile. As we have seen, this included the average shape and size of household; a particular sex and age profile; the shape and size of the labour force; numbers classified as in poverty; the geography of health and ill-health; adult and infant mortality rates, and so on. The demographic profile was also an imagined construct in that the system of social insurance inaugurated by the Beveridge reforms was predicated on particular ideas about the ethnic make-up of the population and the social relations of gender and age by which it was characterized.

This chapter looks at the ways in which this post Second World War welfare state was restructured in the 1980s and 1990s. It considers the ways in, and the mechanisms by, which the four areas of 'settlement' were undermined and restructured as part of an attempt to redefine the terms of state-organized and state-regulated welfare. As with Chapter 1, this chapter provides a general overview of these changes and highlights the points of tension and contradiction which resulted from the restructuring. In offering a picture of the general contours of change, the chapter provides a point of reference against which Chapters 3 to 8 can be read.

2 Crisis and opportunity: general contours of restructured welfare

It is now widely accepted that by the mid 1970s the general conditions underpinning the 'old' or social democratic welfare state had been eroded. As a result, the 1970s marked the beginning of a major shift in the ways in which the welfare state was organized. The foundations of this shift lay in the interplay of declining economic competitiveness, social changes and the political challenges which arose from new or emergent political constituencies, such as those formed by feminism, anti-racism and the gay and lesbian movement. The decline of the UK's relative economic competitiveness (which had become increasingly apparent from the 1960s) was matched by both national and international capital beginning to renegotiate the conditions of employment (Clarke and Newman, 1997, p.9) and, indeed, investment. As capital became more mobile in its pursuit of opportunities for accumulation, new supplies of labour at cheaper prices were sought and established forms of worker protection were broken. In the UK of the 1970s these general trends were accompanied by a reorientation of fiscal and monetary regimes under what was called monetarism. These changes meant that the 'old' welfare state also became a target for radical change as it became the object of attempts at ideological and practical destabilization from the mid 1970s. As Pierson (1994, pp.2–3) has pointed out, under the social democratic consensus social expenditure – including that on welfare services and benefits – was part of both macroeconomic and microeconomic policy. It was seen as a means both to keep the economy working within certain bounds of upswing and downswing and as a means of offsetting the worst effects of downswing and market-produced inequalities.

Economic changes such as these were accompanied by social changes which expressed themselves in the make-up of the labour force and population more generally – for example, more married women entering the labour force; migrants from the New Commonwealth and Ireland; changes in the roles and distribution of power between men and women in families and households, and so on. Moreover, these social changes were increasingly given political expression as constituencies of 'new' political actors became organized around a series of dissatisfactions with the terms of the social settlement in the welfare state and the policies and practices found in many welfare institutions. Thus feminists, disabled activists, black and anti-racist activists, lesbians and gay men, together with squatters, claimants, older people and others, all began to push the boundaries of what has variously been called the 'old', the Beveridgean or the Keynesian welfare state by making demands for recognition of their autonomous welfare needs.

These diverse pressures grew in strength as the 1960s passed into the 1970s and it became increasingly evident that the boundaries of the 'old' or Keynesian welfare state could no longer be maintained. It is generally understood that the shift in the organization of state-controlled welfare involved a breakdown of the political consensus which was central to the Beveridge reforms; that different systems for the delivery of welfare were instituted; that at the heart of this was a radical realignment of the relation between the state, the individual citizen and the private sector; and that the financial and administrative arrangements for the provision of state-controlled welfare were fundamentally altered. **Langan**

(1998a) has written cogently about the ways in which these changes affected the definition of need and the mechanisms for meeting them. In this chapter we will look at some of these changes by considering the breakdown in the four areas of 'settlement' – that is, the economic, political, social and organizational. The chapter employs the term Keynesian welfare state, or KWS, though it should be remembered that this is the same as the 'old' or Beveridgean welfare state.

Before we go on to consider the ways in which the settlements of the KWS have been restructured, it is worth re-emphasizing the point that the welfare state was never conceived to be, nor was, a single, homogeneous entity. It was always a series of complex and varying institutional arrangements and social and political compromises and it always had its critics, from both left and right of the political spectrum. Its distinctiveness lay in the general understanding that the state had a responsibility for ensuring a minimum standard of welfare for all its citizens and the welfare state was the form which emerged as being the most appropriate for implementing this responsibility.

By the late 1970s this distinctive feature was crumbling, with the voices of contestation and opposition gathering strength. This was accompanied by an erosion of the economic growth which had underpinned the Beveridge welfare reforms and together these two factors established the preconditions for a radical attack on the welfare state.

ACTIVITY 2.1

Think back to how the term 'settlement' was defined in the previous chapter and make a brief note identifying the main points.

COMMENT

settlement

The term 'settlement' should not be taken to imply that the frameworks through which state-controlled or state-regulated welfare was delivered were fully fixed and agreed upon by everybody. Rather, 'settlement' is used to convey the sense that a kind of status quo became established which set the limits within which compromises could be made over what, how and to whom welfare services and benefits were delivered. In this sense, then, a 'settlement' is a complex set of positions which construct a series of hierarchically ordered inclusions, conditional rights and responsibilities, dependencies and exclusions. As such, there always were some groups who were marginalized or excluded in the process of negotiation. Such groups either had their welfare needs ignored by the state-organized institutions or had them met to some extent but in a stigmatized or residual way.

■ ■ ■

3 Changing demographics

Chapter 1 suggested that issues of population or demography were important when considering the development of welfare policies and regimes for three reasons. These were that:

1 A particular demographic profile forms part of the basis upon which welfare policies are made.

2 Changes in demographic profiles provide part of the context for political debate and contestation over welfare restructuring.

3 Diversity amongst the population structures welfare needs and demands.

The characteristics of the population and the development and focus of welfare policy are, then, deeply intertwined.

In this section I want to add a few brief points to those you have already considered. First, I want to make a distinction between 'population' and 'demographic profile'. Then I want to introduce you to the idea that demography can be understood as a series of *representations*. In considering these points we are making a link between the social changes referred to above, a specific form of representing – or 'picturing' (see Chapter 1) – them, and the ways in which these changes – as *social facts* – became part of the restructuring of welfare services in the 1980s and 1990s.

3.1 From 'population' to 'demographic profile'

'Population' can be said to refer to the enumeration of people within a specified geographical and/or administrative unit – for example, this unit could be the UK, comprising England, Scotland, Wales and Northern Ireland; or an electoral ward or a district health authority. In contrast, 'demographic profile' or 'demographic structure' refers to the division of this population into separate sub-categories, examples of which you have already seen in Chapter 1.

population

Why might this distinction between 'population' and 'demographic structure' be important in the context of our discussion of the welfare state?

To distinguish between 'population' and 'demographic profile' is useful because it helps to reveal the socially constructed character of the link between the ways in which 'the people' are imagined and the way in which this is then used to underwrite the development and objectives of welfare policy. If 'population' is about the counting of people within a given territory, 'demography' is about the process of classifying and distributing these people into demarcated or bounded sub-categories which are then, either explicitly or implicitly, understood to have implications for state-organized welfare. It is this finer detail on the distribution of population into discrete sub-categories which makes 'demographic profile/structure' a more valuable term when thinking about developments and changes in welfare policy. However, it is important to remember that this 'finer detail' is not indicative of any *essential* characteristics of those included within the sub-group; rather, these groups are to be understood as socially constructed categories. That is, they are groups which are conceived of and represented in particular ways and are also understood to have a particular

demography

relation to, and role in, welfare use, welfare need and welfare care. As such, these sub-categories are not just 'facts', as their recording in official documents might suggest; they are also categories which construct types of people who are then positioned in discourses and relations of welfare.

Let us consider this further by looking at an example from one of the key documents associated with the radical restructuring of welfare which occurred in the 1980s and 1990s.

ACTIVITY 2.2

Try to think about what it means to say that demographic groups are socially constructed categories by working through Extract 2.1 which is taken from the 1989 government White Paper, *Caring for People: Community Care in the Next Decade and Beyond*. As you read, it may be helpful to think about the following questions:

1 Which sub-categories of people are identified in the extract?
2 Which sub-categories is it suggested will have the greatest welfare needs?
3 Which sub-categories are considered as traditional sources of informal care?
4 What demographic changes are indicated?
5 What implications is it suggested will result from these changes?

Extract 2.1 HMSO: 'Demographic change and the challenge for caring'

11.19 Over the next 20 years the number of people over 75 in Wales is expected to increase by 48,000, or 25% and the very elderly – those over 85 – by 26,400, an increase of 65%. Most old people lead fulfilled and independent lives. Nonetheless, there will, as a result of this demographic change, be more people in the population with physical disabilities and with mental illnesses associated with old age. The numbers suffering from other mental illnesses and with mental handicaps are, however, unlikely to change significantly.

11.20 At the same time that numbers in need of care will rise, the number of people in the 45 to 65 age group, which provides a substantial proportion of informal care, are expected to increase by only 19% over the next two decades. Moreover, wider social and economic developments such as the increased mobility of labour, the growing number of women at work, the increasing number of single-parent families, and increased rates of separation and divorce, are all likely to reduce the number of people who can devote significant amounts of time to the care and support of their frail elderly or other disabled relatives. Although these changes have to be kept in perspective – they represent developments in the need for care and a decline in the availability of informal care at the margin of the existing pattern – it is nonetheless an important margin which will represent a major challenge for health and social care.

(HMSO, 1989, pp.92–3)

COMMENT

There are a number of sub-categories of people identified in Extract 2.1: those who are elderly and very elderly; those who are middle-aged (between 45 and 65); those with physical disabilities; and those who are referred to as having 'mental illnesses' and 'mental handicaps'. This range can be further sub-divided into two: those who occupy age categories and those who are defined as having certain 'conditions'. As the extract goes on there is an implicit conflation of these in that there is some suggestion that belonging to particular age categories (the elderly and very elderly) will correspond to having a condition of 'mental illness', 'mental handicap' or 'physical disability'. **Hughes (1998)** has demonstrated the socially constructed nature of 'mental handicap', and this extract provides another example of this. The extract also identifies two more sub-categories of population – working women and 'single-parent families'. These are defined neither by age nor by condition, but they are relevant to the document because they are identified as having implications for the provision of welfare care for those sub-categories which will have the greatest welfare *needs*. It is the *middle-aged* who are identified as the sub-category which will provide traditional sources of care, and the *demographic changes* which are indicated are the increased mobility of labour, the increase in the number of women in paid employment, the rise in the number of single-parent families and the rise in marital breakdown. The suggested *implication* of these changes for the provision of welfare is decline in traditional sources of informal care. There is, however, another suggestion embedded in this last implication and that is that demographic changes are also *social changes* which alter the assumed and actual structure of *roles and responsibilities* which are tied to being a particular kind of person. Thus the increase in the number of women engaged in paid labour suggests that they will not be available to perform caring roles which were assumed to be associated with being a wife and mother.

■ ■ ■

This short extract is taken from a government White Paper which played a key role in the restructuring of health and social care and it illustrates well the continued relationship which is made between demographic structure and the development of welfare policy which we saw in Chapter 1. Our discussion also illustrates a wide range of assumptions and expectations about the relationship of particular categories of people to, their roles in, responsibilities for and needs of welfare services.

3.2 Demography as representation

Once we recognize this it becomes possible to identify in more abstract terms the different elements carried in the notion of demographic profiles or structures when linked to welfare policies. We have already seen that 'population' can be understood as a system of enumeration and recording of the people in a given geographical and/or administrative unit. In this way population counts provide a picture or snapshot of a set of people at a particular moment in time. Demographics provides a more detailed snapshot or image because it divides the 'population' further by grouping it into sub-categories which are said to reflect the distributions of the population according to such factors as age, gender, class, 'race' and/or ethnicity, household type, educational attainment,

occupational status, birth and mortality rates, regional distribution, and so on. It provides images of the composition of the population. I have used the term 'images' here because I want to hold on to the idea that population and demographic profiles are *representations* which construct differences amongst a given set of people as much as they reflect these differences. The term
representation 'representation' here refers to how a particular thing, group or event is projected and the chains of meanings and associations which are then attached to these. We have seen one example of this in the discussion of working women above. This example also allows us to add another element to our understanding of
position the term 'representations'. That is that representations also act to position people in a specific way in social and cultural relations. By 'positioned' we are referring to a double process. On the one hand, we are referring to the ways in which people and behaviours are categorized, classified and normalized in such a way as to produce ideas about their relative social, cultural, economic or moral value. In this sense it is part of what Foucault (1979) termed the 'technologies of power' and is part of a process of normalization. On the other hand, this process of classification and normalization produces spaces – known as subject positions – which people then occupy.

ACTIVITY 2.3

To understand this, look, for example, at the two definitions of the family from the Censuses of 1981 and 1991, given in Extracts 2.2 and 2.3. As you read these, consider the following questions:

1   What shifts in the definitions of the family can you identify between the two extracts?

2   Why do you think these shifts have occurred?

Extract 2.2 Office of Population Census and Surveys: 'Defining a family in 1981'

A *family* consists of:

a)   A married couple with or without their never married child(ren),

or

b)   a father or mother together with his or her never married child(ren),

or

c)   grandparent(s) with grandchild(ren) if there are no apparent parents of the grandchild(ren) usually resident in the household.

In this definition ... Type (a) is a *married couple family* and type (b) a *lone parent family*. Families of type (c) would be classified as a married couple family or lone parent family, as appropriate.

The *head of a family* was taken to be the husband in a married couple family, or lone mother, or lone father or lone grandparent in a lone parent family.

(Office of Population Census and Surveys, 1981, p.23, para. 89)

Extract 2.3 Office for National Statistics: 'Defining a family in 1991'

7.13 For the purposes of statistical output the detailed family unit types identified ... are grouped into one of the following standard types:

(a) *married couple family:* a married couple with or without their never married child(ren) – including a childless married couple;

(b) *cohabiting couple family:* two persons of the opposite sex living together as a couple with or without their never married child(ren) – including a childless cohabiting couple;

(c) *lone parent family:* a father or mother together with his or her never married child(ren);

or

(d) *no family person:* an individual member of a household not assigned with other members to a family; for example, a household containing a brother and sister only would be classified as *no family, two or more persons.*

7.14 Grandparent(s) with grandchild(ren), if there are no apparent parents of the grandchild(ren) resident in the household, are classified as type (a), (b) or (c) as appropriate ...

7.18 The *head of family* is generally taken to be the head of household if the family contains the head of household, otherwise:

- in a couple family, the head of family is the first member of the couple on the form;
- in a lone parent family, the head of family is the lone parent; or
- in some tables a no family person (type (d) in paragraph 7.13) is treated as a head of family.

(Office for National Statistics, 1991, p.36)

COMMENT

These extracts show that the official definition of the family broadened between 1981 and 1991 so that, by the latter date, cohabiting, heterosexual couples, with or without children, were included in the definition. Similarly, who counted as the head of family was opened up to self-definition by 1991. On the other hand, the category 'no family person' implies that to be officially recognized as a family still requires heterosexual relations since sisters and brothers would not constitute a family. Moreover, gay or lesbian couples living together are not mentioned as constituting a family anywhere in the definitions.

We can also see that population and demographic counts are a means of bringing into being types and categories of people who are then said to stand in a particular relation to a given set of resources or to have particular needs. To grasp this, let us return to lone-parent households. In Extract 2.1 we noted that the government White Paper had identified the rise in lone-parent households as having implications for the future provision of welfare services for elderly and very elderly people. What this statement did not discuss was the gender make-up of the lone parents, nor any of the social processes which had precipitated the rise in such households. The vast majority of these households are made up of a lone mother and her child(ren). Some of these will be widows – that is, they will have started as a married heterosexual couple and this will have ended not through choice or marital breakdown but by death. However, many more will have arisen from quite other reasons and in part this will be related to the changes in the gender order which occurred from the late 1960s (see, for example, **Lentell, 1998**).

As a result of complex legal, social, economic and cultural changes, women were increasingly able to establish lives in which they were either independent from men or more equal partners in the relations they had with them. One reflection of this was a rise in the numbers of women choosing to have children alone and, in doing so, they formed families which were different from the traditional nuclear family, with its male breadwinner and dependent wife and children, which was the cornerstone of the KWS. However, the increasing numbers of non-traditional families did not mean that they had no welfare needs and demands. Indeed, to some extent their needs proliferated, as in, for instance, the demand for nursery places or income support benefits. As a result, non-traditional families were the site of conflicting arguments as to the legitimacy and morality of their welfare demands. As Clarke and Langan (1993, p.44) have pointed out, the increase in lone-parent families, births outside marriage and divorce rates have been read by some as indications of the collapse of *the* family and of a growing immorality. Yet for others, including some (at least) of these women themselves, non-traditional families are an indication of the refusal to accept the inequalities structured into the 'old' welfare state, while their demands and needs are an expression of their claims for full citizenship rights.

■ ■ ■

The changing demographic profiles to be found among the population of the UK were, then, a way of both reflecting social change and constructing images of new constituencies of welfare need and the demise of old constituencies of welfare provision (for example, the care provided by women within the home). These changes, presented in the form of demographic tables, form part of the complex web of forces which destabilized the settlements of the 'old' or Keynesian welfare state. As official documents, demographic profiles represented the social changes and political protests which emerged between the 1950s and the 1980s. This can most clearly be seen in the emergence of what we call 'new welfare subjects' and consider below. However, if the changing demographics indicated that the old settlements were no longer tenable, the *direction* of change was not something which was predetermined. It was the outcome of the erosion of the social democratic consensus and the seizure of the political agenda and power by New Right forces embodied in and articulated by the governments of Margaret Thatcher.

4 The rhetoric of attack

It is possible to identify three main strands in the political rhetoric mobilized against the welfare state. I will list these briefly here and then develop them further in relevant parts of later sections which discuss the settlements. The political rhetoric itself argued that the welfare state had become too costly. This argument had already begun to be made prior to the first Thatcher government in 1979, as is evident from the cuts in welfare (and other public) expenditure which were instituted by the Callaghan Labour government in 1976 in accordance with the terms of an International Monetary Fund loan. It was, however, with the coming to power of a series of New Right governments that this argument was honed and deployed with great effect. Moreover, this was not just an argument about cost in the monetary sense – though this was of course part of it;

the welfare state was said to be too costly because of its purported effects on private enterprise. The three principal strands to this rhetoric comprised:

1   The argument that the huge expansion of what was called an 'unproductive sector' – that is, not contributing to the production of national wealth – resulted in a drain on funds and initiative in the private sector.

2   Similarly, welfare benefits were said to be draining personal initiative and individual autonomy and leading to the creation of an 'underclass' of welfare dependants, as **Morris (1998)** has shown.

3   An attack on the bureaucratic character of the welfare state. State-run institutions were said to be too controlling and impersonal and to be depriving 'the people' of their rights to choice. There had been precursors to this argument in the Callaghan government, evidenced in, for example, James Callaghan's statement, in a speech delivered in Cardiff in April 1979, that 'council tenants are entitled to ask the question: why should town hall bureaucrats tell them how to run their houses?' (quoted in O'Shea, 1984, p.23). Here too, however, it was only with the arrival of the New Right to power that statements such as these were to blossom into a fully fledged attack upon the bureaucratic and professional structures of the welfare state, a point we consider at more length in the next section.

5   Political dissensus and realigned 'statecraft'

In the previous chapter it was suggested that there were two key features of the political and economic settlements of the Keynesian welfare state. The first was the general consensus that the state should intervene to regulate the economy and deliver welfare services and benefits. The second was the incorporation of the two sides of industry in the policy-making process. Cross-party agreement did not mean that there was no opposition to the consensus from within both major parties; indeed, such opposition gathered pace from the early 1970s on the part of both the right wing of the Conservative Party and the left wing of the Labour Party. However, it was only after 1979 that a more concerted and sharply targeted attempt at undermining the political consensus was put into operation. The extent to which the Thatcherite project cut a huge ideological swathe through this consensus suggests that it was precisely here that it was most successful. By mobilizing what it had analysed as the popular resentment and discontent with both union power ('they're holding the country to ransom') and state bureaucracy and professional power, the Thatcher governments (and their allies and advisers in the right-wing think-tanks) were able to establish the ground for a radical reorganization of the structure and process of policy-making and implementation. This is why Taylor (1992, p.33) has characterized Thatcherism as fundamentally a set of political actions aimed at restructuring political relations, and it is to a consideration of this that we now turn.

5.1   Setting the scene

The first thing to note is that Thatcherism did not emerge out of nowhere. Hall and Jacques (1983, p.10) make the point that, as a political position, Thatcherism had been anticipated by minority voices on the back benches of parliament and in the constituencies, by the phenomenon of Powellism in the 1960s, and by the arguments associated with Keith Joseph in the 1970s. It was Enoch Powell who, on the grounds of a vociferous and racializing anti-immigration stance, first made the claim to speak for 'the people' and against the prevailing consensus, whilst Joseph was an early architect of what was to become known as New Right thinking. Despite these precursors, Hall and Jacques argue that what made it possible for Thatcherism to emerge as the *dominant* political force in the late 1970s and early 1980s was the combination of factors at ideological, economic and social levels, both nationally and internationally, which meant that the old social democratic consensus was eroded. They write:

> Thatcherism appeared at a historic conjuncture, where three trends converged: first, the point where the long term structural decline of the British economy synchronized with the deepening into recession of the world capitalist economy; second, in the wake of the collapse of the third post-war Labour government and the disintegration of the whole social democratic consensus which had provided the framework of British politics since 1945; third, at the resumption of the 'new Cold War', renewed at a frighteningly advanced point in the stockpiling of nuclear weaponry, and with Britain sliding, under Thatcherite inspiration, into a mood of intense, bellicose, patriotic fervour.
>
> (Hall and Jacques, 1983, p.9)

Thatcherism, then, was able to 'seize the time' and place itself at the helm of a project of root-and-branch transformation of the existing consensus, commitments and understandings about the relationship between the state, the economy and 'the people'. To do this it needed to disorganize the centres of opposition (such as trade unions and Labour-controlled local authorities) and the establishment consensus and shift the terms of political debate. In other words, it had to institute a programme of restructured statecraft, that is: 'the system of governmental procedures and mechanisms by which policy is formulated and implemented' (Martin, 1992, p.128).

statecraft

What was required was a break with the social democratic political culture and this was achieved through a rhetoric which constructed the government as being with 'the people' and against the state. This is why Thatcherism has been characterized as a form of *populism* in the sense argued by Laclau (1977) who suggested that populism was a form of politics which emerged when a fraction of the ruling power bloc attempted to mobilize popular feeling against the state apparatus with the aim of altering the prevailing balance of forces. Thatcherism articulated a crisis in economic and social management by appropriating popular grievances with the bureau-professional regime of the old organizational consensus (O'Shea, 1984). It did so by suggesting that its governments stood for 'the people' against what it presented as the tyrannies of collectivism (Clarke and Newman, 1997). In so doing, this rhetoric constructed a clear divide between the Conservative Party of the 1980s and the Labour Party whose commitment to forms of collectivism characteristic of the old social democratic consensus was constructed as 'alien' and against 'the people'/nation. For example, as early as 1975 – the year she took over the leadership of the Conservative Party – Margaret Thatcher said that the Labour Party held many of 'the voices that seem anxious not to overcome our economic difficulties, but to exploit them, to destroy the free enterprise society and put a Marxist system in its place. Today these voices form a sizeable chorus inside the Parliamentary Labour Party ...' (Margaret Thatcher, speech to the Conservative Party Conference, 1975, quoted in O'Shea, 1984, p.26).

But if the form of populism deployed by Thatcherism was such as to construct the Labour Party, the left more generally and the forms of collectivism associated with the old social democratic consensus, as alien and 'Other' to the interests and impulses of 'the people'/nation, this was not applied wholesale to rank-and-file trade unionists. This is despite the huge ideological and legislative attack directed at trade unions as organizations and at their leaderships (see, for example, Table 2.1 in section 5.3). For, as O'Shea again notes, Thatcher, and the politics and ideology she represented, could present herself as speaking *for* trade unionists:

> Let us not forget. The left opposes any extension of the secret ballot. For the left, democracy means the mass meeting marshalled by the bully boys ... The left knows that the majority [of trade unionists] are not Marxist and will not support Marxists. Conversely, for us Conservatives, an extension of trade union democracy is simply a new version of an Old Conservative maxim. Trust the people. Trust the rank and file trade unionists.

> (Margaret Thatcher, speech at Nottingham,
> 17 November 1979, quoted in O'Shea, 1984, p.28)

The Conservative Party under Margaret Thatcher was, then, constructed as the voice and protector of 'the people' – fundamentally good, patriotic, moral and committed to freedom and justice, all of which were said to be stifled and devalued by the terms of the old social democratic consensus.

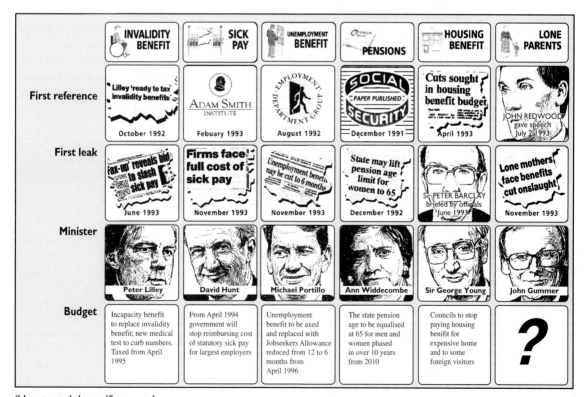

'How to end the welfare state'

5.2 Ideological attack: the argument against the welfare state

The starting-point for the ideological attack on the KWS, and the political consensus it contained, were the problems which were said to accrue to it. As one author sympathetic to the New Right project put it:

> Since 1945 the welfare state in Britain has developed not in accordance with any overall design but in response to the successful importuning of the Government by various pressure groups. The result is a higgledy-piggledy structure which is by universal consent a catastrophe for everyone involved – from the claimants to the almost equally unfortunate ministers and civil servants who have to run and answer for the mess.
>
> The human consequences of the present system are enough to give anyone pause. ...
>
> The underlying fact is the spuriousness of the 'contributory' element. The state has never used the contributions, as a properly defined provident fund would, to finance future payments via investment ... The welfare system which results from these movements can be criticized on at least four main grounds – the cost of the system, its organisation, its effects and its failure to adapt constructively to changed circumstances.
>
> (Davies, 1986, p.13)

By posing what he saw as the issues in this way, Davies made a claim which connects economic with administrative, moral and social elements and this was a common feature of arguments against the Keynesian welfare state which emanated from the New Right. Here I want to explore further the issues that Davies raised about the organization and effects of the welfare state since these were most closely related to the creation of a political *dissensus* about state-organized and state-delivered welfare.

When Davies raised the issue of the organization of the welfare state, he was targeting his criticism on its operation or administration. According to him (pp.14–15) there were four aspects to this problem:

1 it failed to relieve poverty;

2 it had an ineffective system of targeting;

3 it was far too complex – with a variety of administrative agencies, qualification criteria, types of benefit and methods of collecting finance (via tax and national insurance contributions); and yet

4 it lacked any defined or coherent goals.

Moreover, these problems resulted from both 'too much government' and too little rationality.

On the effects of the welfare state, Davies again identified four key features, two of which were central components of the ideological attack on the welfare state and thus were reiterated constantly by a range of commentators. These were the notions that the welfare state had created a dependency culture and that it had created and administered a series of disincentives to paid work. Let us hear Davies in his own voice again:

The creation of a class of permanent state dependants excluded from the normal workings of society and existing in a marginal half-world of surreptitious casual work. ...

Quite apart from the obvious social and political dangers, the waste of talent and degree of unhappiness involved are, quite simply, intolerable. It is clear that several serious errors made by the State have contributed to this human disaster (especially failures in public sector housing and education). At the root of these failures is the creation of a welfare system whose machinery has trapped many individuals in a position where they *cannot* help themselves, and are dependent upon the often capricious workings of an impersonal yet paternalistic state.

And:

The creation of incentives for behaviour and attitudes which are highly undesirable.

Effort, initiative and work are penalised; passivity and lack of will are rewarded. Administration of many benefits is highly paternalistic, undermining individual responsibility for, and control of, many aspects of claimants' lives. People can escape the consequences of actions which are by any reasonable definition irresponsible; yet attempts to act in a responsible manner can lead to loss of entitlement to benefit and of income. A 'nanny' syndrome is created in which individuals surrender their autonomy and become dependants of the state ...

(Davies, 1986, pp.16–17, 15–16)

At the heart of this argument it is possible to identify a series of oppositions:

Old welfare state	*Restructured welfare*
Disincentive	Incentive
Dependence	Independence
Irresponsible	Responsible
Constraint	Opportunity

These descriptors were also applied to the analysis of the economic effects of the Keynesian welfare state indicating that, for the New Right, it was *all* aspects of the social democratic consensus which were in need of reform. In the context of the political settlement, however, they were written through a language of morality and public concern. As such, they also carried a conception of the relationship people should have to the state in terms of their responsibilities in the provision of welfare.

ACTIVITY 2.4

Extract 2.4 is taken from a pamphlet entitled *The Emerging British Underclass*, written by Charles Murray, a well-known American commentator on the issue of the 'underclass' (see also **Morris, 1998**). Read through the extract and identify:

■ the unit or collectivity of people Murray suggests should be the unit of local control;

■ the suggestion he makes about the relationship between these units and central government.

Extract 2.4 Murray: 'Authentic self-government is the key'

The alternative I advocate is to have the central government stop trying to be clever and instead get out of the way, giving poor communities (and affluent communities, too) a massive dose of self-government, with vastly greater responsibility for the operation of the institutions that affect their lives – including the criminal justice, educational, housing and benefit systems in their localities. My premise is that it is unnatural for a neighbourhood to tolerate high levels of crime or illegitimacy or voluntary idleness among its youth: that, given the chance, poor communities as well as rich ones will run affairs so that such things happen infrequently. And when communities with different values run their affairs differently, I want to make it as easy as possible for people who share values to live together. If people in one neighbourhood think marriage is an outmoded institution, fine; let them run their neighbourhood as they see fit. But make it easy for the couple who thinks otherwise to move into a neighbourhood where two-parent families are valued. There are many ways that current levels of expenditure for public systems could be sustained (if that is thought to be necessary) but control over them decentralised. Money isn't the key. Authentic self-government is.

(Murray, 1990, p.34)

COMMENT

The first and perhaps most noticeable point about this extract is that the *individual* person does not appear anywhere in it. The smallest unit is 'the couple', otherwise Murray talks about 'communities'. However, what is important is that these 'communities' are formed around a common value system. It is a shared moral position which forms the connective tissue among them, rather than what he sees as an enforced collectivism imposed by central government and expressed in the taxes taken to provide the services and benefits of the welfare state. This is why 'communities' should be given 'self-government' since their 'natural' morality will ensure that the ills said to be produced by the welfare state – such as crime, illegitimacy and idleness – are prevented from happening. In other words, left to themselves 'communities' will deal with the social ills said to derive from the welfare state.

■ ■ ■

5.3 Undermining the corporatist state: the attack on the trade unions and local government

What was necessary to attain these apparently desirable goals of individual autonomy, responsibility and morality was a series of actions which would rid the UK of its 'nanny' welfare state and the forms of corporatist and professional power which administered and controlled it. Chief among these sites of power were the trade unions and local authorities.

We have already seen that part of the post-war political consensus was a general acceptance of a particular style of government. Central to this style was a high degree of consultation among government; employers' organizations, such as the Confederation of British Industry (CBI); and trade union bodies, such as the Trades Union Congress (TUC). With the advent of the Thatcher governments in 1979, this corporatist style of government was identified as a major obstacle to the radical restructuring which the New Right argued was necessary if the 'British disease' was to be tackled and the country was to re-enter the global economy as a major player. In this context, and despite the rhetoric which constructed a close affinity between the government and trade unionists, *trade unions as organizations* were identified as one of a range of 'enemies within' and accused of 'holding the country to ransom' if, and when, traditional forms of labour struggle, such as strikes, were engaged in. Trade unions within the welfare state were identified as sites of professional and service worker power. (A possible exception to this was the nurses who, despite increasing militancy, were less easy targets for this form of characterization, since they held an enormous amount of public support.) The rhetorical distinction that was made between, on the one hand, the leaderships of the trade unions and their organizational strength, and, on the other, the millions of individual trade unionists, enabled the government to gloss over the contradiction between this rhetoric and the legislative attack on trade unions (see Table 2.1).

Table 2.1 Legislation aimed at curbing trade union activity

1980	Employment Act	Closed shop made unlawful without ballot every five years; secondary picketing unlawful
1982	Employment Act	Lawful to dismiss strikers with selective rehiring after three months; employers can sue unions for damages in cases of industrial action
1984	Trade Union Act	Secret ballots on all proposals for industrial action – later amended to compel postal ballots; members to be balloted on political fund every 10 years; unions liable for damages in official strikes
1988	Employment Act	Legal action against unions possible where strike action not supported by secret ballot; individual workshops within one company to be balloted; postal ballots for political funds; industrial action in support of closed shop unlawful; unions unable to pay fines of their officials; Commissioner for the Rights of Trade Union Members established
1989	Employment Act	Reduced rights to time off for trade union duties
1990	Employment Act	Unions now legally liable for all strike action and they can be sued for unlawful action unless they repudiate it; employers can selectively dismiss workers and any action against it is unlawful
1993	Trade Union Reform and Employment Rights Act	Ballots on industrial action to be fully postal and independently scrutinized; individuals have right to go to court to challenge strikes; employers to be notified before and after ballot on industrial action

Source: adapted from Trades Union Congress/School Curriculum Industry Partnership, 1995, p.13; and *Labour Research*, 1997, p.19

Thus the attack on the trade unions was presented as part of a programme aimed at restoring government authority, democracy and the national interest over sectional interests. The legislation undermined trade union activity in four main areas: individual employment rights; trade union recognition; industrial action; and the organization and administration of trade unions (Trades Union Congress/School Curriculum Industry Partnership, 1995, p.13). In addition, there was a media onslaught on the trade unions and a general contention that trade unions were redundant forms of organization in the modern-day conditions of employment. Moreover, membership of trade unions was rapidly declining as a result of the unprecedented levels of unemployment from the early 1980s.

This attack on the trade unions was in keeping with the Thatcherite attack on collectivist visions and forms of organization. Wilding (1992, p.201) makes the point that 'collectivist approaches to welfare provision are grounded in two beliefs – the virtue and necessity of social rather than individual responsibility for substantial areas of life and the practicality of efficient and effective provision by government.' The approach of Margaret Thatcher and her series of ministers was not, however, one based on ideas of collectivism and in this context trade unions, as a form of collective responsibility and as an element in policy formation and development under the old political consensus, were an obvious and necessary target for attack. Trade unions were sacrificed in the move to a new statecraft and political culture.

Collectivist visions equal national threat?

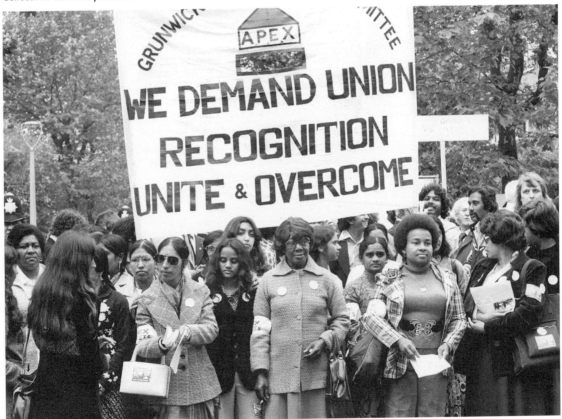

The attack on local authorities

Between 1979 and 1989, 50 pieces of legislation curtailing or redefining the powers and responsibilities of local authorities were passed (Wilding, 1992). Collectively, these reduced the financial independence of local authorities (LAs), limited their functions and circumscribed them as a source of opposition to central government ambitions and practices. Wilding (1992) identifies five main landmarks which express this attack on local government:

1   Restriction of their ability to determine the level of revenue to be raised in order to deliver services.

2   The compulsion, in the early 1980s, to sell council housing, and the demise of their house-building role which had been such a key feature of the Beveridgean attack on 'squalor'.

3   The wide-ranging transfer of power from local education authorities to the Department of Education (later renamed the Department of Education and Employment) in the 1988 Education Reform Act. LAs were further undermined by this Act in the clauses which introduced local management of schools and the ability of schools to opt out of LA control and become grant-maintained.

4   The requirement for LAs to put their services out to compulsory competitive tendering – thus bringing in market mechanisms as a way to denude LAs of their functions. Compulsory competitive tendering can also be seen as having a profound effect on local authority trade unions, since employees in those services put out to tender often found themselves either without a job at all, or employed under new conditions with new employers, some of whom also restricted their trade union rights.

5   The move from LAs as providing agencies to enabling agencies whose functions were redefined as ones of organizing, supervising, contracting and regulating the actions of other agencies who provided services. This was a major effect of the National Health Service and Community Care Act of 1990. Many of the providing agencies operative since that time are in the private and voluntary sectors and therefore outside of any direct electoral responsibility.

5.4   Realigned statecraft

The relative autonomy of local government from control by the centre, expressed in, for example, the ability to raise local taxes, to institute local by-laws and other regulations, and to oversee and provide some welfare services such as education, housing or personal social services, was one of the ways in which the power of the party controlling parliament could be curtailed. Similarly, the bureau-professionalism which characterized the organizational settlement in the KWS provided another potential obstacle to unmediated central control and power. Other 'buffer' mechanisms could be found in the general consensus across political élites about what constituted appropriate and legitimate behaviour and in the existence of a non-political civil service or the autonomy of senior government advisers from overt party allegiance or control (Taylor, 1992). However, because this system of informal control on the power of the governing party was not guaranteed by a constitution, it was always fragile and had the potential of becoming the subject of a sustained attack at any time. According to Taylor (1992), it was precisely such an attack which was inaugurated by successive Thatcher governments. This was led by an extension of the centre, one component of which was the onslaught against Labour-controlled local authorities. But there were additional aspects to this centralization of control and power:

- The abolition of relatively autonomous regulating bodies in the health service, such as the regional health boards and their replacement with management boards made up of representatives from a narrower cross-section of the local population, often resulting in a major shift in the balance of interests.

- The direct intervention in the promotion of senior civil servants.

- The emerging political imbalance of appointments to top positions in otherwise relatively autonomous institutions such as the BBC (Taylor, 1992, p.48).

- The abolition or reformation of institutions such as the National Enterprise Board, the Manpower Services Commission and the National Economic and Development Organisation (Martin, 1992, p.128), all of which had a membership comprising representatives of trade unions, business and central government and were therefore associated with the old corporatist forms of statecraft.

Indeed, such was the assault on the existing ground rules for operation within, and links between, government and semi-autonomous institutions that one commentator has remarked: 'There is no doubt that this abandonment of the reciprocal autonomy stance marked a major break with old Conservative statecraft' (Bulpitt, 1986, p.38). This reference to the break with *Conservative* statecraft is suggestive of the range of the ideological remit of the project of radical transformation and the pursuit of central state power in the process of policy formation and implementation.

As I have already suggested, ideologically this transformation in the political settlement was achieved on the basis of a rhetoric of 'rolling back the state', 'cutting the costs of welfare' and reinstituting enterprise and self-reliance. But Gamble (1988, p.14) has also shown that part of this rhetoric evoked a contest between two images of the nation: 'the nation of the future versus the nation of the past, the nation of independence and self-reliance versus the nation of dependence and subsidy, the nation of the employed and prosperous versus the nation of the unemployed and poor.' This ideological division of the nation, together with the restructured process of policy formation and the centralization of power, established the contexts in which the transformation in welfare was to take place and which are addressed in more detail in later chapters in this book.

6   Changing economics

Just as the Beveridgean or Keynesian welfare state had its economic underpinnings in the form of Keynesian demand management, so too the welfare 'reforms' inaugurated by Margaret Thatcher and continued by John Major had their economic counterpart in a neo-liberal form of supply-side economics. Marquand (1988, p.170) has argued that 'the national traditions to which Thatcherism appeals point not towards a renewal of Britain's old economic supremacy, but towards subordination to stronger economies and multinational forms.' In similar vein, Martin (1992, p.134) has characterized the economic strategy pursued since 1979 as one of *internationalization* in which the economic structure is organized around the import and export of multinational capital and there is 'open recognition ... that the interests of the British state are no longer synonymous with the interests of explicitly domestic capital, but with capital operating in Britain and the operations of British capital overseas.' This has meant an explicit break with the existing relations between the state and economy and redefinition of the meaning of state intervention in the economy. At one level this involved a commitment to restructuring and support for the City and the financial sector (often referred to as the 'Big Bang'); adoption of a market-led strategy for economic regeneration via control of inflation and promotion of entrepreneurialism – both of which included an attack on 'inefficient' firms and sectors, who felt the discipline of the market via the control of the supply of money; and a commitment to undermining 'restrictive practices' in the labour market by breaking trade union power and thereby attempting to increase 'flexibility' in the labour market. The attempt to reorganize state–economy relations also involved an attack upon levels of and a commitment to public expenditure, especially in the nationalized industries, which were subject to progressive waves of privatization; and on welfare services and benefits. In this sense, then, the restructuring of the welfare state was as much a part of a new economic strategy as it was a reorganization of the relation between the state and the citizen:

> In Mrs. Thatcher's Britain free markets, possessive individualism and self-reliance were to replace state intervention and subsidy as the motive forces shaping economic growth and allocation. This move to enlarge the province and agency of free market capitalism was projected not merely as the only sure road to economic prosperity ... but also as a way of increasing the sum of human welfare by extending the scope for individual freedom and expanding consumer choice.
>
> (Martin, 1992, p.126)

A disabled patient who requires help with bathing is having to endure the indignity of having his top half washed by staff from Camden Council's social services department and his lower half by district nurses.

Hampstead and Highgate Gazette,
9 February 1996

This humiliation could happen because since 1994 the NHS provides 'medical' care, and the local authority social services provide 'social' care. Neither is legally allowed to cross the boundary, both are strapped for cash, and no one can agree on which side of the boundary falls many a (much needed) bath. These boundary disputes cause pain to staff as well as users.

(Mackintosh and Smith, 1996, p.144)

However, contrary to the political rhetoric considered above, this move to free up the market was not accompanied by a withdrawal from intervention by the state, but rather by a narrowing and deepening of intervention (Thompson, 1990). The state was not 'rolled back' in relation either to the economy or to welfare services. Indeed, as many commentators have noted, it was not until the third Thatcher government that there was a concerted attempt to restructure welfare provision, attempts which were marked by the systematic introduction of 'market' mechanisms into health, education and the personal social services in 1988, as Chapters 3, 6 and 7 show (see also Le Grand, 1990). Up until that time housing and income maintenance had been the sites subjected to the most radical reform (see Chapters 4 and 8).

One gauge of the relative resilience of the welfare state, in the face of government attempts to reduce its size, is the level of overall state expenditure on it. Table 2.2 shows that these levels remained remarkably high despite the sustained ideological and policy attack on aspects of the welfare state throughout the 1980s.

Table 2.2 General government expenditure: by function, UK, £ billion at 1995 prices

	1981	*1986*	*1991*	*1994*	*1995*
Social security	61	76	83	100	102
Health	26	29	35	40	41
Education	28	29	33	37	38
Defence	25	29	26	25	23
Public order and safety	9	10	15	15	15
General public services	9	10	13	13	14
Housing and community amenities	14	12	10	11	10
Transport and communication	8	6	8	7	9
Recreational and cultural affairs	3	4	4	4	4

Source: adapted from Office for National Statistics, 1997, p.118, Table 6.21

One reason why the levels of state welfare spending remained so high throughout the 1980s and into the late 1990s was the emergence of extremely high levels of unemployment throughout this whole period. As **Gazeley and Thane (1998)** have shown, at times during the 1980s levels of unemployment exceeded those of the 1930s, the decade usually thought of as synonymous with the worst periods of unemployment in the UK since industrialization. Le Grand (1990) makes a link to demography by suggesting that stable levels of spending in some welfare programmes was a result of their use by the middle classes. Thus programmes such as health and education have maintained relatively stable levels of state expenditure in real terms, whilst those of social security and housing benefit have lost in real terms.

However, if successive governments were not able to cut dramatically overall levels of expenditure on welfare benefits and services, this does not mean that they were unsuccessful in radically altering the ethos and practice of welfare finance. Rhetorically this was summed up in the phrase the 'costs of welfare'. At one level, of course, this refers to overall expenditure on welfare, but it also refers to how and where to raise the money, as well as on what it should be spent. Thus,

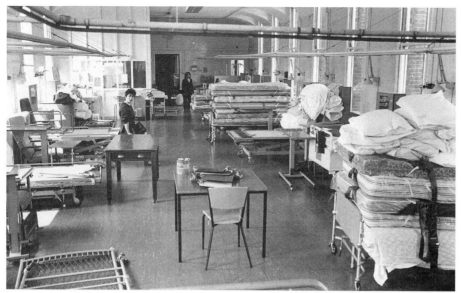

The costs of welfare cuts

alongside a relatively stable level of state expenditure on welfare, there have been major changes which have radically altered the ground rules of welfare provision. For example, the introduction of budget holding for some general practitioners and trust status for hospitals has introduced market-like relationships into the National Health Service (NHS). Similarly, the introduction of local management of schools resulted in budgetary responsibilities being devolved to individual schools via their governing body, which both by-passed the local education authority and led to competition between individual schools. And in local government departments such as social services, the division between purchaser and provider has reorganized relationships between colleagues and departments around market-type axes (Langan and Clarke, 1994).

What this points to is that, alongside its role as the regulator of welfare provision (in the sense of legitimating, legalizing and defining what, how and who provides welfare), there was a reorganization of the role of the state in welfare – shifting from a provider of services to an enabler or purchaser of services. The effect of this was to increase the role of the private and voluntary sectors in the provision of welfare – sectors which had always been present in welfare delivery but were given a much enhanced role.

The central ideological thread binding this enhanced role for the market was the rhetoric of 'consumer choice' achieved by breaking the monopoly power of the bureau-professional power blocs, which were said to characterize the 'old' welfare state, and introducing various forms of privatization. The purchaser–provider split is one form of this privatization and this has carried with it a rising dominance of managerial principles (see Chapter 9). As one commentator has observed: 'the new social services department is designed to promote "cost effectiveness" and to encourage competition among providers, giving preference where possible to the voluntary and private sectors' (Langan, 1993, p.151). The chapters which follow in this book provide a more detailed consideration of this and other changes in specific welfare programmes. What it is important to note here is that the introduction of market mechanisms facilitated a fundamental change in the social relations of welfare provision.

7 'New welfare subjects' and the demise of the social settlement

Earlier in this discussion I referred to the idea that the reconstruction of welfare involved dismantling the social settlement of the 'old' welfare state. Just as the political and economic settlements were destabilized and substituted with newer forms of expression and co-ordination, so too the social settlement of the KWS was subjected to change. This involved redefining the roles and responsibilities of the individual citizen – or more accurately the native-born and descended, white male breadwinner and his family – and the state. In other words, the reconstruction of the welfare state was not just about a realignment of political and economic forces, it was also a realignment of *social* forces.

In this section I want to explore this idea further by considering the ways in which the social figures which characterized the welfare state of Beveridge and Keynes became displaced and replaced by a series of other social figures. To help us consider this I will organize the section into three parts:

1   An exploration of the notion of 'the subject'.

2   An exploration of the forces and challenges which emerged as a result of the formation of collectivities consolidated or formed around social solidarities other than class – such as the disability movement, the feminist movement, the movements of black people and others defined as 'ethnic minorities', and the gay and lesbian movement – and from which new welfare subjects emerged.

3   An exploration of the challenges from 'above' which also contributed to the formation of new welfare subjects – for example, the manager of 'new managerialism', and 'the customer'.

Let us start with the notion of 'the subject'.

7.1   What or who is a 'subject'?

subject

For those involved in any level of formal education the most common association or meaning conjured up by the word 'subject' is perhaps that of an academic discipline – as in 'what subject are you studying?' Alternatively, the word 'subject' is often taken to mean 'issue'– as in, for example, 'in the 1960s the issue of homelessness became a subject of much public concern and controversy.'

It should be clear, however, that in this and the previous chapter, the word 'subject' is not being used in either of these senses. Rather, it has been used in association with the terms 'individuals' or 'groups' and, since this is the case, why, then, replace these two words with those of 'the subject'? I want to begin to answer this question by considering briefly what is implied by the term 'the individual'. An individual is generally thought of as being a person who is formed once and for all at some specified time in their lives – either at birth, or puberty, or on reaching the age of majority. An individual is a person who makes rational decisions and choices, constrained only by their access to resources and their innate abilities. She or he is presented as a unified being, holding all the parts of themselves together in a seamless web (unless they have a mental health problem or a learning difficulty), and, once an adult, having the right and duty to act responsibly and freely. An individual implies a person who exists prior to society – is formed outside of society and is then inserted into it to act in the ways just described. An individual is a product of nature or the human condition rather than of the society into which they are born and/or in which they live out their life.

However, for the social scientist working within a social constructionist perspective, to accord a person this pre-social condition is problematic. Those working within a social constructionist perspective would want, in contrast, to draw attention to and investigate the ways in which people are 'made up' into specific types of person out of the webs of material and discursive relations in which they find themselves at different times and in different contexts (see, for example, **Hughes, 1998; Lewis, 1998a; Saraga, 1998a**). For those working in this kind of framework the notion of 'the individual' is replaced by the notion of 'the subject'.

We can identify a number of key points about the figure of 'the subject':

- Subjects are not pre-social, rational and unified beings which are created in a once-and-for-all fashion. Rather, 'subjects' are constantly 'made up' or constituted during their everyday encounters and over their life course as they move in and out of a series of interlocking webs of relations. For example, a person born as a girl may move over her life course from being a daughter, a lover, a married woman, a mother, a lone mother, a heterosexual, a lesbian, a waged worker, an unemployed person, a patient, and so on. In addition, she may combine a number of these at any one moment and have to negotiate what these mean both personally and socially as she goes about her everyday interactions. In this sense, then, 'subjects' are always being brought into being (in contrast to 'the individual' who is made once and for all).

Can you think of similar examples from your own life?

- Subjects are 'made up' or constituted within a web of intersecting relations. These relations are both material (that is, those relations which are organized around tangible things such as access to resources), and discursive (that is, the ideas and fields of expertise or knowledge by which types of people are recognized, categorized and evaluated). It is from this process of 'recognition', rather than some essential and pre-existing character which is noticed, that subjects are created. The subject emerges from a particular understanding and interpretation of a condition or behaviour and in this sense is formed by specific fields of 'knowledge'. For example, medicine as a field of 'knowledge' creates the sick person or patient out of its identification and classification of particular conditions as illnesses.

- A subject is also a status or position in a field of knowledge or a discourse. This has two aspects: one the one hand, as a subject *of* the discourse – for example, discourses on lone mothers are *about* all those who can qualify for this name; they become the category at the heart of the discussions and policy formations concerned with lone mothers. On the other hand, subjects are also subjected *to* the discourses which make the claim to know the truth about their categories of concern. So, to take the category 'lone mothers' again, those who occupy this position will be subjected to the scrutiny and effects of social policies which are based on this 'truth'. For example, they may be entitled to claim a specific benefit aimed at this category, whilst simultaneously feeling the sharpness of ideas which link lone motherhood with youth crime.

- In this sense, the notion of *power* is integral to the notion of subject. This has two aspects also: on the one hand, those who have the power to make their discourses or knowledges the dominant ones – the ones which become the 'common sense' (see **Clarke and Cochrane, 1998**) – thereby have the power to construct the subject in a particular way. On the other hand, and closely related, the notion of the subject is linked to that of power because subjects are the targets of the social and institutional practices which emerge from these discourses or knowledges.

- Subjects are also psychically constituted in terms of their inner sense of self. We call this the 'subjectivity' of the person and this is also understood to emerge from a given set of complex relations that exist at a given time and place. For example, my sense of myself as a *black* woman is only possible in the context of late twentieth-century Britain after decades of black struggle for self-definition and social justice. In another time in Britain it is likely that I would have a sense of myself as 'coloured', a 'mulatto' or a 'half-caste'.

- Subjects also have identities – a term closely related to that of 'subjectivity', but referring more to the social categories of belonging which a person develops over their life course and through which people construct connections to others.

Subjects, then, are produced through processes of naming which in turn position them in particular ways in fields of knowledge or expertise and the institutional practices which emerge from this. The point to emphasize here is that the way in which people are named affects their own and others' expectations of them in specific sites: so, for example, being a 'customer' positions a person within discourses and practices of health professionals and institutions in a different way to being a 'patient' would.

I have outlined the notion of 'the subject' in this way because it is important for understanding the ways in which the apparently universal subject – the citizen – enshrined in the social settlement of the 'old' welfare state became eroded and replaced by a whole series of 'new welfare subjects'. On the one hand, there is a series of such subjects which has emerged from the challenges of the new social movements and has exposed the class, racial, gendered and ablist character of the earlier social settlement. These 'new' subjects have challenged the 'false universalism' (Williams, 1993) of the KWS and expressed new demands and welfare needs at the same time as they have demonstrated how complex are the social relations of power in welfare. On the other hand, the New Right has also constructed a range of 'new welfare subjects' in the form of 'customers', 'managers' and the 'underclass' (as opposed to the 'citizens' and 'clients' of the old organizational settlement) whilst simultaneously attempting to reimpose the triangle of nation, family and work, albeit in tandem with the introduction of market principles and ideas of 'self-reliance'. Let us consider each in turn, beginning with the new welfare subjects which emerged from the challenges from the 'margins'.

7.2   Challenges from 'below': marginal subjects

Earlier it was stated that the *subject* of the KWS was the British-born and descended, white male breadwinner. As a citizen, he was constructed as having a set of rights which provided a direct and autonomous relation to benefits and services associated with (what in 1945 was) the new welfare state. His responsibilities were to engage in paid work, pay his taxes and national insurance contributions and look after his family. The state was to meet its obligations by using macroeconomic policy to ensure that the economy (and therefore employment) was in good order and to organize and deliver a package of welfare services and benefits. Drawing on the work of Williams (1989), Chapter 1 pointed out that this set of reciprocal rights and responsibilities was organized around a triangle of nation, family and work.

If this was the dominant and direct relation of the citizen to the welfare state, a series of subordinate and marginal forms of inclusion were constructed for those who could not occupy the subject position of native-born and descended, white male breadwinner. What linked those people whose position within the social settlement was one of subordination and marginalization was their status as 'minors' within the social relations of welfare. However, if their 'minority' status was what linked them, it is important to note the distinctions between the various forms of subordinated inclusion. Here I want to note three such subordinated positions (though no doubt others could be added – such as gay men and lesbians who were not recognized as having any specific or legitimate welfare needs) and to give brief illustrations of the ways in which these subordinations were challenged and led to the creation of a series of 'new welfare subjects'. I am referring to these as 'new welfare subjects' not because the people who came to occupy these positions did not exist before. Rather, they are categorized as 'new' because, in the wake of the politicization of difference which accompanied the rise of the new social movements, activists within these movements made demands for recognition of their independent and self-defined welfare needs. As such, they constructed a new set of social subjects through and to which welfare services and benefits could be legitimately distributed.

The three types of subordinated and marginalized inclusion within the social relations of the KWS I want to highlight are:

1   That of the indirect and dependent status/relation. Married women had this status (this is discussed further in **Lewis, 1998b**) and it was this which became progressively challenged by the rise of feminism from the late 1960s.

2   The status/relation of being 'alien' and 'Other'. Those who were legally and/or socially defined as 'immigrant' had this relation and, again, this position began to be progressively challenged as those whose origin and/or descent was in the New Commonwealth began to identify the assumptions and practices of welfare professionals and institutions as racist.

3   The status/relation which accrued to those constructed as minor and dependent because of a physical or mental impairment. The rise of the disability movement challenged the subordinated inclusions which arose from this position.

As these positions were progressively challenged by a range of newly created political constituencies, the boundaries of the social settlement of the KWS were increasingly destabilized. The demands for recognition of the specific and self-defined welfare needs which were expressed by these constituencies required that they be accepted as legitimate and, therefore, that resources be allocated to meet them. The political pressure this exerted on the KWS meant that, in the end, some radical change was necessary. That this change took the direction it did in the New Right reforms was neither expected nor desired by many of the activists associated with these movements. However, before going on to consider the ways in which the New Right appropriated the dissatisfactions with the KWS expressed by these movements, we should take some time to consider some illustrations of the challenges they posed. To do this we will look at the challenge from anti-racism and that posed by the disability movement.

subordination
marginalization

new welfare
subjects

The challenge from anti-racism

This challenge emerged in opposition to the construction of black peoples' welfare needs as 'alien' and their mere presence as a danger to the 'British people'. As 'immigrants' not only were their welfare needs seen as subordinate, they were also represented as a risk to the welfare of the indigenous population. For example, in 1966 the British Medical Association (BMA) published *The Medical Examination of Immigrants* in which they stated that: 'The BMA has for some time past been concerned about the possible risk to the health of the people of this country of the increasing flow of immigrants from overseas …' and that, in contrast to 'the view held by some that Commonwealth citizens should have completely free access to this country … such a policy carries obvious health risks to the indigenous population' (quoted in Brent Community Health Council, 1981, p.9). While in the 1979 edition of Bradford Council's annual statistical report *District Trends*, it was said that: 'One of the worrying problems in Bradford is the high rate of some handicaps – such as congenital deafness and severe mental handicaps among Asian children. The number is increasing as the number of Asian children increases' (quoted in Brent Community Health Council, 1981, p.21).

Statements such as these provide clear examples of the ways in which people whose origin or descent was in the New Commonwealth were constructed as both 'alien' to and a drain upon the resources of the welfare state. Such constructions and the subjects which they produced were to become the target of black and anti-racist activists, the effect of which was to push the boundaries of the social settlement of the KWS.

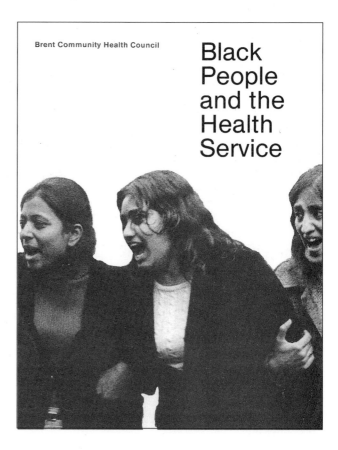

Challenging the terms of racialized subordination

Think back to the quotations from the British Medical Association and Bradford Council and then read through Extract 2.5 which illustrates the kinds of challenge issued from this new political constituency. As you do so, identify:

- how the authors reconstruct the issues;
- what part they attribute to NHS professionals and structures in the issues.

Extract 2.5 Brent Community Health Council: 'Exposing institutional racism'

Among NHS professionals racism is a taboo word. If you suggest to one of them that he or she is behaving in a racist way they are likely to respond with outrage as though you had used a dirty word about something sacred.

Professionals, people are led to believe, are above racism. ...

The studies which have been done so far of black people and the NHS all focus on black people as the problem. In this report the NHS and not black people is the object of study. We have looked first at the racism which has been institutionalised within the NHS and secondly at the way in which the NHS itself is involved in perpetuating racism.

The NHS is often presented as a warm caring arm of the state ... Similarly doctors, nurses and other NHS professionals are presented as people with a vocation, immune to political pressures – the health service is there, we are told, to heal the sick irrespective of class, sex or colour. But if we look at people's actual experience of the health service a very different picture emerges. ...

As the evidence we present shows, racism permeates every aspect of the NHS, from its recruitment policies to its assumption of the superiority of white diets, family systems, traditions of healing and approaches to child rearing; from mythologies about black 'pain thresholds' to eligibility for NHS treatment. The structures the NHS has established and the attitudes it has nurtured are closely intertwined with wider policies which have led to exploitation of black workers, the exclusion of their dependants throughout the sixties and seventies and now to an attempt to 'encourage' them to leave Britain. ...

What black patients and black workers in the NHS are up against is not just a few individuals with nasty attitudes but a health service which in its policies and institutional practices continually makes assumptions about black people which serve to justify and perpetuate their continued exploitation.

(Brent Community Health Council, 1981, p.2)

Whereas the British Medical Association and Bradford Council constructed the problem as the presence of people from the New Commonwealth and their descendants, the authors of this extract reverse the terms and identify the institutional practices and assumptions of NHS professionals as the issue to be addressed. In so doing, Brent Community Health Council both challenges the processes by which black people's welfare needs are constructed as subordinate and marginal, and makes a claim for the legitimacy of black people's experiences and demands. As such, they illustrate the ways in which racialized groups began to reconstitute themselves as subjects who have legitimate and specific welfare needs which could not and should not be mediated through the old social settlement.

■ ■ ■

The challenge from disabled citizens

Since the late 1970s the disability movement has shown how the social construction of disability leads to the social exclusion and enforced dependency of those who are defined as disabled (see **Hughes, 1998**). For the disability movement this dependency is the product of a series of discriminations which result from the constructions of what it is to be 'normal'. As Barnes (1991) has noted, the effect of these normalizing constructions is to transform impairments into a series of complex and interlocking social restrictions and discriminations. As with black people, disabled people have identified welfare policies, structures and professionals as having a central role in infringeing the privacy, autonomy and independence of disabled people. The latter have challenged 'the traditional philanthropic and welfarist attitudes towards people with disabilities' (Liberty, 1994, p.10). Disabled activists have placed a shift in the balance of power between welfare professionals and disabled people themselves at the centre of their challenge to the dependencies and marginalizations produced by the KWS. Strongly influenced by the North American experience, the disability movement in the UK has increasingly challenged the organization of welfare services by professionals in ways which create dependency and offered alternative conceptions located in discourses of rights and active citizenship. As the European Network on Independent Living has put it: 'We demand social welfare systems which include personal assistance services that are consumer controlled, and which allow various models of independent living for disabled people, regardless of their disability and income. We demand social welfare legislation which recognises these services as basic civil rights' (quoted in Clarke *et al.*, 1996, p.67).

Demands such as these resulted in a radical challenge to the boundaries of the KWS as they intersected with similar challenges emanating from other political constituencies and destabilized the deeply embedded notions about who the independent subject of the social settlement was. Thus when we talk of 'new welfare subjects' we are referring to the ways in which diverse groups of people from a wide range of social positions began to challenge the terms of their inclusion within the social settlement of the KWS. In so doing they made claims for independent, direct and self-defined status within the social relations of welfare, seeking to displace the singular and universal subject of welfare which was represented by the native-born and descended, white male breadwinner.

These intersecting challenges had a profound effect on official and popular discourses of the welfare state and their impact is in part reflected in the increasing recognition of the diversity and plurality of contemporary UK society. One gauge of this recognition and the impact of the political demands expressed by the new social movements can be found in the rise of equal opportunities policies and procedures which were adopted by welfare agencies working within the state and voluntary sectors. However, the spread of equal opportunities policies and procedures did not represent any simple or wholesale acceptance of the critiques of and challenges to the social settlement of the KWS. For a start, there was a huge variation in the principles underlying different equal opportunities approaches. Similarly, the extent to which they effected fundamental disruptions to the processes which constructed a whole array of subordinated and marginalized inclusions in the terms of welfare relations is debatable.

Despite this ambiguity, it is clear that these challenges contributed to a substantial destabilization in the social settlement of the KWS. Given this, the paradoxical appropriation by the New Right of the dissatisfactions articulated by these movements is even more stark. For, on the one hand, the New Right attempted to harness these criticisms as part of its attack on the collectivist and redistributive visions of the welfare state; while, on the other, it was to use some of the responses to these challenges by, for example, Labour-controlled local authorities, as a means by which to attack them and claim that they had lost touch with 'the people'. Thus the claims made by the new social movements both for a recognition of diversity and for the legitimacy of equal access to welfare services and benefits were used by the New Right but in opposite ways. It was from within the tensions between these two that the Thatcher and Major governments were to embark on the project of substituting the market and its 'subject' – the customer – as the new figure of restructured social relations of welfare. It is to this that we now turn.

7.3   The challenge from 'above': the citizen as customer

Without implying a homogeneity within and across the diverse range of organizations, actions and debates which comprised what we call the new social movements, it is possible to trace out some general lines of direction which are common to at least parts of all these movements. Three such general lines come to mind, these are that they:

1   argued for group rather than individual rights;

2   sought greater redistribution and not just greater individual opportunity;

3   sought an expanded, rather than a narrowed, version of the welfare state.

These general themes stand in stark contrast to those which characterized the general political direction of the New Right, as we have already seen. This is why we have talked of the *appropriation* of the challenges posed by new social movements.

One place to begin to explore this contrast is the Citizen's Charter (HMSO, 1991) introduced by the Major government in July 1991. On its introduction the Charter was billed as the first in a series of initiatives aimed at making public services more responsive to the needs and wishes of their users and, thus, stressed the themes of quality, standards, choice and value for money (Farnham, 1991/92). As such, the government claimed it was responding to the concerns and wishes expressed by users of public services, such as the NHS or the railways, in a way which combined the attempts to make these services more efficient and effective. The themes of quality, choice, standards and value formed the basis of the following principles, as Oliver (1993) has pointed out:

(1)   Clear published standards: the setting, monitoring and publication of explicit standards for public services.

(2)   Information and openness: the provision of full, accurate and easily understandable information on public services.

(3)   Choice and consultation: the public sector should provide choice between competing providers wherever possible.

(4)   Courtesy and helpfulness: an emphasis on greater responsiveness and accessibility.

(5)   Redress of grievance: the provision of effective complaints procedures.

(6)   Value for money: efficient and economical delivery of public services within the resources the nation can afford.   (Oliver, 1993, p.26)

What is the relationship between the citizen of this Charter and the citizen of the Keynesian welfare state?

As we have seen, the rights to welfare which accrued to the citizen of the Beveridge reforms did so because 'he' (*sic*) was a member of a political community whom the state had a duty to protect from the worst excesses of a capitalist economy. The 'citizen' of this welfare community had the duty to contribute 'his' share to the collective fund for social protection in the form of national insurance contributions and by being a 'good' father and husband. In contrast, the 'citizen' of the welfare community encapsulated in the Citizen's Charter was only an autonomous individual who could protect her or his personal interests and have the right to do this guaranteed by the Charter. The 'subject' embodied in the notion of the citizen has become reconstituted in the move away from the social settlement of the KWS.

We can see this more clearly if we return again to Oliver and note the points she makes about the key mechanisms for guaranteeing the rights of the autonomous individual embodied in the Charter:

(1) Privatization ...

(2) Further contracting out and competitive tendering.

(3) More performance related pay in the public sector.

(4) Published performance targets and the publication of standards achieved ...

(5) More effective complaints procedures: a strengthening of public utility regulators ...

(6) Tougher and more independent inspectorates ...

(7) Better citizen redress. Citizens will gain the right to challenge unlawful strikes.

(Oliver, 1993, p.26)

All of these mechanisms had more to do with guaranteeing the rights of the 'consumer' than those of the citizen, if the latter is understood as a subject who stands in a particular relation to the state both in terms of electoral aims and affinities, and in terms of a collectivist consensus about the state's role as organizer, provider and regulator of welfare services. The mechanisms above resonate with echoes of the market and address the relationship between the provider and the consumer of services. In this way we can see a correspondence between the reconstituted 'subject' of welfare/public services and the restructuring of the economic and political settlements we have already discussed. Moreover, the market was portrayed as the most efficient means by which to recognize diversity and respond to particularistic needs. Thus 'better management' and 'greater efficiency', which are contained in the Charter, have been expressed through the fostering of the belief that 'freedom from being over-taxed is premised on individuals making their own choices rather than having them foisted on them by the state' (Lewis, 1993, p.317). The Charter introduces the market as the mediator

customer

of the relationship of people to welfare services by its emphasis on 'customers', competition, privatization and contracting out.

ACTIVITY 2.6

Extract 2.6 is taken from the Patient's Charter, which applied the general philosophy of the Citizen's Charter to the NHS. Read through this extract and consider whether this is a Charter for 'citizens' or one for 'customers'.

Extract 2.6 Department of Health: 'The patient's charter'

The rights and standards set out in this leaflet form *The Patient's Charter*.

The Charter is a central part of the programme to improve and modernize the delivery of the National Health Service to the public, while continuing to reaffirm its fundamental principles.

The Patient's Charter puts the Government's *Citizen's Charter* initiative into practice in the health service. ...

Three new rights

From 1 April 1992, you will have three important new rights:

- to be given detailed information on local health services, including quality standards and maximum waiting times. You will be able to get this information from your health authority, GP or community Health Council;

- to be guaranteed admission for virtually all treatments by a specific date no later than two years from the day when your consultant places you on a waiting list. Most patients will be admitted before this date. Currently, 90% are admitted within a year;

- to have any complaint about NHS services whoever provides them investigated, and to receive a full and prompt written reply from the chief executive of your health authority or general manager of your hospital. If you are still unhappy, you will be able to take the case up with the Health Service Commissioner.

National Charter standards

There are nine standards of service which the NHS will be aiming to provide for you:

- respect for privacy, dignity and religious and cultural beliefs;

- arrangements to ensure everyone, including people with special needs, can use the services;

- information to relatives and friends about the progress of your treatment, subject, of course, to your wishes;

- an emergency ambulance should arrive within 11 minutes in an urban area, or 19 minutes in a rural area;

- when attending an accident and emergency department, you will be seen immediately and your need for treatment assessed;

- when you go to an outpatient clinic, you will be given a specific appointment time and will be seen within 30 minutes of it;

- your operation should not be cancelled on the day you are due to arrive in hospital. If, exceptionally, your operation has to be postponed twice you will be admitted to hospital within one month of the second cancelled operation;

- a named qualified nurse, midwife or health visitor responsible for your nursing or midwifery care;

- a decision should be made about any continuing health or social care needs you may have, before you are discharged from hospital.

(Department of Health, 1992)

COMMENT

What is noticeable is that what are termed the three additional 'rights' are posed as those which arise between parties to a business contract rather than those we might associate with a social contract between state and citizen. Similarly, 'difference' is equated with individual choice and preference, with the one exception of respect for religious and cultural beliefs. However, like the respect for privacy and dignity, this respect is only an *aim* and not a right. The rest of the Charter returns to the language and imagery of the business contract where guarantees are about efficient management and co-ordination of time and information. At the centre is a 'customer' of a business, the 'patient' is hidden from view, as is the cluster of social relations which are organized around this subject and that of manager, professional and all those other 'subjects' who run the NHS.

■ ■ ■

manager

If the reconstruction of welfare carried with it the creation of a new subject of welfare in the form of the 'customer', so too it created another new subject in the form of the 'manager'. As Clarke and Newman (1997, p.92) have noted, this figure allowed those who previously understood themselves as 'administrators', 'public servants' and 'practitioners' to see themselves anew – as 'purchasers', 'business managers' and 'leaders'. Moreover, the 'manager' as subject was emotionally involved in the organization so that, in contrast to the *rational* distance said to be created by bureaucracy, *feelings* were deployed as a means of motivating, controlling and co-ordinating the operational processes (du Gay, 1994) of the welfare agency.

NHS red tape threatens care

Too many chiefs
NHS 'market' fails the carers

Management dynamism frees resources? (Source: The Herald, *18 January 1996)*

Thus the move to a model of the 'customer' as the subject of welfare use had its counterpart in the 'manager' as the efficient co-ordinator and motivator of welfare production. This is illustrated by the Patient's Charter. As such it provides a clear example of the way in which the New Right reconstruction of the welfare state led to a range of new welfare subjects. Whether these were the same subjects envisaged by the new social movements is debatable. Similarly, whether this was the most appropriate way to guarantee rights – of redistribution, autonomy and self-definition – for those who were included within the terms of the old welfare state in subordinated and marginalized ways is equally open to question. Moreover, any doubts about this are further compounded by the *re-emergence* of a well-known welfare subject from the past: that of the 'undeserving' or 'welfare scrounger'. This terminology emerged again in the 1980s as a way to characterize many of those who were recipients of certain welfare benefits, such as housing benefit, income support and other forms of income maintenance payment. It indicated that a hard divide was being constructed between those whose use of welfare services was seen as legitimate and those who were seen as illegitimate and a drain on national resources. The discourse of 'customer' was reserved for the former. Together these changes indicate that the old social settlement was fundamentally destabilized. The place where this is most keenly apparent is on the site of what we have called the organizational settlement and it is to this that we now turn.

8   The crisis of the organizational settlement

In this and the previous chapter the organizational settlement of the KWS was said to comprise two general features – bureaucratic rational administration and professionalism – often referred to in combined form as bureau-professionalism. We also suggested that, like the other settlements, this became an object for transformation by the New Right. Thus, as a set of organizational values and a means of structuring the relationships between groups of people engaged in the production, delivery and use of welfare services and benefits, this fourth settlement was also destabilized. It is to this that we refer when we talk of the crisis of the organizational settlement.

One dominant strand in this destabilization has been managerialism, as both a discourse and as a mode of institutional practice, and in Chapter 9 Janet Newman provides a sharply focused analysis of this. But the changes in the organizational arrangements within welfare institutions cannot be reduced to managerialism alone and in this section I want briefly to consider two points. First, I want to look at the way in which attacks upon collectivist versions of 'the public', which were contained in the KWS and articulated through notions of 'public service' (Clarke and Newman, 1997, p.4), were used as a means of undermining bureau-professionalism. In this sense there are links to the New Right populism of the Thatcher governments and managerialism as a discourse (see above and Chapter 9). Here I want to focus on this in terms of the promotion of 'change' as both necessary if the hold of bureaucratic and professional self-interest was to be broken, and as a 'good thing' in itself – that is, as an organizational value. I then want to consider the ways in which relationships within and between welfare institutions were organized around new forms of co-ordination and distributions of responsibilities, which were effected through a shift in the balance between the state and private- and voluntary-sector activity in the provision of welfare services. This shift was not evenly distributed across all the areas of the welfare state and as you read through the following chapters it is worth thinking about the comparisons and contrasts between sectors. In this chapter I simply raise some points which indicate the unevenness and complexity of the process.

Before I go on to consider these issues briefly, I want to make two further points. First, I have focused on these two aspects of the promotion of change because they illustrate that it was at the level of the organizational settlement that the tensions and disruptions within the other three settlements played themselves out. In this way the organizational settlement became the site upon which the forces of destabilization of the KWS coalesced. Second, when we talk about the disruption of the organizational settlement we are not suggesting that a totally new institutional culture and set of social relationships came into being. Professionals continue to operate within the NHS, social services, housing and education, for example; so too do bureaucratic methods of co-ordinating the links within and between welfare agencies and, indeed, both of these points will be evident as you read through the chapters which follow. Rather, it is as the *dominant* means of organizing institutional methods and relationships that we have seen a shift in the organizational settlement.

8.1   Articulating the need for change

Earlier I suggested that the New Right project represented by successive Conservative governments in the 1980s and 1990s was populist because it attempted to appropriate and mobilize popular dissatisfactions with an array of state institutions. Nowhere was this more marked than the attack on the bureau-professional settlement of the KWS. Clarke and Newman (1997, p.16) have suggested that the organizational forms and practices of the welfare state were marked out in this way by the New Right 'because they constituted a field of relationships and symbolism that embodied (in bricks and mortar as well as "vocations") an alternative social formation to that being pursued by the New Right.' Central to this process of displacement and marginalization of an alternative social formation was the construction of new set of ideological values organized around the notion of change.

The Citizen's Charter and its specific versions, such as the Patient's Charter, provide examples of this ideology of change. In general terms the ideology of change spoke a number of shifts which had been identified as necessary if the ossified and oppressive structures and practices of the KWS were to be overcome. Thus change was necessary if:

- welfare providers were to be responsive to 'customer' needs and demands;
- staff initiative and energy were to be released and mobilized;
- the potential for autonomy, dynamism and choice which the market can offer was to be realized;
- new ideas about the relation between employer and employee, and state and citizen, were to be allowed to take root and flourish.

'Change', then, became the narrative through which to articulate the destabilization of the bureau-professional regime which had characterized the organizational settlement of the KWS.

8.2   Shifting balances

Shifts in the organizational settlement were also effected through changes in the modes of co-ordination within and between agencies and through a shift in the balance between services provided by the state and those provided by the private and voluntary sectors. Deeply intertwined with this rebalancing was an attempt to increase the extent to which women within the home – symbolized through the figure of 'the mother' – provided care. Privatization in this sense, then, should be taken to include the increase in informal care within families and households, as well as an expanded role for private- and voluntary-sector provision of services which accompanied the purchaser–provider split.

Of course, the Keynesian or Beveridgean welfare state was never completely a state-dominated set of institutions and practices. Many aspects of the welfare state were outside the direct control of the state, both within the voluntary sector (in many cases a legacy from nineteenth-century forms of philanthropy) and in the private sector. As now, 'the private' always included the informal care provided (mainly) by women within the home and, as we have seen, this was an assumption built into the terms of the Beveridge reforms. But to say this is not to deny that the balance between the state, private and voluntary sectors radically shifted as a result of the restructuring of welfare which began in the 1980s. Thus the delivery of welfare became increasingly organized through independent and semi-independent agencies within the private and voluntary sectors and co-ordinated and regulated through the formal institutions of the state. 'Managers' and 'customers' were the subjects of the social relations of this new form of co-ordination, and 'markets' (or what are sometimes called 'quasi-markets') were the mechanisms through which control of budgets and resources was attained. Thus the expertise of the professional, and the rational and distanced control of bureaucratic administration, were to *some extent* displaced. And it is to 'some extent', for the old exists alongside the new. Thus internal markets within, for example, the NHS created a system of health care which was neither the 'old' state model nor a completely privatized alternative. The mixed economy of welfare did not equate to a simple split between the state, on the one hand, and the market, on the other. An expanded role for the private and voluntary sectors still left public-sector agencies with key responsibilities in, for example, assessing needs and purchasing care packages, and therefore retaining the 'expertise' of professionals or care managers. Finally, it was the case that welfare benefits and services remained predominantly publicly *funded* even if not publicly provided.

9   Conclusion

By the late 1990s much of what had generally come to be understood as something called 'the welfare state' remained in place; the state still played a central role; people still received many services free at the point of delivery; and the private and voluntary sectors had a greatly expanded role, but were not the only means of access to or provision of welfare services.

Having said this, it is equally clear that the New Right project of fundamentally shifting the ground upon which assumptions about and expectations of the welfare state were made was largely successful. It could no longer be generally expected that the state would be the main *provider* of services, or indeed would guarantee full (male) employment or support from 'cradle to grave'. The election to government of New Labour under the helm of Tony Blair in 1997 made it clear that there had been a radical shift in the ways in which the relationship between the state and the citizen was imagined. The responsibilities, *rights and outcomes* which characterized the language of the KWS were replaced by a language of *responsibilities and opportunities*, as was clear from a speech given by Peter Mandelson (Minister without Portfolio at the time of writing) and generally understood to have been a chief architect of the successful Blair campaign. New Labour, he said, is 'about building a fairer society – where we all owe a responsibility to each other; where every individual has a sense of their own intrinsic worth and has the opportunity to fulfil the potential that lies uniquely in them; where every family can feel it has a stake in society' (Mandelson, 1997). Moreover, this language of responsibility was central to the 'welfare-to-work' programme which was at the core of Blair's first government. As part of the 'contract' between the recipient of welfare benefits and the providing agency, these recipients would only retain their eligibility if they committed themselves to one of a number of routes to employment. This was made clear by Gordon Brown, Chancellor of the Exchequer, in the first budget issued by the Blair government, and the element of compulsion for young people was equally clear:

> With those new opportunities for young people come new responsibilities. There will be no fifth option – to stay at home on full benefit. So when they sign on for benefit, they will be signing up for work. Benefits will be cut if young people refuse to take up the opportunities.
>
> (Gordon Brown, Budget speech, *Hansard*, 2 July 1997, vol.297, no.31, col.308)

If the first New Labour government seemed to indicate that a new consensus had emerged, it was also noticeable that there were some differences between them and the New Right governments of Thatcher and Major. This was perhaps most apparent in the stated commitment by New Labour to tackling the material inequalities which widened enormously over the 1980s and 1990s. Mandelson made this point in his speech to the Fabian Society quoted above when he announced the establishment of a unit to tackle social exclusion. Again, however,

Welfare to work?

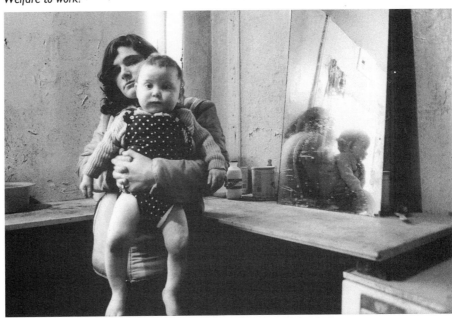

the language in which this announcement was made indicated a radical shift away from the underlying principles of the old social democratic consensus and an acceptance of the discourses characteristic of the New Right. Thus the much needed economic 'flexibility' would not be possible without finding 'ways of getting people off dependency' and a more equal society would not result from 'the redistribution of cash from rich to poor' (Mandelson, 1997). All this would be achieved through the promotion of economic flexibility, plus 'welfare to work'; partnership with business in developing the infrastructure; standards of fair treatment, and so on.

In broad terms, then, all we can say for certain is that the settlements which characterized the social democratic consensus of the post Second World War era were radically destabilized, if not completely overturned. The impact of these changes within and across specific sites of welfare was uneven and complex. As you read the other chapters in this book you will become more keenly aware of this. One question that might guide your reading is to consider to what extent and in what ways the old settlements associated with the Keynesian or Beveridgean welfare state were 'unsettled'.

Further reading

Two books which are particularly useful for a further consideration of the process of the reconstruction of welfare in the 1980s and 1990s are Hills (1990 and 1993). Nancy Fraser's *Justice Interruptus* (1997) also provides some interesting essays which explore the connections between welfare regimes and women's status within them. The essay by Williams (1993) offers a similar analysis of the connections between British welfare policy and the 'differences' of class, gender and 'race'. Several pamphlets published by the Institute of Economic Affairs provide examples of New Right arguments against the 'old' welfare state and their ideas for its reformulation. The references to Davies (1986) and Murray (1990) are two such pamphlets.

References

Barnes, C. (1991) *Disabled People in Britain and Discrimination*, British Council of Organizations of Disabled People, Calgary, Hirst.

Brent Community Health Council (1981) *Black People and the Health Service*, London, Brent Community Health Council.

Bulpitt, M. (1986) 'The discipline of the new democracy: Mrs. Thatcher's domestic statecraft', *Political Studies*, vol.34, pp.19–39.

Clarke, J. (ed.) (1993) *A Crisis in Care: Challenges to Social Work*, London, Sage.

Clarke, J. and Cochrane, A. (1998) 'The social construction of social problems', in Saraga (ed.) (1998b).

Clarke, J. and Langan, M. (1993) 'Restructuring welfare: the British welfare regime in the 1980s', in Cochrane and Clarke (eds) (1993).

Clarke, J. and Newman, J. (1997) *The Managerial State*, London, Sage.

Clarke, J., Cochrane, A., Collins, R., Graham, P., Harris, P., Langan, M., McLaughlin, E. and Saraga, E. (1996) D211 *Social Problems and Social Welfare. The Hitchhiker's Guide to D211*, Milton Keynes, The Open University.

Cochrane, A. and Clarke, J. (eds) (1993) *Comparing Welfare States: Britain in International Context*, London, Sage.

Davies, S. (1986) *Beveridge Revisted: New Foundations for Tomorrow's Welfare*, London, Centre for Policy Studies.

Department of Health (1992) *The Patient's Charter*, London, HMSO.

du Gay, P. (1994) 'Colossal immodesties and hopeful monsters: pluralism and organizational conduct', *Organization*, vol.1, no.1, pp.125–48.

Farnham, D. (1991/92) 'The Citizen's Charter: improving the quality of the public services or forthcoming market values?', *Talking Politics*, vol.4, no.2, pp.75–80.

Foucault, M. (1979) *The History of Sexuality*, vols 1–3, London, Penguin.

Fraser, N. (1997) *Justice Interruptus: Critical Reflections on the 'Post Socialist' Condition*, New York and London, Routledge.

Gamble, A. (1988) *The Free Economy and the Strong State: The Politics of Thatcherism*, London, Macmillan.

Gazeley, I. and Thane, P. (1998) 'Patterns of visibility: unemployment in Britain during the nineteenth and twentieth centuries', in Lewis (ed.) (1998c).

Hall, S. and Jacques, M. (1983) *The Politics of Thatcherism*, London, Lawrence and Wishart.

Hills, J. (ed.) (1990) *The State of Welfare: The Welfare State in Britain Since 1974*, Oxford, Clarendon.

Hills, J. (1993) *The Future of Welfare: A Guide to the Debate*, York, Joseph Rowntree Foundation.

HMSO (1989) *Caring for People: Community Care in the Next Decade and Beyond*, Cm 849, London, HMSO.

HMSO (1991) *The Citizen's Charter: Raising the Standard*, London, HMSO.

Hughes, G. (1998) 'A suitable case for treatment? Constructions of disability', in Saraga (ed.) (1998b).

Labour Research (1997) 'Eighteen years of feathering their nests. Election special', *Labour Research*, vol.86, no.5.

Laclau, E. (1977) *Politics and Ideology in Marxist Theory*, London, New Left Books.

Langan, M. (1993) 'New directions in social work', in Clarke (ed.) (1993).

Langan, M. (1998a) 'The contested concept of need', in Langan (ed.) (1998b).

Langan, M. (ed.) (1998b) *Welfare: Needs, Rights and Risks*, London, Routledge in association with The Open University.

Langan, M. and Clarke, J. (1994) 'Managing in the mixed economy of care', in Clarke, J., Cochrane, A. and McLaughlin, E. (eds) *Managing Social Policy*, London, Sage.

Le Grand, J. (1990) 'The state of welfare', in Hills, J. (ed.) *The Future of Welfare: A Guide to the Debate*, York, Joseph Rowntree Foundation.

Lentell, H. (1998) 'Families of meaning: contemporary discourses of the family', in Lewis (ed.) (1998c).

Lewis, G. (1998a) 'Welfare and the social construction of "race"', in Saraga (ed.) (1998b).

Lewis, G. (1998b) 'Citizenship', in Hughes, G. (ed.) *Imagining Welfare Futures*, London, Routledge in association with The Open University.

Lewis, G. (ed.) (1998c) *Forming Nation, Framing Welfare*, London, Routledge in association with The Open University.

Lewis, N. (1993) 'The Citizen's Charter and next steps: a new way of governing?', *The Political Quarterly*, vol.65, no.3, pp.316–26.

Liberty (1994) *Access Denied: Human Rights and Disabled People*, London NCCL/RCODP.

Mackintosh, M. and Smith, P. (1996) 'Perverse incentives: an NHS notebook', *Soundings,* issue 4, pp.135–48.

Mandelson, P. (1997) Speech to the Fabian Society, 14 August.

Marquand, D. (1988) 'Paradoxes of Thatcherism', in Skidesley, R. (ed.) *Thatcherism*, London, Chatto and Windus.

Martin, R. (1992) 'The economy', in Clarke (ed.) (1993).

Morris, L. (1998) 'Legitimate membership of the welfare community', in Langan (ed.) (1998b).

Murray, C. (1990) *The Emerging British Underclass*, London, The IEA Health and Welfare Unit.

Office for National Statistics (1991) *Census Definitions, G.B.,* London, HMSO.

Office for National Statistics (1997) *Social Trends 27*, London, The Stationery Office.

Office of Population Census and Surveys (1981) *1981 Census Definitions,* London, HMSO.

Oliver, D. (1993) 'Citizenship in the 1990s', *Socialist Review*, pp.25–8.

O'Shea, A. (1984) 'Trusting the people: how does Thatcherism work?', in *New Foundations, Foundations of Nations and People*, London, Routledge and Kegan Paul.

Pierson, P. (1994) *Dismantling the Welfare State? Reagan, Thatcher, and the Politics of Retrenchment*, Cambridge, Cambridge University Press.

Saraga, E. (1998a) 'Abnormal, unnatural and immoral? The social construction of sexualities', in Saraga (ed.) (1998b).

Saraga, E. (ed.) (1998b) *Embodying the Social: Constructions of Difference*, London, Routledge in association with The Open University.

Taylor, P. (1992) 'Changing political relations', in Clarke, P. (ed.) *Policy and Change in Thatcher's Britain*, Oxford, Pergamon.

Thompson, G. (1990) *The Political Economy of the New Right,* London, Pinter.

Trades Union Congress/School Curriculum Industry Partnership (1995) *Trade Unions in the Modern World*, London, Trades Union Congress.

Wilding, P. (1992) 'The British welfare state: Thatcherism's enduring legacy', *Policy and Politics*, vol.20, no.3, pp.201–12.

Williams, F. (1989) *Social Policy: A Critical Introduction,* Cambridge, Polity.

Williams, F. (1993) 'Gender, "race" and class in British welfare policy', in Cochrane and Clarke (eds) (1993).

CHAPTER 3

The Restructuring of Health Care

by Mary Langan

Contents

1   Introduction

This chapter aims to throw new light on the transformation of the health service in the 1990s and, by focusing on the renegotiation of the post-war settlement, to deepen your understanding of that complex and contested resolution of the problem of how to deliver welfare in a modern industrial society. The chapter includes several extracts, which have been selected to illustrate particular viewpoints which were influential in the complex conflicts through which the process of re-negotiating the post-war welfare settlements proceeded.

The reforms enacted in the NHS and Community Care Act 1990 – which introduced the internal market into the health service – were the culmination of nearly two decades of turbulent change. This process of transformation was triggered by the breakdown, in the course of the 1970s, of the complex set of arrangements that made up the post-war welfare settlement (see Chapters 1 and 2). Just as the different aspects of that settlement were the product of protracted conflicts, so the new framework that began to emerge in the mid 1990s was the outcome of often intense contestation.

settlement

The chapter begins by outlining the transformation of the health service in terms of the familiar dimensions of the post-war settlement:

■ *Political: the eclipse of social democracy*
Though the first departures from social democratic commitments – to full employment and rising public spending – came under the Labour governments of the late 1970s, it was the offensive of the Conservative governments after 1979 against collectivist traditions in all their forms that inflicted a decisive defeat on the social democratic tradition.

■ *Economic: the end of the Keynesian welfare state*
The introduction of the internal market and its associated commercial values of competition, efficiency and value for money in the early 1990s signalled the final abandonment of the principles of state welfare proclaimed by Keynes and Beveridge and embodied in the post-war welfare state.

■ *Social: from collectivism to pluralism, from doctor/patient to provider/ consumer*
Just as the early NHS was powerfully symbolic of the egalitarian and collectivist social values of the post-war era, the reformed NHS reflected the more individualistic, fragmented and pluralist outlook of the 1990s. Both the 1990 reforms and the 1991 White Paper, *The Health of the Nation*, which emphasized health promotion and disease prevention, assumed welfare subjects who were active participants in their own health.

■ *Organizational: the rise of managerialism*
The infusion of managers and management-speak into the health service was one of the key features of the reforms of the 1980s and 1990s. Though medical autonomy was reduced, it was far from destroyed, as doctors retained considerable power under the new arrangements.

In the succeeding sections we shall examine more closely each of the different aspects of this process of change.

What were the key features of the post-war welfare settlement that came into question from the 1970s onwards?

2 Renegotiating the settlements

In the early 1990s the health service in the UK underwent the most drastic changes for half a century. The scale of this transformation, which turned hospitals into trusts and GPs into fundholders, and subjected the whole system to the rigours of the 'internal market', was all the more remarkable given the long-standing prestige and stability of the National Health Service. Yet, just as the NHS had been central to the settlements of the 1940s – the complex arrangements on which the post-war welfare state had been established – it also had a crucial place in its restructuring in the 1990s.

2.1 The eclipse of social democracy

The social democratic consensus began to crumble in the second half of the 1970s under the impact of recession, the return of mass unemployment and the Labour government's squeeze on public spending. However, Labour's attempts at reform of the health service proved controversial and largely unsuccessful. Measures to curb costs and to increase efficiency provoked mass demonstrations against 'the cuts' and recurrent industrial action by health service workers. Turmoil in the health service was a major element in the wave of strikes which become known as the 'winter of discontent' and which heralded Labour's defeat in the 1979 election, in which Margaret Thatcher first came to power.

The election of the Conservative government committed to rolling back the state from its involvement in both the economy and welfare and to the wider promotion of the values of the free market, marked a decisive break with post-war traditions. Yet the government's early reforming initiatives in the health service were as ill-fated as those of its predecessors. It was not until after their third election victory in 1987 that the Conservatives began to make much progress in reforming the NHS. By the early 1990s a decade of Tory rule had demoralized the social democratic tradition to such an extent that a growing consensus around distrust for the state and approval for the market now provided the framework for restructuring health care. It was left to John Major, who replaced Mrs Thatcher as prime minister after a Conservative Party revolt in November 1990, to push through the reforms of the NHS drawn up by his predecessor.

2.2 The end of the Keynesian welfare state

In the 1980s expressions of dissatisfaction with the health service came from all sides: from striking nurses and ambulance workers protesting over stagnating pay levels, from medical bodies demanding more resources, from public opinion inflamed by media accounts of inordinate delays, waiting-lists and other manifestations of inefficiency. At the same time, the collapse of the Soviet Union, undermining the legitimacy of state socialist policies internationally, provided an ideological boost to the notion that market forces were a more efficient means of delivering everything (including health care) than state bureaucracies.

Squeezed between the chronic stagnation of the real economy and the apparently relentless demand for higher public expenditure, the 'Keynesian welfare state' gave way to the new 'mixed economy of welfare' in which private

Health workers on the march: members of the moderate Royal College of Nursing swelled the ranks in trade union protest in the 1980s

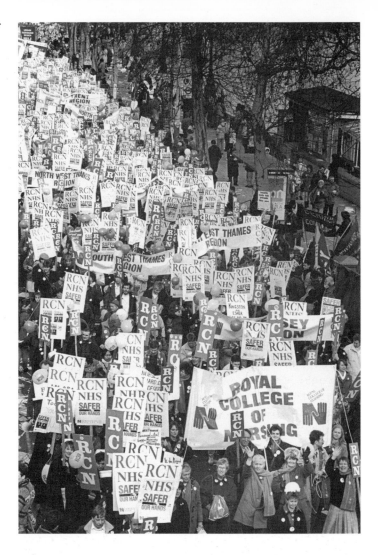

and voluntary initiatives were required to compensate for public parsimony. The values of consumerism, managerialism and competition displaced the fraying ethos of public service.

consumerism
managerialism
competition

2.3   The unravelling of the social settlement

Though the early NHS was celebrated at home and abroad as a free and universal service, imbued with the collectivist and egalitarian principles of the post-war Labour government, it was often perceived as a hierarchical and paternalistic system. The triad of images of the heroic/authoritarian doctor, the dutiful/wonderful nurse and the stoical/deferential patient was promoted from the Ealing comedies to *Emergency Ward Ten* (Britain's first medical soap, launched by ITV in 1957) (Karpf, 1988). These images reflected both the dominant representations and the reality of a health care system that was, for all the radical rhetoric, still influenced by inequalities in class, gender and 'race' relationships that prevailed in UK society.

Doctors were drawn virtually exclusively from the upper middle classes, often from medical families, and they were overwhelmingly male. Nurses, apart from an elite in the teaching hospitals, were largely of working-class origin, and almost exclusively female. Patients – like the mass of hospital workers engaged as cleaners, porters, kitchen staff and so on – were also largely working-class. But, despite these differences, harmony prevailed, reflecting the considerable degree of collective commitment to the provision of public health care.

The strains in the social fabric of UK society and its health service began to appear from the 1960s onwards. Doctors, like other professions, expanded their ranks and drew on wider layers of society; though they included more women, the career ladder remained forbidding, especially in surgical specialties. Nursing also became a more diverse profession. The shift from matron to manager was accompanied by an influx of men who were soon much better represented in administrative offices than on the wards. From the 1950s onwards, shortages of nurses and other hospital staff led to a policy of direct recruitment from Ireland, the Caribbean and other former colonies. The character of patients changed too: as the memory of pre-war poverty and post-war austerity faded and living standards rose, a younger generation emerged that was less deferential to authority and more demanding of higher standards of health care. In place of harmony, there was now growing strife; in place of consensus, increasing conflict.

By the mid 1990s the old images could no longer be sustained, any more than could the old assumptions about class, gender and 'race' that underpinned them. In the 'primary care led' NHS, the doctor no longer wore a white coat, the nurse had long forsaken her uniform and her 'angelic' demeanour, and the patient was now a customer, demanding value for money. Viewers of contemporary hospital television dramas, such as *Casualty* and *Cardiac Arrest*, now saw a health care system under pressure, its diverse staff torn by conflicting demands and internecine tensions.

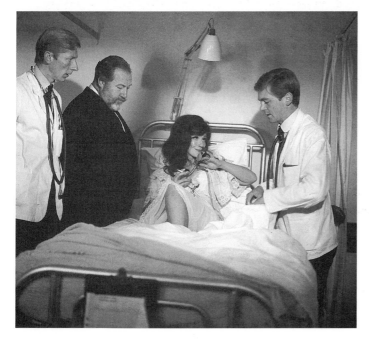

The supreme consultant: James Robertson Justice presides at the bedside in the film comedy, Doctor in Clover, *1965*

2.4 The professional imperative

In driving a hard bargain with the Labour government in 1948–49, the doctors set the standard for other professional groups eager to bolster their public prestige through a formal relationship with a state-administered bureaucracy. In the 1950s and 1960s the leaders of the medical profession were in close contact with government ministers, senior consultants effectively controlled the purse-strings in the hospitals and, though GPs had little access to resources, they enjoyed virtually complete autonomy in their disposal. Inevitably, the ascendancy of the market and the managers, not to mention the patient as consumer, in the reforms of the 1990s meant the partial displacement of medical power from some crucial areas of decision-making and greater constraints on professional autonomy. Yet, though the profession as such was weakened by the reforms, doctors still retained considerable power at every level of the health care system. This was in marked contrast to the loss of prestige of other public service professionals such as teachers and social workers.

By the late 1990s, and the return under Tony Blair of the Labour Party to government, the breakdown of the old welfare settlements was unmistakable. What was more difficult to discern was the shape of the new welfare regime emerging from a protracted process of reform and conflict. However, a closer look at the process of transition from the old welfare settlements can help to reveal the emerging character of the health service for the UK into the next century.

What were the key factors that influenced the health service reforms of the 1990s? Can you identify how these were different from the factors that decided the settlements of the 1940s?

3 The end of the social democratic consensus

Do you know there are still people in Britain who believe in consensus? I regard them as quislings, traitors.

(Margaret Thatcher, 1979)

I have always regarded it as part of my job – and please don't think of it in an arrogant way – to kill socialism in Britain.

(Margaret Thatcher, 1984)

The reforms first proclaimed in 1989 in the White Paper, *Working for Patients*, and subsequently codified in the NHS and Community Care Act 1990, were finally implemented in April 1991. The introduction of the internal market into the NHS marked the culmination of nearly twenty years of strife, beginning from the ancillary workers' pay disputes of 1972–73 and the subsequent conflicts between the doctors and the government.

Historians have revealed that the consensus in support of the principles of the NHS never went unquestioned, and was periodically challenged by influential conservative politicians and neo-liberal economists throughout the post-war period (Webster, 1994). From the early 1950s onwards there were recurrent complaints about excessive public spending on health care and demands to curtail it. There were also persistent tensions between the medical profession and the government and simmering unrest among other workers in the health service over poor pay and conditions.

Yet there can be little doubt that in the 1970s a qualitative shift took place. Whereas in the 1950s and 1960s industrial action in the health service was virtually non-existent, after 1972 it became commonplace. By 1975 even doctors were becoming militant: while consultants threatened to resign en masse from the NHS, some junior hospital doctors actually went on strike, demonstrated and set up picket-lines. In June 1974 hospital workers at London's Charing Cross Hospital took industrial action, not for more pay, but in an explicitly ideological campaign to force private 'pay-beds' out of NHS hospitals. Meanwhile, across London at the Royal Free Hospital, feminists were challenging the right of a traditional male obstetrician to dictate how women should deliver their babies. Similar protests took place in Scotland, Wales and Northern Ireland and in other regions of the United Kingdom.

By the late 1970s the health service had acquired the aura of permanent crisis which was to persist through the next decade. The Labour government's imposition of cash-limited budgets on the health authorities and strict wage controls on health service workers in response to the public expenditure crisis of 1976–77 provoked a rising tide of discontent both outside and inside the NHS. One effect of the spending curbs, exacerbated in London and the south

public expenditure crisis

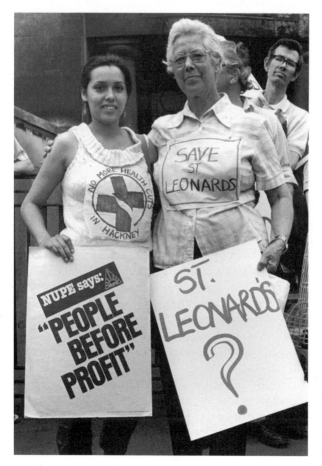

St Leonard's Hospital in Hackney was one of many closed as a result of the Labour government's redistribution of health care resources in the late 1970s

by the redistribution of resources imposed by the government's Resources Allocation Working Party (popularly known by its acronym, RAWP) was a wave of hospital and bed closures, provoking numerous local campaigns, demonstrations and even hospital occupations. Another was the series of strikes and protests that culminated in the wider public sector revolt in the winter of 1978–79.

Despite the change of government in May 1979, militancy and conflict carried on unabated under the Conservatives into the 1980s. The government continued to wrangle with the doctors, suppressing the 1980 Black Report, prepared by a prestigious committee chaired by the eminent physician Sir Douglas Black; the Report implicitly blamed the government for presiding over growing social differentials in health standards and demanded more resources for a wide range of social services in order to tackle them (Black, 1992). The government also continued the squeeze on public sector pay, and ambulance workers and nurses were soon back on the picket-lines.

By the mid 1980s, however, the government was beginning to succeed in imposing its authority in the health service as in other areas of British society. Despite opinion polls revealing high levels of public sympathy for striking nurses, in December 1982 the government forced them and other health service workers to accept pay rises below the rate of inflation. Hospitals were now legally required to introduce compulsory competitive tendering (CCT) for hospital cleaning, catering and laundry services. Though many of these tenders ultimately were awarded 'in-house', the process effectively neutralized union organization in the health service and often resulted in redundancies and pay cuts.

compulsory competitive tendering

Though the doctors appeared at first to fare better than the unions, they too were faced down by the government. The managerial reforms proposed by Sir Roy Griffiths, seconded from J. Sainsbury in 1983 to introduce some commercial rigour into the workings of the NHS, proved largely ineffectual in face of the entrenched power of the medical profession (Hunter, 1994). Yet, there were early indications that the doctors' power could be curtailed. The imposition in 1984 of the 'limited list' of drugs available on prescription, against concerted resistance from the doctors and the drug companies, was a significant, though little recognized, victory for the government. As Timmins (1995, p.413) observes, this affair was 'a watershed in the relations between the government and the BMA, demonstrating once and for all that ministers could defeat the association'. This victory undoubtedly gave Conservative ministers increased confidence for the higher profile confrontations five years later.

The government's increased authority in the health service was part of the wider success story of the Conservative government under Mrs Thatcher in the 1980s. Triumphant over their enemies at home (most notably the unions – a category in which ministers included the BMA) and abroad (in the Falklands War), the Conservatives inflicted an even heavier defeat on Labour in 1983. Yet an incident in the autumn of 1982 revealed a continuing diffidence about taking on the social democratic tradition in the sphere of health care, generally regarded as its greatest stronghold.

In September a report from the Central Policy Review Staff, a think-tank that reported directly to the Cabinet, proposed a series of radical reforms that amounted to dismantling the welfare state: it included plans for replacing the NHS with a system of private health insurance. Though favoured by some ministers, most were appalled at such drastic proposals, and the report provoked what Nigel Lawson (1992, p.303) later described as 'the nearest thing to a Cabinet riot in the history of the Thatcher administration'. Leaked to *The Economist*, it was seized on by opposition politicians as revealing the Tories' hidden agenda for privatizing the welfare state. Yet, speaking at the Conservative Party Conference less than a month later, Mrs Thatcher made her celebrated statement that 'the National Health Service is safe with us'.

The tension between the government's public commitment to the NHS and its private inclinations towards a drastic reduction of state involvement in health care revealed its continuing lack of confidence about carrying through the free market strategy in the area of welfare that enjoyed greatest public popularity and political prestige. Events over the next few years were to strengthen the government's hand and reduce its ambivalence about subordinating the NHS to the imperatives of the marketplace.

By the late 1980s the balance of forces in UK society had swung decisively to the advantage of the government. The defeat of the prolonged miners' strike of 1984–85 marked the end of an era of trade union militancy. Though in retrospect the Thatcher/Lawson boom of the late 1980s came to be regarded as superficial and speculative, at the time it was hailed as the end of a long recession (Le Grand, 1990). The expansion of share ownership, particularly in the newly privatized public utilities, appeared to inaugurate a new era of popular capitalism.

Perhaps the most revealing indicator of the new climate was the shift of the Labour Party, especially after its third consecutive general election defeat in 1987, to adopt the policies of 'new realism'. Under Neil Kinnock, Labour repudiated the strategy of seeking to restore the state of affairs prior to 1979 by reversing the innovations of Thatcherism. There was now no question of a return to the socialist programme advocated by left-wingers such as Tony Benn and Arthur Scargill through the 1980s. Labour too, in other words, abandoned the social democratic consensus, and shifted away from measures of state intervention and public expenditure towards a greater emphasis on individual initiative and private and voluntary provision.

Labour's retreat from the strategy of raising welfare standards through high public spending and redistributive taxation was confirmed by the publication of *Social Justice: Strategies for National Renewal* (Commission on Social Justice, 1994), a major review of welfare policy by a think-tank closely aligned to the party leadership. Not surprisingly, this gave the Conservatives new confidence in bringing the hidden agenda of market reform of the NHS out into the public domain.

ACTIVITY 3.1

In the course of the 1970s and 1980s defenders of the social democratic traditions of the post-war welfare state fought a protracted rearguard action against the ascendant forces of the pro-market conservatives. There follow representative accounts of each of these points of view by David Green and John Lister. As you read these extracts, make a list of Green's arguments in support of a market-led approach to the provision of health care. Make another list of Lister's defence of state provision. Why do you think Green's case for the market carried greater weight than Lister's defence of the state?

David Green of the Institute of Economic Affairs, one of the leading right-wing think-tanks of the Thatcher era, provides in Extract 3.1 a summary of the New

Right's critique of the NHS, drawing attention to the influence of US models of health care. Marginalized by the influence of the social democratic consensus in the post-war decades, the free marketeers became increasingly influential in the 1970s and 1980s.

Extract 3.1 Green: 'Lessons from the US market in health provision'

In Britain intellectual opinion remains predominantly socialistic and this is especially true of thinking about the NHS. The new liberal criticism of the NHS has aroused much passionate denunciation and has resulted in defenders of the NHS coming up with new arguments in its support, but few minds have been changed. The chief reason is that support for the NHS is rooted more in emotion than in reason. Some are attached to it because of their commitment to compulsory equalisation, but more are devoted to it because they associate the NHS with elementary decency or fair play.

At one stage, this view that the NHS represented the very utmost in altruism was the main argument used in support of it. Against this demand-side case that the NHS was necessary to ensure that the poor received adequate health care, the new liberals successfully argued that this could be accomplished in more than one way – by subsidies, or by vouchers. Such alternatives could protect the poor whilst also enhancing their ability to direct their own affairs by increasing the power of the patient *vis-à-vis* professionals and administrators.

Against this argument supporters of the NHS countered with a supply-side case for the NHS. The consumer, they said, could not exercise the choices that are essential to the market process. This was partly because the consumer was too ignorant, and partly because of professional monopoly power. In addition, the health market is distorted by the insurance mechanism which means that, unlike a normal market, competition promotes neither efficiency nor effectiveness. The choice on the demand side, writes Mr Nick Bosanquet in his critique of the new liberalism, 'is not between a market system and a government monopoly free at the point of consumption', it is between 'a national system of health care and a system of third party payment with quite extensive subsidies to those who cannot get coverage' (1983, p.151). He then makes the extraordinary claim that 'in reality there are only two possible budgetary contexts for medicine'. One is a cost-plus system in which 'doctors decide what is best for the patient ... then simply send in the bill for the best treatment to the third party'. The other is 'to set an overall budget within which individual decisions have to be contained'. This, he says, could be done through the NHS or a national health insurance scheme like Canada's. But the 'essential choice is between a cost plus system or one that introduces budget constraint' (ibid., pp.151–2).

His error is to assume that a market cannot provide pressures for cost-containment. But developments in the American health market in recent years show this claim to be wholly false. During the late 1970s and early 1980s there has been a great flowering of competition in the US health marketplace (Green, 1985a; 1986). Government programmes to promote cost-containment have played their part. Both Medicare and Medicaid have frequently been restructured to encourage cost-consciousness.

More important still have been the developments in the private sector. Cost-effective alternatives to hospital inpatient care have developed rapidly, especially ambulatory (or day) surgery centres. Home care backed by specialist nursing agencies also competes with hospital inpatient care, not only because it is cheaper but also because patients often prefer a less institutionalized environment. Hospital outpatient departments face equally strong competition from emergency centres as well as from group practices. Health maintenance organisations (HMOs) have a long history, but have begun to expand rapidly in recent years. Instead of charging for every visit to the doctor, the HMO receives a fixed payment per month in return for which the patient receives all necessary medical services without further payment …

More recently, preferred provider organization (PPOs) have emerged, largely as a reaction to the success of HMOs. The PPO is an effort to secure the advantages of the HMO without the necessity for the subscriber to confine his choice of doctor to a fixed panel. When an individual joins an HMO he or she pays a monthly premium and the HMO is fully at risk for any health care required by the subscriber. The HMO also 'locks-in' its subscribers, that is, if they go to a doctor outside the HMO panel they have no insurance cover. The PPO is different in two main respects. First the PPO itself bears no financial risk for the medical expenses incurred by subscribers. These are borne by the insurer, whether an insurance company or a self-insured employer. The providers are paid on a fee-for-service basis, at negotiated discounts, not by the individual patient, but by the insurer. Second, the PPO does not lock-in subscribers. If consumers choose to use the services of a PPO doctor they are of course covered, but if they use an outside hospital or doctor they still enjoy cover, though at a lower level (perhaps 80% or less).

…

The implication of these developments is this. Health economists have been quick to interpret evidence from America about skyrocketing costs (during a period when governments were pumping millions of dollars into the demand side) as evidence that the insurance mechanism, generated perverse incentives, and particularly an incentive to over-consume. Recent developments suggest that this conclusion has been arrived at too hastily. The market in the last few years has shown a tendency to adjust over time. And in the last few years there has been a great flowering of inventive mechanisms for cost-containment without cutting corners at the patient's expense.

These developments contradict the supply-side case for the NHS, a view which rests on the belief that competition – which ordinarily puts the consumer in the driving seat – cannot work in health care. The producer is said to be too powerful due to professional monopoly power and due to the unavoidable ignorance of consumers about medical matters. Events in the US market show this conclusion to be false. The producer's monopoly power has been undermined by government action to eliminate legal barriers to competition. Today the US market is no longer dominated by the producer. One of the main reasons is that federal and state governments no longer reinforce professional power to the extent they once did. The Federal Trade Commission (FTC) has been particularly effective in outlawing the restrictive practices of the American Medical Association, such as its advertising ban. A turning-point came in 1982 when the Supreme Court ruled in the FTC's favour. Advertising by American doctors is now growing.

The consumer's lack of knowledge has been overcome in a variety of ways, by third-party endorsements, by counselling and by the emergence of approved panels of doctors. Such panels simplify the consumer's choice, because he or she knows that every doctor on the panel acts in accordance with the rules of the organization, whether it is an HMO or a PPO. These rules lay down fees, and provide for the review of each doctor's performance by professional colleagues as well as by administrators acting on the consumer's behalf.

Thus, the 'inevitable monopoly' thesis which lies at the root of the supply-side case for the NHS fails to find support in the US market. Historical evidence from Australia (Green and Cromwell, 1984) and Britain also refutes it (Green, 1985b). It cannot therefore be argued that the market is unavoidably incapable of supplying health care.

References

Bosanquet, N. (1983) *After the New Right*, London, Heinemann.

Green, D.G. (1985a) 'American health care: the re-awakening of competition', *Economic Affairs*, vol.6, no.2, pp. 22–3.

Green, D.G. (1985b) *Working-class Patients and the Medical Establishment*, Aldershot, Gower/Temple Smith.

Green, D.G. (1986) *Challenge to the NHS: A Study of Competition in American Health Care and the Lessons for Britain*, London, IEA.

Green, D.G. and Cromwell, L. (1984) *Mutual Aid or Welfare State*, Sydney, Allen and Unwin.

(Green, 1987, pp.179–83)

John Lister, a veteran radical journalist and leading campaigner in the largely union-financed pressure group, London Health Emergency, offers 'an answer to the NHS crisis' in the course of an account of the trade union disputes and other conflicts in the health service in the 1980s reprinted as Extract 3.2. In response to the government's drive to subordinate the NHS to the dictates of the market, Lister upholds the commitment to collective state provision on which the NHS was founded.

Extract 3.2 Lister: 'An answer to the NHS crisis'

... [A]s Thatcher's review seeks to roll back the wheel of history, further reducing the proportion of national wealth spent on health services while maximising the involvement of the private, commercial sector, there *is* an alternative approach, which would build on the principle of collective, social provision of health care that were [*sic*] embodied in the formation of the NHS. It is particularly important to fight against any renewed imposition of charges or means-testing for health care.

[We] have argued against the conventional Tory myth that demand for health care is necessarily 'infinite', and tried to show how capitalism itself (and especially Thatcherite policies of deepening poverty and widening class divisions) actually *increase* demand for health services by generating avoidable illness. A systematic approach to health services would follow the alternative logic of the Black Report, and seek to *reduce levels of illness,* by eradicating poverty, poor housing and inadequate diet at the same time as improving health education, developing preventive medicine and primary care, and establishing an occupational health service as an essential complement to improved NHS services.

Alongside steps to minimise the creation of new 'patients' a serious health policy would set out to *measure* the real levels of need for the various forms of health care and treatment both for acute specialities and for the more chronic conditions of the mentally ill, mentally handicapped and the elderly – many of whom need not hospital or institutional care but effective support in the community. A proper costing of these services must include provision for substantial pay increases for all grades of health workers to enable the NHS to recruit and retain a stable, skilled workforce.

We also need a detailed national inventory of the hospital and other building stock available to the NHS, together with details of its physical condition. This would enable an overall estimate to be made of the need for new building, upgrading and repairs to achieve minimum acceptable standards of hygiene, accessibility and comfort for patients and staff. Once the actual level of demand for services and the required amount of capital investment and additional staffing costs are known, it becomes relatively simple to calculate the resources needed to offer patients a legal *right* to treatment, and ensure that every health authority is financed to provide at least a basic minimum level of services.

With these legal rights and obligations laid down as a safety net, the way would be open for the regular *election* of health authorities, comprising local representatives of health workers, the electorate, and patients and user groups. These new, accountable bodies should be given control of an integrated service comprising hospitals, community services, community care, family practitioner services and an occupational health service.

This type of properly-resourced NHS, with management held accountable to elected authorities – and under legal obligation to provide services rather than merely balance the books – would once again begin to squeeze out costly and inefficient private competition. Private medicine should be completely separated from NHS premises, ending all of the unofficial, under-cover subsidies; and part-time consultant contracts should be ended, promoting junior doctors to fill any posts left vacant if consultants resign in protest.

Of course extra money won't solve everything; but it would solve many of the problems of the NHS. Just as it is necessary to invest to generate wealth, we must invest to protect our health. A crash programme of backlog maintenance, and speeding up new building programmes would create valuable new jobs for the unemployed and liberate fresh NHS resources. Ending the contracts of all private cleaning, catering and laundry firms, and returning these services 'in-house' with a restoration of previous staffing levels and bonus payments would bring dramatic improvements in hygiene and patient care, relieve poverty among NHS ancillary staff and create useful new jobs.

Pumping this kind of increased investment into buildings and staffing would help restore nursing morale: and additional measures, including provision of crèches and flexible contracts offering part-time working with full employment rights to experienced and trained nurses who have left to have children, would help to tempt them back and resolve the nursing crisis.

Systematic investment in community care facilities for the mentally ill and mentally handicapped would not only improve their quality of life and that of their families, but also enable many to find or return to useful employment, regain their dignity and care for themselves. It is typical of short-sighted 'devil-take-the-hindmost' Thatcherism that it condemns tens of thousands of such individuals to an institutionalized scrapheap rather than allow then to realise their own potential and contribute to society.

Of course the implicit values of such a plan for health services are socialist: but the policies themselves could in theory be implemented even within a capitalist framework. Indeed they are the most efficient way of delivering health care – and Nigel Lawson's 1988 Budget showed that spare billions could be found to pay for such policies – except that he prefers to hand this cash to the wealthy in tax cuts.

However, a thoroughgoing *socialist* approach would provide not only the framework for a comprehensive service, but also liberate the *resources* for it, through the nationalization of the major drug firms, monopoly suppliers, banks and finance houses. A socialist plan would also facilitate the coordination of research programmes between the NHS, the universities and the drug industry, thus ensuring increased resources for research on issues such as AIDS and cancer.

The financial resources are available: and the gains and lessons of 40 years of the NHS offer a valuable starting point for a model system of health care. Yet Thatcher prefers to cut the lifeline to millions of men, women and children who depend on the NHS. If the labour movement, health campaigners, patients and relatives do not take up the fight now to defend our hospitals, the very notion of health care free at the point of use and available to all on the basis of medical need could be destroyed before our very eyes.

(Lister, 1988, pp.132–5)

COMMENT

While New Right theorists demanded that welfare services be exposed to the full rigour of market forces, the activists of the traditional Left demanded more public resources for a more accountable health service. However, at a time when the main opposition party linked to the unions was moving away from such policies (and when the major international model of state socialism, the Soviet Union, was on the verge of collapse), it was not clear how Lister's alternative might be implemented.

■ ■ ■

4   The internal market

Once you say 'we want the good features of competition, with independent bodies competing, in a service that remains publicly funded', then the internal market just falls out as a conclusion ... for us 1988, with the Education Reform Act, the NHS review, the Griffiths report [on community care] and the Housing Act, was the *annus mirabilis* of social policy.

(David Willetts, Conservative policy advisor, quoted in Timmins, 1995, p.433)

Returned for a third term in 1987, the Conservative government was in a powerful position to implement the free market agenda in welfare services. Yet, within weeks of Thatcher's election victory, the NHS was once again in a financial crisis. According to one authoritative account, 'the 1980s were a decade of financial austerity for the NHS ... there is little doubt that the rate of growth of public spending on the NHS was lower in the 1980s than in the 1970s' (Day and Klein, 1991, p.42). There was also little doubt that, though there had been some improvements in the efficiency of the service, the demand for health care had grown much faster than the resources supplied to the health service. As a result 'the rise in the provision of services in the 1980s went hand in hand with a mounting perception of inadequacy' (Day and Klein, 1991, p.43). By the end of the decade nearly one million people were on hospital waiting-lists for elective surgery.

Towards the end of 1987, health ministers were thrown on the defensive by a series of sensational media exposures of apparent shortcomings in the hospitals.

Reports of shortages of intensive care beds and of babies being denied heart surgery were transparently manipulated by a medical establishment demanding more resources for health care. In December a joint statement by the presidents of the Royal Colleges of Physicians, Surgeons, Nursing and General Practitioners warned that the NHS was on the brink of ruin unless 'additional and alternative funding' was found: 'We call on the government now to do something to save our National Health Service, once the envy of the world' (quoted in Timmins, 1995, p.457).

In response, in January 1988 Mrs Thatcher announced (on television) a top-level review of the NHS. Thatcher's NHS review broke with tradition in style as well as in the substance of its recommendations. It was a lean and efficient working party, which included five ministers, mainly from the Treasury; it met in secret and conspicuously ignored the representations of the doctors. Exactly twelve months later the White Paper, *Working for Patients*, was launched – at a cost of £1m – with a staff video and a laser-lit, closed-circuit telecast (Timmins, 1995, p.465). In her foreword to the White Paper Mrs Thatcher proclaimed that 'taken together the proposals represent the most far-reaching reform of the National Health Service in its forty-year history' (Department of Health, 1989). Though many mocked her characteristic bravado, within a short time few would dispute the impact of the reforms.

The White Paper proposed three key reforms, which came into effect in 1991. It recommended the creation of an internal market in the health service, by separating the purchasing function from health authorities from the provision of services by hospitals and GPs – the purchaser–provider split. It proposed that hospitals should become self-governing trusts, from which health authorities and GPs could purchase services. And it proposed that GPs should be allocated their own budgets, with which they could purchase services on behalf of their patients from hospital trusts. (GPs who opted in to this scheme subsequently became known as fundholders.) In addition, it proposed measures to improve performance and efficiency and to enhance managerial autonomy and the voice of the consumer. It recommended decentralizing management and abolishing lay representation on health authorities.

internal market
purchaser–
provider split
self-governing
trusts

fundholders

With the support of the opposition parties, the medical profession campaigned vigorously against the introduction of the internal market reforms (see below). But as the government pursued a combative approach to implementing its plans, divisions soon appeared in the medical ranks: key hospital consultants signalled approval for forming trusts and prominent GPs opted for fundholding. Labour's fourth consecutive general election defeat in 1992 confirmed that the Conservative government's reforms were there to stay. Resistance crumbled and by 1996 hospital trusts were firmly established and more than half the population was registered with a fundholding GP.

In the latter half of the 1990s a new consensus began to take shape around the concept of a 'primary care-led NHS', first officially sanctioned in a report from the NHS executive in 1994. This approach pursued the logic of the internal market reforms by further encouraging the initiative of GPs in both rationing services to patients and in imposing a degree of market discipline on their hospital colleagues: 'The aim is for decisions about purchasing and providing health care to be taken as close to the patient as possible by GPs working closely with patients through primary health care teams' (NHS Executive, 1994, p.5). The publication of the White Paper, *The New NHS*, in December 1997, six months after New Labour's landslide election victory, confirmed the ascendancy of the primary care-led NHS.

The convergence of different trends around the new consensus was most apparent in the evolution of GP fundholding. In the mid 1990s there was a sharp division between fundholding GPs (mainly in rural and suburban areas) and non-fundholders (mainly in poorer inner-city areas). Rival camps were organized in the National Association of Fundholding Practices and in the National Association of Commissioning GPs, formed in 1994 to promote 'locality commissioning', a process of contracting hospital and other services by GPs in a particular area, according to collective judgements about needs and priorities (Singer, 1997, p.22). Though sharply antagonistic at first, these factions were dramatically reconciled in the run-up to the 1997 general election.

A number of factors encouraged convergence. While the first wave of fundholders was subsidized to cover management and computer costs, later converts were less substantially rewarded and experienced greater difficulties. An Audit Commission survey concluded that, despite the investment of substantial resources, 'the majority of fundholding practices do not appear to be especially good at management and networking or achieving a large number of benefits for patients' (Audit Commission, 1996, p.87). Meanwhile in a number of areas groups of GPs began to pursue alternative models – including 'locality commissioning' and 'multifunds' through which budgets were allocated to a number of GPs. As the political tide turned decisively towards New Labour, the initiative shifted to the commissioning model.

Many commentators drew attention to the gap between rhetoric and substance in the December 1997 White Paper. In deference to Labour's tradition of hostility to the Tory reforms, *The New NHS* proclaimed that the internal market was to be abolished and GP fundholding replaced. 'In fact', as the social policy experts Glennerster and Le Grand noted, 'the key elements of the old internal market will be retained' and the proposed GP-led commissioning amounted to 'the ultimate extension of fundholding' (*The Guardian*, 10 December 1997). The key element in the new plans – a central role for 'primary care groups' in commissioning health care services for local populations of around 100 000 people – marked the triumph of the locality commissioning model. However, by making participation by GPs in primary care groups compulsory and by introducing stricter mechanisms of monitoring and control, the new scheme had a distinctly authoritarian dynamic.

The most striking difference between the 1989 White Paper that launched the reform process and *The New NHS* in 1997 was the public response. Whereas *Working for Patients* provoked a storm of protest from the medical profession, opposition politicians and the media, New Labour's document was very quietly received. Even leading fundholding GPs and Conservative politicians could scarcely raise a protest. If the public attitude was more one of resignation than of enthusiasm, this perhaps reflected exhaustion with a decade of hectic change in the NHS and a general acceptance of the terms of a primary care-led, market-ruled NHS. It was left to the minority Liberal Democrats to point out that the key problem for the new NHS was the acceptance by the New Labour government of public spending projections by the outgoing Tories which meant a drastic squeeze on resources for health. According to the Institute of Fiscal Studies, this squeeze was 'more stringent than anything the Conservatives managed in their 18 years in power' (*The Guardian*, 4 July 1997).

Written while a journalist on *The Independent* during the period of the NHS reforms, Nicholas Timmins provides a revealing account of the conflict between Kenneth Clarke, the Conservative minister responsible for implementing the NHS reforms, and the medical profession, represented by the British Medical Association. Clarke's distant predecessor, Aneurin Bevan, famously claimed that he stopped the top consultants from protesting over the introduction of the NHS by 'stuffing their mouths with gold'. Clarke's technique of what he called 'mud-wrestling' proved just as effective – and much cheaper.

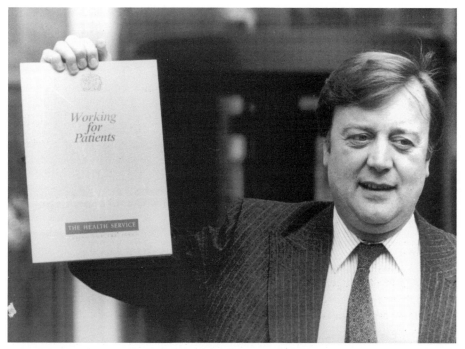

A smiling Kenneth Clarke presents the Conservative government's health service reforms to the public; behind the scenes he engaged in what he called 'mud-wrestling' to overcome medical opposition

ACTIVITY 3.2

Timmins provides a lively journalistic account of events in Extract 3.3. As you read it, try to identify the main outcome for the BMA.

Extract 3.3 Timmins: 'Introducing *Working for Patients*'

On publication day … Dr John Marks, the BMA's chairman of council, was careful to state only that the association would consult its members. Clarke did the opposite: he assaulted the BMA for attacking the plans before they had even done so. 'The BMA, in my unbiased opinion, has never been in favour of any change of any kind on any subject whatsoever for as long as anyone can remember,' he told his television audience [*Independent*, 2 February 1989].

This attack, according to Clarke, was deliberate. 'Margaret was very annoyed with me when I presented the White Paper to Cabinet, for I told colleagues there was going to be one hell of a political row. I told them we were going to Tavistock

House [BMA headquarters], lifting most of the tablets of stone and smashing them on the pavement in front of their eyes. These guys are going to mount one hell of a campaign.' The decision to get his retaliation in first was based on Clarke's experience of the BMA as

> a very powerful, Imperial Guard-type organisation in politics … the one thing we had to do was knock the BMA off its pedestal … so long as the BMA emerged as the spokesman for the savers of lives and the healers of the sick, and the people whose only concern was for the welfare of the poor and the elderly, we were in a no-win situation – we had to pull them into the mud with us and make it clear that this was just another trade union, actually one of the nastiest I had ever dealt with, and battle it out. [Interview with author]

Without that, he believes, the reforms would not have happened.

The BMA for its part argued that the reforms not only fragmented the service but 'lay the groundwork for the future dismantlement of the NHS' [*British Medical Journal*, 1989, vol.298, pp.340–1]. There were, as Clarke believed, good trade union issues here. The BMA knew that the review had looked long and hard at rewriting consultants' contracts, a move it finally backed away from when it realised that the existing contract, if actually enforced, was not so bad. Furthermore, Clarke had decided that with the government already at loggerheads with GPs over their terms and conditions, a similar battle with the consultants might actually, even for him, be one battle too many. He had insisted, however, that self-governing hospitals would be free to set their own terms and conditions of service for doctors, a move which could crucially undermine the BMA's role and would in time produce new and varying consultant contracts.

The BMA did indeed want to stop that. But their self-interest was married to a genuine attachment to an NHS which they believed the reforms would break up. Their fears were not assuaged by cheerful admissions from Clarke a good six months into the process that he was still effectively 'making it up as he went along' [*Independent*, 28 July 1989] nor by suggestions from Willetts that the reforms were intended to 'destabilize' the existing NHS in order to produce change [*Independent*, 9 February 1989]. In all the furore about what the reforms would mean, it was barely noticed that a review triggered by a financial crisis had in fact done nothing about financing the NHS. Rather, it had become almost a celebration of the service's success, with the 1948 settlement reaffirmed by Mrs Thatcher in the foreword where she had promised to preserve a tax-funded system largely free at the point of use. Money had, however, been a chief cause of the problem, and Clarke's formidable skills as a spending minister, along with Lawson's conviction that this time the money would buy real benefits, soon saw the NHS in 1988 enjoying the first of a series of relatively generous settlements after the years of financial drought.

As Clarke and the BMA slugged it out, the atmosphere was further poisoned by the GPs' contract remaining unresolved. The new contract had only indirect links to the other changes, but family doctors saw it would increase their workload, make them compete with each other, and subject them to central direction about what types of screening and other procedures they would have to carry out. There was enough overlap for the contract negotiations and the NHS reforms to become hopelessly entangled. Clarke threatened to impose a new contract in an attempt to get it out of the way while meetings of GPs up and down the country were attended on a scale not seen since the 1960s charter negotiations. Repeated threats of resignation from the NHS were uttered, though whether over the NHS reforms or the new GP contract, or both, was often as confused as was the concept that doctors would somehow protect the NHS by leaving it [*Independent*, 9 March, 11 March 19 April 1989]. Clarke successfully inflamed the situation by saying at a dinner of the Royal College of General Practitioners: 'I do wish the more suspicious of our GPs would stop feeling nervously for their wallets every time I mention the word reform.' In the next breath he equally upset the consultants by pointing out, entirely correctly, that fund-holding would profoundly change GPs' relations with them to the family doctor's advantage. Fund-holding would ensure, he said, that 'some consultants pay more attention to GPs than they do now' [speech to Royal College of General Practitioners, 9 March 1989]. As Clarke delivered his speech, Professor Sir Dillwyn Williams, chairman of the conference of medical Royal Colleges, was seen to go white with anger [interview by author with John Marks]. 'Feeling for their wallets' became a phrase that would haunt Clarke. As the temperature rose, the BMA launched the start of what was finally to be a £3 million advertising campaign. The message on its posters was that the NHS was 'underfunded, undermined and under threat'.

By now, the informal channels between the BMA and the Department of Health which had so eased negotiations in the past had virtually gone. Almost all talks, now, had to be formal talks. The one attempt at an informal resolution was a secret dinner for four in a private room in the Carlton Club organized by Sir Arnold Elton of the Conservative Medical Society. Marks and Dr John Havard, the BMA secretary, urged Clarke to introduce the reforms as a trial in one region. 'If I do that,' Clarke replied with a grin, 'you buggers will sabotage it' [interview by author with John Marks]. For by far the biggest row over the NHS since its inception, the Conservatives had found themselves their own Nye Bevan, but one who on the major NHS reforms found no need this time to compromise at all.

Marks's great fear was that the GPs would indeed resign over their contracts. 'The government,' he says, 'would have yodelled from the roof-tops. The NHS would have been finished and whose fault would it have been? The grasping doctors reaching for their wallets' [interview by author with John Marks]. Negotiations were in the hands of Dr Michael Wilson, a quiet, Boycott-like Yorkshireman, and the antithesis of Clarke's ebullient brashness. In hindsight, colleagues judged of the GPs' chairman that 'he tended to negotiate by repeating himself. He didn't finally know when to give and take' [unattributable interview]. In early May, however, a deal was finally struck over ten hours of sandwiches, low-alcohol beer and Kenneth Clarke's cigar smoke during which Wilson and his colleagues won some significant concessions and agreed to commend the package to their members. Clarke that night was at his most hectoring, behaving, on his own account 'extremely badly' as he missed the Prime Minister's tenth anniversary dinner in order to achieve a settlement.

Five weeks later, a special GPs' conference called to ratify the deal threw it out on the narrowest of margins, 160 votes to 155, and a subsequent ballot in which 82 per cent of GPs rejected it by three to one [*Independent*, 21 July 1989]. For the first time in the history of the NHS, the troops had proved more militant than the BMA's leaders. The vote, however, proved merely to be a defiant gesture. Clarke's exasperated response was finally to impose the contract, this government having ceased to be one that allowed professional opposition to stand in its way. A few isolated further calls for resignation from the NHS gained no momentum. Wilson had spoken no less than the truth when he had warned his members at their special conference that the Secretary of State for Health 'holds all the aces' [*Independent*, 22 June 1989].

(Timmins, 1995, pp.466–9)

In 1948 the medical profession – led by the BMA – fiercely opposed the introduction of the NHS and fought for key modifications in the new service. Government ministers in the late 1980s were not slow to point out to the doctors' leaders the irony that, though they had fiercely resisted the introduction of the NHS, forty years later they had become its most doughty defenders. Another contrast was even more painful. The BMA campaign in the late 1940s succeeded in preserving independent contractor status for GPs, in ensuring a structure of health care administration independent of local government and in generally consolidating medical power at every level of the service. The outcome of the BMA's campaign against the reforms proposed in the 1989 White Paper was a substantial setback to medical autonomy and authority within the NHS.

■ ■ ■

5   The new public health and the new patient

welfare subject

new public health

health promotion

One of the wider themes in the restructuring of welfare is the reconstitution of the welfare subject, through the transformation of welfare discourses along with the relationship between the individual in society and the agencies through which welfare is delivered (see Chapter 2). In the sphere of health, the rise of what has become known as the 'new public health' and the associated practice of health promotion have effectively redefined 'the patient' as the entire population and in the process have transformed the relationship between patient and doctor that lay at the heart of the traditional health care system.

Discussions of the restructuring and reform of the NHS have tended to focus on the 1989 White Paper, *Working for Patients,* and the subsequent legislation, while neglecting the 1991 White Paper, *The Health of the Nation*, which is often regarded as having quite separate concerns. In fact, these two initiatives are closely linked and complementary.

Emphasizing prevention rather than cure, the promotion of health rather than the treatment of disease, *The Health of the Nation* aimed to improve the health of the population by setting targets in five distinct areas: coronary heart disease and stroke; particular cancers (breast, cervix, lung, skin); mental illness (particularly suicide); HIV/AIDS and sexual health; and accidents (especially among children and young people) (Department of Health, 1991). To further these objectives, the White Paper identified 'risk factor targets' in four areas: smoking, diet and nutrition, blood pressure, and HIV transmission by injecting drugs.

The Health of the Nation indicated official endorsement for the policies of a new generation of public health doctors. Advocates of the new public health had long been calling for a whole population approach to the prevention of the chronic degenerative and malignant diseases which had become the main problem of Western societies no longer much troubled by the old enemy of acute infectious diseases. Whereas traditional doctors focused on the disease process as it was manifest in the individual patient, the specialists of the new public health were concerned with the role of social, environmental and lifestyle risk factors in the health of populations (Lupton, 1995; Nettleton, 1995). The rise of the new public health took place in parallel with the imposition of market disciplines in the wider NHS, with important implications for the health care system and for the relationship between doctor and patient.

lifestyle risk factors

The shift from a curative to a preventive approach had a number of consequences for medical practice. It led to a greater emphasis on 'primary' health care by GPs, nurses and other health professionals working 'in the community' rather than on the 'secondary' (hospital) sector. In general practice, financial incentives encouraged a dramatic improvement in rates of childhood immunization, cervical smear tests, health checks and an explosion of well woman, well man and other health promotion clinics. The combined effect of the new contract for GPs introduced in 1990 and the 1991 White Paper was a dramatic increase in the proportion of GPs' time spent on prevention and health promotion.

preventive approach

Reports of GPs telephoning patients to invite them to attend for screening tests or other preventive measures revealed both the impact of incentive bonuses to achieve certain targets and the transformation of the patient. The patient was no longer somebody who presented with a particular symptom that required assessment, investigation or treatment; the patient was now anybody registered with a particular doctor. Or to put it another way, everybody was now a patient, as the category expanded to include the entire population. The proliferation of workplace-based health promotion activities, extending from general check-ups, cholesterol screening and cervical smear tests to various forms of counselling, was another illustration of this trend (May and Brunsdon, 1994).

The contrast between the discourse of the new public health and that of traditional medical practice was striking. In the early decades of the NHS, the hospital doctor enjoyed high prestige, boosted by the development of powerful new drugs and dramatic surgical techniques. A skilled practitioner of scientific medicine, the doctor was concerned with diagnosis and treatment, aiming to restore the patient to health (and, it was generally assumed, to work). The patient's role as the passive repository of the disease process was poignantly symbolized by the old consultants' habit of referring to the individuals in hospital beds by their diagnostic labels rather than by their names.

It is worth recalling the privileged status of the 'doctor–patient' relationship in the old NHS. Everybody else in the health service was either peripheral and supportive of that relationship, or invisible. The use of the labels 'auxiliary' and 'ancillary' for much of the hospital staff indicated their subordinate status. The rigid hospital hierarchy reflected wider differentials in status according to class, gender and 'race'. The world of general practice was distinctly inferior, conducted by failed hospital doctors in shabby premises.

The new public health appropriated the radical critique of mainstream medical practice in the 1960s and 1970s. The American microbiologist René Dubos (1960) challenged what he regarded as the narrow and mechanical approach of 'biomedicine' in favour of a more holistic approach to the diseases of modern society. The British epidemiologist Tom McKeown (1979) emphasized the much greater contribution of social and environmental factors, rather than medical interventions, in the conquest of infectious disease and proposed a similar approach to the modern epidemics of heart disease and cancer. Others criticized the medical profession as elitist, hierarchical, patriarchal and paternalistic (Illich, 1976; Navarro, 1976; Doyal, 1979). Feminists challenged medical control over childbirth, abortion and contraception, and other movements asserted the rights of black people, people with disabilities, and people with specific health problems or needs (Oakley, 1980).

Elements of the radical critique of biomedicine were subsequently taken up by different professional groups and other agencies. Thus, for example, the Royal College of General Practitioners from the early 1980s adopted the cause of prevention as a means of overcoming GPs' historic sense of living in the shadow of the hospitals. As Nettleton (1995, p.229) writes, 'in effect, GPs used prevention to establish their professional identity'. Radical doctors in the new public health movement sought to transcend the individualistic focus of early health promotion with their emphasis on the links between health and social deprivation and their demands for radical social change and 'community empowerment' as the key to improving the health of society (Martin and McQueen, 1989). This message was reinforced by international initiatives in health promotion, notably the World Health Organisation conference in Ottawa in Canada in 1986 which launched a charter for health promotion as part of the campaign 'Health For All By The Year 2000' (Dines and Cribb, 1993) (see Extract 3.6 below).

The adoption of the programme of the new public health by government in the UK was a fitful and prolonged affair. It first appeared in a discussion document produced on the authority of David Owen when he was Labour health minister in 1976. The central theme of *Prevention and Health: Everybody's Business* was bluntly stated: 'much of the responsibility for ensuring his [*sic*] own good health lies with the individual' (DHSS, 1976, p.95). The government White Paper published the following year, under the same title, adopted an even sterner tone and indicated the widening scope of individual responsibility: 'Much ill health in Britain today arises from over-indulgence and unwise behaviour ... The individual can do much to help himself [*sic*], his family and the community by accepting more direct personal responsibility for his own health and well-being' (DHSS, 1977, p.39). *Eating for Health*, published by the Department of Health in 1979, observed that an unhealthy lifestyle resulted from ignorance and irresponsibility and emphasized the need for information and education to change behaviour. The Health Education Council's *Look After Yourself* campaign took the message to the public – and the media took up the cause with what one authoritative commentator describes as 'unbounded enthusiasm' (Karpf, 1988, Ch. 1).

The slogan 'Look after yourself' expressed well the ambivalent tone of government health promotion. On the one hand, it sounded like a positive encouragement to greater well-being. On the other, it could be interpreted as both 'victim-blaming' and as a caution: if you become ill through your own fault, then don't expect anybody else to look after you. The government's endorsement of health promotion fitted well with its wider concern to shift more of the burden of health care from the state onto the individual (for more on these issues see **Langan, 1998a, 1998b**).

Though the government's encouragement of preventive medicine in the late 1970s had little effect, the campaign for a more systematic approach to health promotion gathered momentum through the 1980s until it was given a prominent place in the health reform package of the early 1990s.

One striking feature of *The Health of the Nation* campaign was that it was

individual responsibility

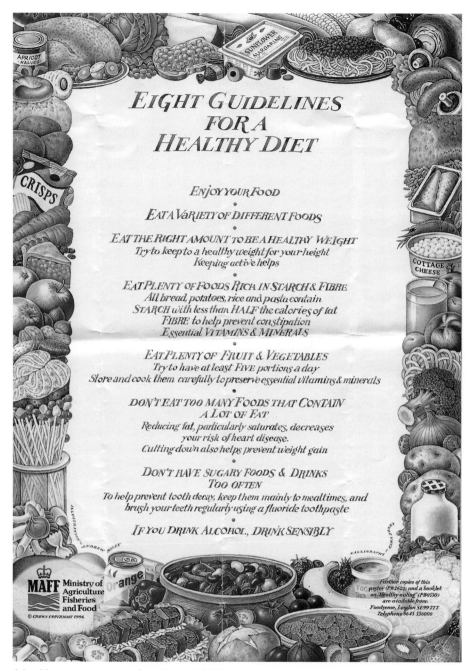

A health promotion poster from the mid 1990s

the first major initiative in the sphere of health which did not include proposals for spending any more money on health care. Indeed, the White Paper contained an implicit echo of the Beveridge fallacy: the notion that promoting better health could ultimately save resources on health care. However, the effect of encouraging health checks and screening procedures was inevitably to reveal more occasions for medical intervention, many of which, such as the long-term treatment of raised blood pressure or cholesterol levels, could prove highly expensive.

Some sociologists have criticized the ascendancy of health promotion for creating a 'vast network of observation and caution', a system of 'surveillance over individuals' and a 'creeping medicalization of lives' (Lupton, 1995; Nettleton, 1995). But there has been relatively little discussion of its paradoxical effect on the construction of need: a set of measures designed to enhance individual responsibility and reduce demand for health care may in fact create new needs and renewed demands for resources.

As Labour health minister at the time of the 1970s public expenditure crisis, David Owen, himself a former hospital doctor, was quick to recognize that 'preventive health measures' could be cost-effective. His emphasis on the need for individual lifestyle change as the key to improving health, though now familiar, was then a novel approach.

ACTIVITY 3.3

You should now read Extract 3.4, noting Owen's key points in his argument that health is improved by lifestyle.

Extract 3.4 Owen: 'Patient, help thyself'

The National Health Service cannot be the sole provider of health in this country. Each of us must develop a responsibility for our own health, and so I welcome the Lifespan series on "The art of body maintenance" which begins in the [*Sunday Times*] Magazine this week as a guide for everybody to follow in cultivating a healthy life.

The scope for improvement is there in the statistics for anyone to see. In many ways, of course, things have greatly improved. A hundred years ago a boy at birth could expect to live 41 years and a girl to 45. Only six babies out of ten survived to adulthood. Since the last century improved health measures, housing, nutrition and other factors have reduced deaths for tuberculosis, typhoid, diphtheria, scarlet fever, whooping cough and measles by 99 per cent.

Today, however, there are new killers – and they are increasingly striking down people who have survived their formative years. A man aged 50 in 1841, when reliable records begin, could expect to live for a further 20 years; by 1972–74 a man aged 50 could expect to live another 23 years. So despite the vast improvements in health care in the intervening time, life expectancy had increased by just three years.

What has changed is that TB and pneumonia are no longer the primary causes of death. Today during the working years, coronary heart disease, cancer, especially lung cancer, strokes, accidents and bronchitis are the biggest killers of men. Cancer, especially breast cancer, and strokes are the main causes of death in women in this age range.

Coronary disease causes 43 per cent of all deaths among men aged 45 to 64. The risk factors are becoming better known; cigarette smoking, obesity, lack of exercise, high blood pressure, high blood-fat levels and a family history of heart trouble. It is also known that people who take regular and vigorous exercise usually enjoy better health and have lower blood pressures and blood cholesterol levels. Reducing the consumption of animal fat and sugar is helpful, and these are all actions which lie within the control of individuals.

Many of the diseases that are most difficult to prevent depend on individual behaviour. Over 95 per cent of young people are now aware that smoking causes lung cancer, yet the change in behaviour implied by this knowledge has been slight. The number of male cigarette smokers fell from 59 to 49 per cent between 1961 and 1973, yet the figure for women stayed at 43 per cent.

It is still not sufficiently appreciated that about half a million people in England and Wales, and proportionately more in Scotland, have a serious drink problem. Twenty-five years ago a bottle of whisky cost 45 per cent of the average man's disposable weekly income; today the cost is less than 20 per cent and consumption has quadrupled.

...

There is a general feeling that exercise is a good thing, but few of us recognise the startling changes that have occurred in the average person's lifestyle over the last few decades. Ninety-three per cent of homes now have televisions. The average adult spends more time on watching TV than on anything else except sleep and work. This, with mechanization of industry, more cars and labour-saving devices, leads to the lack of exercise which is one of the besetting sins on modern men and women.

The costs of preventive health need to be carefully considered. Polio immunization has saved twelve times its cost in twenty years. Fluoridation of all water supplies could cut dental decay by 50 per cent and enable resources to be transferred to other services. Seat belts, universally used, could save £50m a year overall by reducing road deaths and serious injury.

...

Breast cancer caused 11,775 deaths in 1970. One in twenty young women will develop it if they live long enough. One in thirty will die from it. Screening is by clinical examination and X-ray (or thermography or ultrasonography, which have no radiation hazards). Using one method alone misses 25 per cent of cases. Breast cancer screening once a year for women in their fifties could reduce the annual deaths by 3,000 and cost between £20m and £30m. The possibility of specially trained nurses doing the examinations and radiographers reading the X-rays is being explored.

As a country we have grown used to believing that money spent in hospitals and pills dispensed by doctors hold the key to good health. We have appeared to encourage individuals to ignore responsibility for their own health and we have progressively allowed the emphasis of the NHS to become that of a sickness service.

Any government initiative in these areas inevitably raises difficult problems of balance between liberty and welfare. Some habits hurt others – for example, drinking and driving – and society now accepts that it is reasonable to curb these, but even ten years ago the public outcry over the introduction of breathalyser tests revealed a very different climate of opinion.

Government alone cannot be held responsible for prevention, and government interference in all these areas raises sensitive issues relating to individual freedom. Governments prefer to be seen to react to public opinion, or, at least, not to be too far in advance of public opinion. To change public opinion much more needs to be done by individuals, local communities and Government. We urgently need a radical reorientation of our attitude to health and I am in no doubt that prevention must be given a far greater priority than hitherto.

(Owen, 1976, p.16)

Extract 3.5 is the text of a leaflet distributed in the mid 1990s in hospital and GP waiting-rooms, in schools and community centres, and at similar points of contact between the state and its welfare subjects. It well illustrates some of the key themes of *The Health of the Nation* campaign of the early 1990s. Problems of health are implicitly attributed to familiar lifestyle factors – notably diet and exercise, smoking and drinking – and everybody is exhorted to do something to reduce their risks and improve their health.

Extract 3.5 Calman: 'The Chief Medical Officer's challenge'

I am issuing a challenge to every person in the country to take one small step to improve their own health.

There should be something that you can do from this list of suggestions and you may have some ideas of your own.

- Take the stairs instead of the lift or escalator
- Exercise – cycle, jog, swim or dance
- Walk – don't ride. Get off one stop early and walk
- Give up smoking or set a date to stop
- Protect your child from tobacco smoke – particularly if you're pregnant
- Grill rather than fry your food
- Cut the fat off meat
- Change to skimmed or semi-skimmed milk
- Watch how much you eat – think twice before seconds
- Eat your greens – make sure you have plenty of vegetables or salad each day
- Try fresh fruit instead of cake or biscuits
- Have fish instead of meat once a week
- Be sensible about how much you drink – have at least two alcohol free days a week
- Fit a smoke alarm – its [*sic*] only the price of a pint and two packets of cigarettes and it could save your life
- Is your home safe from accidents? Check it tonight
- Don't drink and drive
- Kill your speed not a child. Make sure your children know about road safety
- Protect your child from sunburn – with lightweight clothes, a hat and use a sunscreen
- Reduce your stress – take a ten minute time-out every day.

(Calman, n.d.)

Petr Skrabanek, a medical commentator who originated in Czechoslovakia and settled in Dublin (and whose last book was published posthumously), was a trenchant critic of health promotion from an individualistic, right-wing libertarian perspective. In Extract 3.6, in a characteristic passage, he challenges the approach of the new public health as intrusive and authoritarian.

ACTIVITY 3.4

Read the critique of health promotion by Skrabanek in Extract 3.6, noting the key features of his challenge to the new health projects.

Extract 3.6 Skrabanek: '"Positive" health and its promotion'

In 1926, the President of the American Medical Association, Wendell Phillips, announced that

> Physicians must give a new significance to the word patient, for in the new order of things both sick and well people must and will be recorded in the lists of their physicians.

Just to be well would not be enough.

> Too many of our inhabitants worry through life with only fairly good health and while they accomplish their daily duties, these fairly well persons may never know the exuberance and happiness of perfect health. Hence, one goal of the future practitioner of medicine will be the attainment and maintenance of exuberant health, which is the inherent right of every person. A higher average of overflowing good health means a higher average of happiness, comfort, usefulness and economic value of the individual. The superman will never materialize without superhealth. [Phillips, 1926]

This instructive passage, though written nearly 70 years ago, sounds surprisingly modern. It has all the ingredients of today's health promotion rhetoric. Health must be more than the absence of disease, it must be exuberant health, super-health. Health is happiness and happiness is health. All healthy people must be under constant supervision. It does not omit to mention the 'economic value of the individual' and the nonsense of the 'inherent right' of everyone to super-health. The superman idea is distinctly American. Is the function of medicine to turn people into economically useful, happy robots?

Phillips' idea of superhealth was incorporated into the Constitution of the World Health Organisation in 1946, where health is defined as 'not merely the absence of disease or infirmity' but 'a state of complete physical, mental and social well-being'. The sort of feeling ordinary people may achieve fleetingly during orgasm, or when high on drugs.

In 1975, Dr Halfdan Mahler, Director-General of the WHO, addressed the Organisation's Regional Committees and he chose as his subject 'Health for All by the Year 2000!' (the exclamation mark is his). He acknowledged that one has to be realistic since 'it will take another generation for the world's population to achieve an acceptable level of health *evenly distributed throughout it'* (emphasis added). At the end of his speech, Mahler confessed that he had not 'the slightest doubt that we shall reach this goal before the year 2000' [Mahler, 1975]. The catchy title 'Health for All by the Year 2000' was subsequently adopted by the World Health Assembly in 1977 as its goal.

Anyone sick or, God forbid, on their deathbed, anyone not experiencing the euphoria of positive health, as defined by WHO, would spoil this objective. Old people drifting into the oblivion of dementia, sour spinsters, jilted lovers, ruined gamblers, wives of drowned fishermen, victims of violence, or immured lunatics would also spoil the picture. Even Christians, in their boundless optimism, have been more realistic in deferring the promise of complete happiness to the afterlife.

In 1978, at the Lenin Palace in Alma-Ata, WHO assembled representatives of 134 countries, who unanimously adopted the Alma-Ata Declaration, reaffirming WHO's definition of health, and declaring such health to be a 'fundamental human right'. The delegates applauded the message from their host, Mr Leonid Brezhnev, who emphasised that 'questions of national health are constantly in the forefront of the activities of the Communist Party and the Soviet State' [WHO, 1978a, 1978b]. The delegates, including those from the Haiti of Baby Doc, the Uganda of Idi Amin, and the Central African Republic of Bokassa, besides representatives from scores of other murderous regimes, totalitarian state and military dictatorships, were confident that 'Health for All by the Year 2000' was an attainable goal.

...

The first WHO conference on health promotion took place in Ottawa, Canada in 1986 and resulted in the Charter for Health promotion ...

The signatories of the Ottawa charter pledged:

> to acknowledge people as the main health resource; to support and enable them to keep themselves, their families and friends healthy through financial and other means, and to accept the community as the essential choice in matters of its health, living condition and well-being.

The signatories expressed their hope that by the year 2000 the WHO objective of Health for All would become a reality [WHO, 1986] ...

...

Health promotion is big business. Because it deals with universal happiness it is immune to criticism, which, anyway, could only come from misanthropists or fools. The theory is provided by academics in university departments and by experts and consultants employed by government, the practice is implemented by entrepreneurs running health shops, health clubs, health farms, health promotion magazines, holistic centres, and screening clinics (some for 'executives', some for 'well women', some for just anyone). Food industrialists and manufacturers of pills have already joined the health promotion bandwagon ...

Serious doubts about the motives and value of the health promotion movement have been expressed by medicine watchers, philosophers, and doctors themselves. An editorialist in *The Lancet* called the movement a bandwagon, and described the evidence for the effectiveness of 'health checks' as 'extremely limited', since they neither reduce morbidity nor mortality, while they contribute to an increase in the cost of health services [*Lancet*, 19897]. The promissory notes issued by the prevention clergy (indulgences for non-indulgent behaviour?) are unlikely to be cashed in for real gold in the future.

...

The US Professor of Public Health, Marshall Becker, described health promotion as based on wishful thinking since the domain of personal health over which the individual has direct control is *very* small, when compared with heredity, culture, environment, and chance.

> We are bothering and frightening people about far too many things, we campaign under the banner of denial of pleasure, and we cannot even agree of the scientific validity and importance of most of our recommendations. [Becker, 1986]

Gill Williams in the *Journal of Medical Ethics* pointed out that health promotion 'experts' use unfounded claims as the basis of their 'expertise in health' and leave the public prey to sharp practices and naive beliefs [Williams, 1984]. The aims of the health promotion movement are so vague (such as, 'any combination of health education and related organisational, political and economic interventions designed to facilitate behavioural and environmental adaptations that will improve health') that the field is wide open to administrative empire-building on a vast scale ...

Cosmopolitan's observer of human follies, Irma Kurtz, recognised the self-centred character of the new health religion. Writing in the *Journal of Medical Ethics* she described it as a paltry faith, which has nothing to do with improving the lot of one's fellow men, but which worships only Self [Kurtz, 1987]. Who would like to be remembered as someone who spent every day of his life 'keeping fit', avoiding the sun (jogging in a wide brimmed hat?), cholesterol and smoking friends, and depositing daily bulky stools (bran is good for you)?

References

Becker, M.H. (1986) 'The tyranny of health promotion', *Public Health Review*, vol. 14, pp.15–25.

Kurtz, I. (1987) 'Health educators – the new puritans', *Journal of Medical Ethics*, vol.13, pp.40–41.

Lancet (1987) 'Primary health care: Government's worthy words amid the gloom', Editorial, vol.ii, pp.1307–08.

Mahler, H. (1975) 'Health care for all by the year 2000', *WHO Chronicle*, vol.29, pp. 457–61.

Phillips, W.C. (1926) 'The physician and the patient of the future', *Journal of the American Medical Association*, vol.86, pp. 1259–65.

Williams, G. (1984) 'Health promotion – caring concern or slick salesmanship?', *Journal of Medical Ethics*, vol.10, pp.191–5.

World Health Organisation (1978a) *Primary Health Care*, Report of the International Conference on Primary Health Care, Alma-Ata, USSR, 6–12 September, Geneva, WHO.

World Health Organisation (1978b) 'Alma-Ata Conference on Primary Health Care', *WHO Chronicle*, vol.31, pp.409–30.

World Health Organisation (1986) *Ottawa Charter for Health Promotion*, Charter endorsed at the First International Conference for Health Promotion, Ottawa, WHO.

(Skrabanek, 1994, pp.41–3, 45, 48–50)

ACTIVITY 3.5

We have all become very familiar with the discourse of the new public health illustrated by these extracts. Everybody today knows about the importance of risk factors, screening tests and other preventive measures. What lifestyle changes have you made in the past ten years in the interests of improving health or preventing disease (for example, stopping smoking, going on a diet, cutting down on fatty foods, taking more exercise)? What does this tell you about the impact of health promotion on individual behaviour?

COMMENT

One of the striking features of the new public health is the way in which it reveals the blurring of the familiar distinctions between left and right in matters of health policy. While it embodies a radical critique of established medical practice, it received its first official endorsement from Dr Owen, a Labour minister whose main concern was to curb public spending on health. It finally became government policy, in the form of *The Health of the Nation* campaign, under a Conservative government, in parallel with the imposition of market reforms on the health service. While radicals criticized particular aspects of the health promotion programme, by far the most comprehensive condemnation came from commentators, like Skrabanek, in pamphlets published by free market, neo-liberal think-tanks. The critical sociologists (such as Lupton and Nettleton) provide a clue to the convergence of right and left in the new public health through their thesis that health promotion offers a mechanism for regulating behaviour.

■ ■ ■

6   The managerial imperative

> If Florence Nightingale were carrying her lamp through the corridors of the NHS today, she would almost certainly be searching for the people in charge.
> (Department of Health, 1983)

Commissioned directly by Mrs Thatcher from the managing director of the Sainsbury food retail chain, the Griffiths Report (Department of Health, 1983) synthesized a decade of mounting criticism of the managerial structure of the NHS. For the critics and their allies in the Conservative government, the top-heavy administrative framework, the conciliatory management style, the privileged position of the medical profession, the recognition of a special place for the unions – these were all the legacy of a post-war settlement that had become an obstacle to a more efficient and effective health care system.

The set of problems that the managerial revolution in the NHS was designed to tackle – and the broad outline of its response – can be briefly summarized as follows:

1   From consensus management to executive direction

We have seen how Mrs Thatcher abhorred the post-war tradition of compromise and conciliation, in the NHS as elsewhere. Her objective was to replace administration by consensus with executive direction. Though she favoured devolving responsibility, she wanted centralized power to push through the reform programme. In place of the weary spirit of public service so central to the post-war organizational settlement in the welfare state, she sought to unleash the entrepreneurial and competitive vigour of the private market.

managed competition

Though the final result was dubbed a 'quasi-market' and 'managed' competition appeared to play a greater role than the real thing, nobody could dispute the commercializing dynamic that permeated the health service in the early 1990s.

2   Making doctors cost-conscious

The problem that doctors enjoyed great power and autonomy in the allocation of NHS resources, but could not be readily held to account for how the money was spent, was a focus of growing concern in the 1980s. Dramatic variations in medical practice – for example, in the prevalence of different operations in different areas – could only be explained by the idiosyncrasies of different surgeons, revealing a lack of accountability and rigour in the allocation of resources. The managerial solution was to decentralize responsibility for spending money and to hold its recipients to account by setting targets. The

accountability decentraliz- ation

110

only way to make doctors accountable was by making them responsible for their own budgets.

Though the doctors retained considerable power in the new NHS, and fundholding GPs believed that they were more powerful than previously, their prestige was undoubtedly damaged in their long-running conflicts with the government. They were not consulted; indeed they were disparaged and fragmented. The medical profession in general found itself in considerable conflict with the new managers, who were keen to share the blame for distributing shrinking resources with doctors.

3 Ensuring effective treatments

Pressures to ration scarce resources, as well as the question of variations in medical practice, also raised questions about techniques for evaluating the efficacy of different treatments. These pressures encouraged the proliferation of methods of measuring outcomes as well as inputs, the expansion of audit **audit** and other measures of quality, performance and effectiveness.

4 Maximizing the potential of human resources

Though it was an employer of more than a million people, the NHS lacked mechanisms for motivating staff, encouraging competition and improving quality. The spirit of the reforms was to promote incentives and to encourage a shift towards 'performance-related pay'. Though the unions clung on to national collective bargaining, the managerial dynamic was to break out of the old framework and its associated rigidities, to remould the NHS in the shape of the 'flexible firm'. According to one authority, some of the most dramatic labour market changes in the 1980s took place in the public sector, including the health service (Mohan, 1995, Ch. 6).

5 From patient to customer

It may be argued that the low expectations and deferential outlook of the traditional NHS patient gave full scope to professional autonomy, and helped to ensure that low standards were tolerated. However, by the 1980s the rising consumer consciousness of the public was paralleled by the growth of a managerial approach that emphasized the need to consult and involve the public and to make health care services more responsive.

But did the 'customer' get any better service than the 'patient'? Discussion around this key question of the reforms was – not surprisingly – intense. Patients certainly had more rights and could (and did) make more complaints. But the **patients' rights** slogan 'the money follows the patient' with which Kenneth Clarke once tried to popularize the reforms, was soon revealed as meaningless. In cash-strapped health authorities, non-fundholding GPs faced even more restricted choices for hospital referrals than in the past.

In what ways does the health service show greater 'customer-awareness' today compared with the past?

7   Conclusion

The NHS is about more than simply producing health; it acts as a mechanism, and a symbol, of reassurance and social stability.

(New and Le Grand, 1996, p.69)

The managerial revolution in the NHS was the culmination of a long process of negotiation and conflict. The 1979 White Paper, *Patients First,* signalled the general direction of legislative reform which was given a sharper managerialist edge in the 1983 *NHS Management Inquiry* (the 'Griffiths Report'). These initiatives succeeded in streamlining the bureaucracy (notably by the abolition of the area health authorities) and in establishing a central management body to oversee the devolution of budgetary responsibility to local managers.

However, though the reforms of the early 1980s created the organizational framework for a more efficient health service, most commentators agree that, in practice, results fell some way short of aspirations (Hunter, 1994; Mohan, 1995). Like all bureaucracies, the NHS was resistant to change, and its distinctive combination of professional autonomy and collectivist traditions made it particularly reluctant to conform to the demands of what most health service staff had come to regard as a hostile government. The continuing furore around the health service that continued through the election year of 1987 confirmed the unfinished character of the Conservative revolution in the NHS. Perhaps the most important consequence of the earlier reforms was that they paved the way for the major reforms of the third term.

In the 1980s the government attempted to impose commercial management on the health service, but without introducing its essential prerequisite – commerce, the dynamic of market forces. As we have seen, the centrepiece of the reforms of the early 1990s was the introduction of the internal market into the health service. This was the common thread running through the 1989 White Paper, *Working for Patients,* and the subsequent White Paper (dubbed 'Griffiths II') on community care. The same spirit of individualism and enterprise was evident in 1991 in *The Patients' Charter* and *The Health of the Nation* documents. Though the White Paper, *The New NHS,* published by the New Labour government in December 1997, proclaimed the end of the internal market reforms, in practice it marked their consolidation. While commercial principles were now balanced by the need to plan the distribution of health resources, GPs were given a central role in rationing services to patients and in negotiating contracts with hospitals.

A number of factors, operating both inside and outside the health service, contributed to the success of this package of initiatives. The government's success in facing down militant protests from different sections of NHS staff, from nurses and ambulance workers to GPs and consultants, strengthened its authority in pushing through the reforms. Its wider victories – over the unions and the Labour Party – contributed to a decisive shift in the balance of forces in the NHS. Not least, the collapse of socialism internationally dealt a terminal blow to the notion of state intervention as a viable alternative to the capitalist system. It provided a timely boost for one of Mrs Thatcher's most powerful slogans, 'TINA: There Is No Alternative' – to the capitalist market.

Looking back on the settlements of 1945 from the perspective of the late 1990s, there can be little doubt that a fundamental transformation has taken place. Yet, it is still easier to see the destruction of the old order than to discern

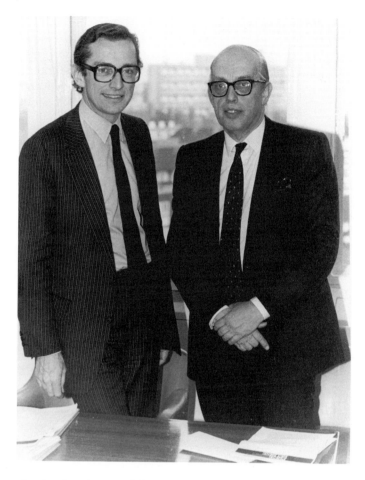

The minister brings in the manager: Secretary of State at the Department of Health and Social Security, Norman Fowler, with J. Sainsbury's Roy Griffiths who set about introducing commercial principles into the NHS

clearly the shape of the new. Blair's New Labour reflected popular concerns about the corrosive effect of the Conservative market-led reforms in health as in other areas of welfare, and indeed in society at large. New Labour's approach to the health service incorporates a recognition of the point made by New and Le Grand, that the NHS is not merely a health care system, but a bulwark of British society itself. At the same time, New Labour has acquiesced to TINA: it too believes that there is no alternative to the market, and has endorsed the spirit of the consumerism that now pervades the health care system. The resolution of these conflicting principles will determine the shape of the health care system in the next millennium.

Further reading

Nicholas Timmins' book, *The Five Giants,* takes its title from the social evils – 'Want, Disease, Ignorance, Squalor, Idleness' – identified by William Beveridge as the targets of the programme of welfare reforms he recommended in the 1940s. It is subtitled 'a biography of the welfare state' and provides a comprehensive account, combining historical rigour with journalistic flair, of each of the main areas of welfare from the era of the post-war Labour government to that of the Conservative governments of the 1980s and 1990s.

Robinson and Le Grand's *Evaluating the NHS Reforms* is an excellent, brief account of the reforms of the 1990s from the perspective of two influential social policy academics broadly sympathetic to the approach of New Labour. In *A National Health Service?*, John Mohan, a social geographer, takes a more critical attitude to the introduction of the internal market, advancing the view in response to the question-mark in the title, that an integrated national health care system no longer exists.

The Australian social anthropologist, Deborah Lupton, is one of the few commentators to question mainstream sociological interpretations of the rise of the new public health and health promotion. Her book, *The Imperative of Health,* mounts a spirited challenge both to the medicalization of life and to medical sociology. Ann Karpf's *Doctoring the Media* is a fascinating and highly entertaining survey of the changing presentation of the world of medicine in print, film and television. It takes in everything from medical soaps through documentaries to health propaganda.

References

Audit Commission (1996) *What the Doctor Ordered: A Study of GP Fundholders in England and Wales*, London, HMSO.

Black, D. (1992) 'The Black Report' in *Inequalities in Health*, Harmondsworth, Penguin.

Calman, K. (n.d.) *The Chief Medical Officer's Challenge (The Health of the Nation)*, Leaflet, London, Department of Health.

Commission on Social Justice (1994) *Social Justice: Strategies for National Renewal*, London, Vintage.

Day, P. and Klein, R. (1991) 'Britain's health care experiment', *Health Affairs*, vol.10, no.3, Project HOPE, Millwood, VA, pp.39–59.

Department of Health (1979) *Eating for Health*, London, HMSO.

Department of Health (1983) *NHS Management Inquiry* (The Griffiths Report), London, HMSO.

Department of Health (1989) *Working for Patients*, Cmnd 555, London, HMSO.

Department of Health (1991) *The Health of the Nation*, Cmnd 1523, London, HMSO.

Department of Health and Social Security (1976) *Prevention and Health: Everybody's Business*, Discussion document, London, HMSO.

Department of Health and Social Security (1977) *Prevention and Health*, Cmnd 7047, London, HMSO

Department of Health and Social Security (1979) *Patients First*, London, HMSO.

Dines, A. and Cribb, A. (1993) *Health Promotion: Concepts and Practice*, Oxford, Blackwell.

Doyal, L. (1979) *The Political Economy of Health*, London, Pluto.

Dubos, R. (1960) *Mirage of Health*, London, Allen and Unwin.

Green, D. (1987) *The New Right: The Counter-Revolution in Political, Economic and Social Thought*, Brighton, Wheatsheaf.

Hunter, D. (1994) 'Managerial challenge' in Gabe, J., Kelleher, D. and Williams, G. (eds) *Challenging Medicine*, London, Routledge.

Illich, I. (1976) *Medical Nemesis: The Expropriation of Health*, London, Calder and Boyars.

Karpf, A. (1988) *Doctoring the Media: The Reporting of Health and Medicine*, London, Routledge.

Langan, M. (1998a) 'The contested concept of need' in Langan (ed.) Ch. 1.

Langan, M. (1998b) 'Rationing health care' in Langan (ed.) Ch. 2.

Langan, M. (ed.) (1998) *Welfare: Needs, Rights and Risks*, London, Routledge in association with The Open Unviersity.

Lawson, N. (1992) *The View From Number Eleven*, London, Bantam.

Le Grand, J. (1990) 'The state of welfare' in Hills, J. (ed.) *The State of Welfare: The Welfare State in Britain since 1975*, Oxford, Oxford University Press.

Lister, J. (1988) *Cutting the Lifeline: The Fight for the NHS*, London, Journeyman.

Lupton, D. (1995) *The Imperative of Health: Public Health and the Regulated Body*, London, Sage.

McKeown, T. (1979) *The Role of Medicine*, Oxford, Oxford University Press.

Martin, C.J. and McQueen, D.Q. (1989) 'Introduction' in Martin, C.J. and McQueen, D.Q. (eds) *Readings for a New Public Health*, Edinburgh, Edinburgh University Press.

May, M. and Brunsdon, E. (1994) 'Workplace care in the mixed economy of welfare' *Social Policy Review*, no.6, Canterbury, Social Policy Association.

Mohan, J. (1995) *A National Health Service? The Restructuring of Health Care in Britain since 1979*, London, Macmillan.

Navarro, V. (1976) *Medicine Under Capitalism*, New York, Prodist.

Nettleton, S. (1995) *The Sociology of Health and Illness*, Cambridge, Polity.

New, B. and Le Grand, J. (1996) *Rationing in the NHS: Principles and Pragmatism*, London, King's Fund Institute.

NHS Executive (1994) *Developing NHS Purchasing and GP Fundholding: Towards a Primary Care-led NHS*, Leeds, NHS Executive.

Oakley, A. (1980) *Women Confined*, London, Martin Robertson.

Owen, D. (1976) 'Patient, help thyself', *Sunday Times,* 3 October, p.16.

Robinson, R. and Le Grand, J. (eds) (1994) E*valuating the NHS Reforms*, London, King's Fund Institute.

Secretary of State for Health (1997) *The New NHS*, London, The Stationery Office.

Singer, R. (1997) *GP Commissioning: An Inevitable Evolution*, Abingdon, Oxon, Radcliffe Medical Press.

Skrabanek, P. (1994) *The Death of Humane Medicine and the Rise of Coercive Healthism*, London, Social Affairs Unit.

Timmins, N. (1995) *The Five Giants: A Biography of the Welfare State*, London, HarperCollins.

Webster, C. (1994) 'Conservatives and the NHS, 1951–64' in Oakley, A. and Williams, A.S. (eds) *The Politics of the Welfare State*, London, UCL Press.

CHAPTER 4

Thinking Social Policy into Social Housing

by Michael Pryke

Contents

1   Introduction

The main aim of this chapter is to consider housing policy – specifically housing policy enacted in the period since 1980 – in relation to wider social policy and to suggest something of their combined effects. In this way it can be seen how housing policy, particularly that affecting people housed in the public sector, became enmeshed in processes of social disadvantage. It will then be possible to consider whether these changes were connected with an emergent new settlement of social welfare (see Chapters 1 and 2 in this volume).

In trying to achieve this aim there is a need to be aware of four issues. *First*, it is important to be sensitive to the influence of past housing policies on those housing outcomes in the period under focus in this chapter. Past policy and trends that began way before the 1980s can reappear in the present in quite unexpected ways; outcomes experienced in the 1980s are thus not simply the sole result of policy enacted in the 1980s. For instance, a lack of housing choice is differential in its distribution and effects, being felt far more intensely in certain parts of the country and within particular urban areas. In Scotland, for example, the post-war dominance of the public sector means that in Glasgow there are areas around the periphery of the central city – Castlemilk, Drumchapel, Easterhouse and Pollok – where comparatively little owner-occupied or private-rented housing is available (see Inquiry into Housing in Glasgow, 1986). This is no accident: it has a history.

The *second* point to note has just been hinted at above: although the chapter is talking about social housing and welfare policy, neither set of policies took

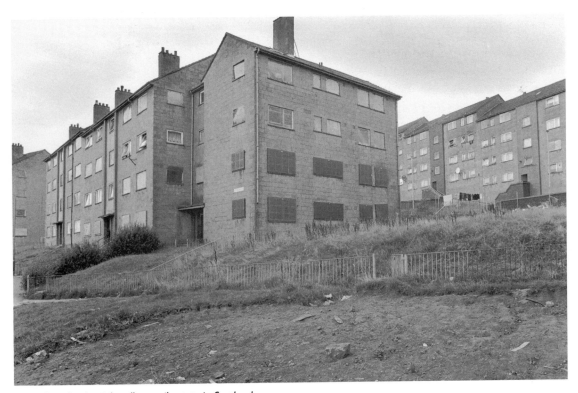

Drumchapel: a 'peripheral' council estate in Scotland

place in isolation. They were enacted through a highly uneven *economic geography* which makes up the UK. This means that cutbacks in social housing expenditure, and the shortage of new social housing that results, were felt far more severely in areas such as Liverpool and parts of the Midlands where the economic restructuring that occurred in the early 1980s (and again in the early 1990s) resulted in areas where unemployment rates were well above the national average. For these unemployed people, a policy initiative that promoted owner-occupation offered no real alternative route to decent, affordable housing.

The *third* point to bear in mind is that in housing policies enacted since 1945 there has been quite a substantial degree of agreement about policy direction. For example, Labour as well as the Conservatives came to view owner-occupation as a 'good thing' – a policy aim adopted well before the 1980s: '[owner-occupation] reflects a long-term social advance which should gradually pervade every region' (Labour Government White Paper on Housing, 1965, quoted in Malpass and Murie, 1994, p.70). But, equally, there was – until 1979 – consensus amongst the parties in support of a 'significant' role for the public sector. There were party differences, however, about whether the private sector rather than the public sector was best suited to deliver policy. The changes initiated in housing policy after 1979 by consecutive Conservative governments were thus notable for their break with the existing consensus (in the case of social housing) but were also predictable (in the case of owner-occupation).

Finally, it is also worth bearing in mind the ways in which those people caught up in the processes noted above (in the peripheral estates of Glasgow, the areas of high unemployment in Liverpool, and so on) are actually talked about and categorized in the (social housing) policy process. Thus the changes to the previously consensual role of social housing that came in 1979 should in part be interpreted as the beginning of a discourse that put in play a new vocabulary for talking about and understanding this tenure, its 'problems' and how to remedy them. In the process, new 'welfare subjects' came to be defined and addressed. This point will be returned to in later sections.

The chapter is organized in the following way:

- Section 2 introduces the area of housing tenures and the framework in which housing policy is developed.

- The next section looks at the types of thinking that have informed housing policy since the start of the 1980s.

- Section 4 then relates social housing policy to wider social policy and examines the process of social disadvantage working through particular housing tenures.

- Section 5 deals specifically with the rise of housing associations as the new providers of social housing.

- Finally, section 6 sets out the issues of homelessness and marginalization in the context of housing and welfare policy change enacted since the beginning of the 1980s.

2 Social housing and social policy

2.1 Locating social housing within housing

If you looked through newspapers dating from the beginning of the 1980s and searched for articles about 'housing in the United Kingdom', you might well find yourself reading, year in, year out, different accounts of a recurring theme: the ups and downs of the owner-occupier housing market. You would find articles about spiralling house prices, the cost and availability of mortgages, the collapse of house prices in the late 1980s, the rise of 'negative equity', building society repossessions, and so on. For sure there would be plenty of coverage of all aspects of owner-occupation. The focus would be on the private sector.

In some senses this focus is unsurprising as owner-occupation has become the dominant tenure in the UK since the early 1980s. Yet it is only one of several housing tenures, and it certainly has not always been the predominant way in which housing in the UK has been provided and consumed. So let us take a look at the main housing tenures and see how they changed in relative and absolute importance in the period between the early 1980s and the mid 1990s.

tenure
social housing

By the end of 1994 there were 23.7 million dwellings in England, Wales and Scotland (Wilcox, 1995, p.92, Table 16a). These dwellings divide unequally into three main tenure types: owner-occupation, privately rented, and social housing, comprising both housing association and local authority rented. The private-rented sector has declined to around 10 per cent of the total UK housing stock. The focus here is on the *overall trend* affecting all tenures. One of the most remarkable features of housing in Britain over this period has been the rise of owner-occupation and the demise of local authority housing. Britain now has the largest percentage – around 75 to 80 per cent – of owner-occupiers under the age of 30 of any industrialized western country (Joseph Rowntree Foundation, 1991). This trend has affected England, Wales and Scotland equally. In Britain owner-occupation represented just over half of the total dwelling stock in 1987 but by 1994 its share of the total stock had grown to around two-thirds. By that date the number of houses rented from either local authorities or new town corporations had fallen to its lowest level for 31 years (Central Statistical Office, 1996, p.176). The same trends have also affected housing in Northern Ireland, where the growth of owner-occupation rose from 54 per cent of all dwellings in 1981 to reach 67.8 per cent by the end of 1993; local authority dwellings declined from 37.9 per cent to 26.7 per cent of all dwellings during the same period (Wilcox, 1995, p.95, Table 16d). Despite the decline in public sector housing completions and the increasing dominance of the private sector (CSO, 1996, Table 10.6, p. 178; Gibb, 1996, Table 1.5) and the regional variations in completions (Office for National Statistics, 1996, Table 6.1, p.98), overall the stock of dwellings in the UK has increased.

If this is the case, it may seem surprising to find a string of problems associated with the housing system in Britain, such as homelessness, poor housing conditions, a concentration of poor tenants and minority ethnic groups in unsatisfactory council estates (Joseph Rowntree Foundation, 1985). The Joseph Rowntree Foundation, an independent philanthropic body supporting research into many areas of social policy, sponsored research which resulted in an influential report, *Inquiry into British Housing, Second Report* (1991). This found that there had been 'substantial withdrawal of expenditure on council housing' and a 'heavy reliance on the private sector to deliver homes', and that the concomitant inadequate investment in rented housing and 'heavy financial bias towards owner-occupation' had resulted in aggravation of the underlying problem of homelessness, which almost doubled between 1980 and 1990. The findings and conclusion of this report serve as useful qualifications to the overall trend in housing stock noted earlier and throw up a number of points and issues that we need to consider in relation to housing policy generally and the relationship between social housing and welfare policy more broadly. The points raised also help to demonstrate the limitations of an approach to housing which focuses on the types and distribution of housing tenures, as will soon become clear. But more immediately, it may be useful to consider what is meant by 'housing policy'.

1.2   Housing policy: its meaning and implementation

As Malpass and Murie (1994) note, housing policy 'is used in different ways and covers a multitude of activities'. Any policy 'implies a process, involving an initial formulation of a problem, a planning or policy-making stage, followed by execution or implementation of the policy, which may itself be followed by an appraisal or evaluation of the success of the policy' (Malpass and Murie, 1994, p.6). Arguably the most important word in this definition is 'process': policy as a process. For what the aggregate figures for housing stock and completions discussed above miss are the policy changes initiated by governments that helped to produce those outcomes. The rise in owner-occupation, for example, did not happen of its own accord; it was produced by general macro-economic policies that saw a rise in personal disposable incomes in the 1980s (see Maclennan, 1994, 1997); it was also produced by specific policies, including the re-regulation of mortgage lending in 1986; perhaps most significantly, owner-occupation became the tenure to aspire to and was a significant element in the 'feel-good' boom years of the 1980s. This was seen not only in the pressure for young people to get into the housing market but in long-term council tenants changing their tenure status. It was this shift in aspiration and attitude to housing that created new social meanings for housing tenures.

The term tenure, it should be noted, has its analytical limitations too. First, however neat a tenure label may appear, it actually hides a good deal of heterogeneity. Second, tenure is 'a mere consumption label'; it leaves out the system of provision: for example, the methods of financing a particular dwelling type and all the implications (such as subsidies) and outcomes (like unequal access to finance) involved in such arrangements (Malpass and Murie, 1994). Traditionally, four measures of housing – its quality, quantity, price and ownership/control – have established the boundaries to thinking about UK housing policy (Malpass and Murie, 1994, p.9). It has been around these four elements of housing that successive UK governments have spoken about and formulated housing policy: 'a decent house for every family at a price within their means' is an objective shared by all the main political parties in the United Kingdom. While parties have agreed about the *objective*, differences have, however, emerged about the best means to achieve it.

housing policy

*Divide and rule –
rules OK*

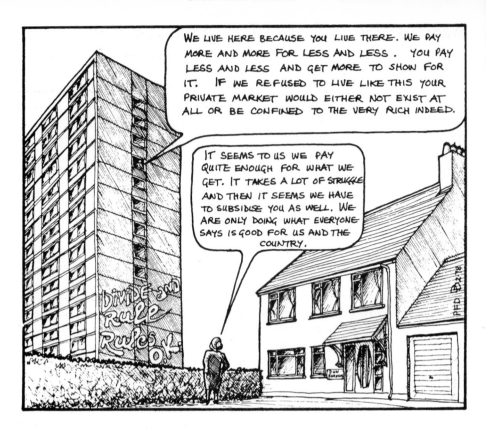

Different emphases might involve the role of the private sector as builders, as financiers, as managers of housing and so on, as opposed to the role of central and local government bodies in the system of provision, financing and management of housing. Central government housing policy has to be mediated through a wide and diverse range of organizations, and involves less than straightforward links between central and local government (Malpass and Murie, 1994, p.10). Moreover, further tensions may arise because central and local government often do not share the same aims and objectives about housing policy: while the centre may be more concerned with economic regulation, local government is more preoccupied with the day-to-day management of housing stock, the setting of rents, building programmes, and homelessness, for example.

The above points suggest that there is ongoing tension in the establishment of a framework for housing policy. Central government cannot easily get its own way and the outcomes of a policy initiative may be quite varied across the UK, due as much to pre-existing local economic and social variations as to the ability of local government to innovate around central government directives.

ACTIVITY 4.1

This section has discussed briefly some of the elements, agents and channels for thinking about the implementation and direction of housing policy. Can you think of a few general – or analytical – points that can be extracted from this discussion which will help to make useful links between social policy and social housing?

For me, the following points begin to emerge. First, at different times particular interests will predominate and influence the direction of housing policy which will affect all tenures, although probably unequally. Second, the importance and social meaning of tenures is open to change over time – witness the rise in owner-occupation noted earlier. Third, there is a wide range of people and organizations involved in the formulation and implementation of housing policy. Central government's ability to control the actions of each varies. Did you think of any more?

■ ■ ■

3 The emergence of a new social housing policy

The relative and absolute changes amongst the main housing tenures in the UK since the late 1970s, outlined in the previous section, did not come about by chance. Prior to the implementation of policies that were to impact upon owner-occupation, local authority housing and the private-rented sector, a series of arguments were taking place, particularly amongst those on the right of the Conservative Party, that were to be influential in the way in which housing tenures would be thought about in the 1980s and beyond. The change in thinking about housing – notably the ideological emphasis on owner-occupation as against council housing – dates back to ideas that were being developed from the late 1960s.

Upon its election in 1979 the first Thatcher government lessened much of its radical rhetoric towards restructuring the welfare state, with the exception, that is, of local authority housing which was subjected to the brunt of 'an anti-welfarist ideology' (Sullivan, 1992, p.166). This 'anti-welfarist' approach had stark effects on public sector housing in particular in the period from the early 1980s. These included sharp declines in both the building of new housing and the reduction of stock of local authority housing as a consequence of the right-to-buy policy, a fall in subsidies to council tenants and an increase in local authority rents in real terms for the first time since 1945.

Central to these changes is the privatization of social housing provision and management. The right-to-buy scheme, which allowed existing council tenants to purchase their homes at a substantial discount to market value, was a significant part of the first of four phases of government housing policy implemented after 1979 (Malpass and Murie, 1994, pp.97–8). The remaining three phases involved the deregulation of housing finance in the early to mid 1980s, which had significant impacts on the private sector, owner-occupied markets. This was followed after 1986–87 with policy intended to *re-regulate* the private-rented sector and change the role of housing associations. The final phase was the outcome of the unintended results of earlier phases, particularly that of financial deregulation; this required a phase of thinking up new initiatives to unpack and ease the problems of such market imperfections as negative equity, created by the rush to buy and the resulting insupportable boom in property prices.

The remainder of this section summarizes the privatization in the housing sector over the course of the 1980s, with specific reference to the right-to-buy legislation and its implementation. The context was the promotion of the market as the optimal allocation mechanism and the promotion of home ownership.

right-to-buy

3.1   A new model of welfare provision?

It is helpful to think about this 'rightward' movement in terms of a switch away from a so-called social democratic model to a market model of welfare provision, a model that informed explicitly the formulation of housing policy from 1979 to 1997. The emphasis on the market model highlights the ideological drive informing policy change during these years of Conservative government.

Before considering the key features of the market model, let us relate the shifts in thinking to what are key elements of the social democratic model and its ideology. Very simply, the *social democratic model* mistrusts the market as the best provider of welfare. The market, and the ways it operates, leads to inequality which must be redressed by state intervention. Citizenship is about the right to full membership in the community, a status that needs to be ensured by the state. At all these levels and more, the social democratic model views state intervention as strategically important to comprehensive and equal welfare provision (see Clapham *et al.*, 1990, pp.28–30).

market model   The market model, on the other hand, is underpinned by neo-liberal economics *and* traditional Toryism (family values, altruism and so on) and thus places great emphasis on market competition and limitation of the role of the state. In this view, individuals should be free to compete in the market and the rights of citizenship are linked closely with 'the rights of individuals to accumulate rewards through individual effort' in the market-place. The proponents of the market model accept that inequality will follow such market-based activity but see this as a positive outcome, as it will promote 'initiative and effort'. Those failing to compete will be supported through kinship ties rather than support from state benefits; the latter are viewed as impediments to the operation of the market. State subsidy, if it is relied upon, should not impede economic liberalism (Clapham *et al.*, 1990, pp.24–6).

ACTIVITY 4.2

What approach to social policy and housing policy might flow from the points emphasized by the market model? In thinking about this question you might like to refer back to Chapter 2 and in particular its emphasis *first* on the ideological attack on the welfare state (in section 5.2) and the key words that have been at the heart of 'restructured welfare' and, *second,* the construction of 'new welfare subjects' (in section 7).

COMMENT

For me, the market model very obviously suggests the centrality of 'markets' in all spheres of economic and social life. The implications for housing policy that arise from this type of thinking, particularly when it is combined with the limited role of the state, include the almost total withdrawal of the state from the provision of many 'social' services including housing. The state is seen as having no role in such areas: the private sector can provide more efficiently and a greater range of choice. Individuals should be able to acquire private sector housing as a result of rewards for their own endeavours in the job market; the more effective they are in competing in the job market, the better quality the housing they should, 'by right', be able to afford and to obtain. With such a view, social housing becomes highly stigmatized accommodation, provided for those either unable or unwilling to compete in the job market. As a result, the funding of this type of housing becomes the target for cutbacks.

■ ■ ■

3.2 The right-to-buy and privatization

Privatization was thus a central process in Thatcherite social policy. As Cole and Furby (1994, p.197) remind us, privatization may take a number of forms such as the *reduction* of public expenditure and subsidies, the *regulation* of provision within a sector to allow entry to the private sector, and the straightforward *private provision* of services. Each form was employed in different degree with the overall aim of realigning housing policy, first, to fit with government ideology (as much as changing macro-economic events allowed) and, second, towards the market model of welfare provision. For instance, whilst tax subsidies to owner-occupiers were increased in the 1980s, subsidies to council tenants were reduced. New building programmes by local authorities were severely curtailed at the same time as council house sales were enthusiastically promoted.

It is worth lingering on the last point – the sale of council houses – as this policy, according to many writers (such as Forrest and Murie, 1985, 1991; Balchin, 1995), lay at the heart of the Thatcherite strategy towards social housing. In brief, under the Housing Act 1980 council house tenants were given the right to buy the house or flat in which they were living. This was a measure promised in the 1979 Conservative Party Manifesto with the aim being to make real '… Anthony Eden's dream of a property-owning democracy' (quoted in Forrest and Murie, 1985, p.19). Buoyed by discounts of up to 70 per cent of market value, the total public housing stock of around six million in 1980 was reduced by one and a half million as houses and flats were transferred from the public to the private sector.

The dream in fact fell flat for many people encouraged to take on mortgages for the first time: repossessions steadily rose through the later 1980s, running at around 30,000 per annum from 1985–89, but then rising rapidly to peak at 62,000 in 1992 (Central Statistical Office, 1996, Chart 10.15); many more new home-owners found themselves trapped in negative equity, having bought at the top of the market. The tax subsidies to owner-occupiers also began to be cut in the 1990s – since such subsidies were seen as interfering with the workings of a free market.

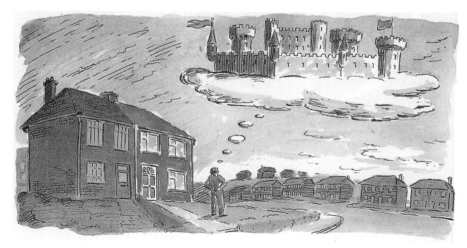

The right to buy a castle

But what was the impact of this form of privatization on social housing and what might be some of the welfare impacts of the policy? The sale of council property was uneven: houses rather than flats made up the greatest proportion of sales; sales were high in the regions enjoying prosperity at the time, such as the south-east of England; sales in the main were to middle-aged tenants and to the skilled working class. The remaining stock thus moved more towards a concentration of 'pensioners', the 'young', the 'unskilled' and those 'dependent' in some form on state benefits. The new market ideology began to have marked material effects in the social housing tenure. Those unable or unwilling to participate in the market for the right-to-buy were quickly left behind and were not always in a position to rely on 'kinship' and 'family' for support. Moreover, some might argue, the categorization of those left behind – the pensioners, the unskilled, and other groups noted above – made it easier for them to be represented as the problem of social housing rather than to think in terms of how a restructured social housing sector, evolving in a wider, uneven socio-economic context, was failing these and other groups. (Again, you might like to refer back to Chapter 2 to form some useful links with the points raised here.)

The introduction of the ideology of the market, of the (supposed) withdrawal of the state, the rhetoric of the individual, and so on, was stepped up around the right-to-buy policy through other forms of privatization. These included the reduction in financial support to local authorities resulting in a rise in council rents. In the first six years of Conservative government, subsidies to council tenants were cut by 31 per cent – while subsidies to owner-occupiers (through mortgage tax relief) rose by some 212 per cent. Housing benefit, which would have helped many tenants to cope with rising rents, was readjusted seven times in four years from 1983, leading to around one million households losing their eligibility for this form of subsidy (see also Wilcox, 1995).

As the rate of right-to-buy sales decreased in the mid to late 1980s, attempts to privatize what remained of the public sector continued. In particular, control of the sector needed to be pulled further away from local authorities. Local authority provision, quite simply, was seen as at odds with the market model. The task was now to transfer ownership – both *management* and *control* – away from local authorities to tenants themselves. As the then Housing Minister John Patten put it, '... continuing as a tenant should not mean being a pawn in the hands of bureaucratic management' (quoted in Cole and Furby, 1994, p.199). Policy initiatives in England, such as the Priority Estates Project and Estate Action, all contained measures to coax local authorities into rethinking the management of their stock (Cole and Furby, 1994; see also Williams, 1997).

The Housing Act 1988 and the Local Government and Housing Act 1989 – both of which came out of the government's thinking expressed in the important White Paper, *Housing* (DoE, 1987) – shared the common goal of further reshaping the rented sector. The key to this process was the demotion of local authorities from providers to enablers in the provision of social housing. In parallel with this initiative was thinking and policy concerned to 'revive' the private-rented sector. This in effect involved the re-regulation of the sector – another form of privatization. The introduction of new *assured* and *assured shorthold* tenancies aimed to promote the growth of *private* landlordism (see Kemp, ed., 1988; 1993). Other measures such as Housing Action Trusts had as their goal the wresting of management and control away from the public sector (see Power, 1987).

3.3   Unequal outcomes

As a result of the Conservative government's ideologically driven social *re*valuation of housing tenures, some (groups of) people have found themselves faced with a limited choice of accommodation and with rising rents, while those in owner-occupation have benefited from its 'increased social valuation'. As Whitehead (1984, p.131), a leading British housing economist, wrote in the mid 1980s, one effect has been to 'redistribute wealth by luck': 'Those unable to take up their option to buy, who live in less suitable public sector accommodation or who have not yet gained access to that sector lose out.'

For some, this outcome might sit uncomfortably amongst the intended consequences predicted in the market model of (welfare) provision. But it is actually about more than being unlucky. Luck in this case, some would suggest, is very heavily influenced by the group in society in which people find themselves positioned. Class, gender and ethnicity all have an important bearing on whether an 'individual' throws a pair of sixes every time. As the following section suggests, these processes of social differentiation need to be entwined with tenure if we are to forge a meaningful link between 'housing' and 'social policy'.

While the ideological drive was for owner-occupation, seemingly at any cost, successive Housing Acts began to have very real social impacts during the 1980s and beyond. These impacts can be understood in terms of the way in which housing tenure plays an important part in shaping social disadvantage. For, as a recent report by the Royal Institution of Chartered Surveyors concludes, following an examination of the social costs of poor housing on two council housing estates in Tower Hamlets in London, 'the cost of poor housing goes beyond bricks and mortar' (RICS, 1997). The social impact of restructuring housing tenure needs also to be located in the wider arena of the significant readjustment in public expenditure on welfare. The following section takes up these themes in more detail.

social disadvantage

4   Social housing and welfare

The main aim of this section is to think about the place of housing – specifically social housing – within the broader framework of social policy, particularly as at the beginning of the 1980s it was already the 'wobbly pillar under the welfare state' (see Harloe, 1995; Kleinman, 1996a). What we want to try to understand are the wider welfare implications that might arise from the restructuring of social housing provision – the actual restructuring of which is looked at more closely in section 5. This section thus examines how economic disadvantage, social disadvantage and marginalization work through housing tenure (see also Forrest and Murie, 1991, pp.73–81). Specific examples will be addressed in section 6, where issues of gender, class and 'race' will be investigated through the impact of government policy on homelessness and the right-to-buy policy. However, in order to make more sense of the effects on social disadvantage of Conservative housing policy in the 1980s, it is helpful first to look at what has been happening to spending on the welfare state since the early 1980s.

'I'll say it's a tough area
– the social workers walk
around in threes!'

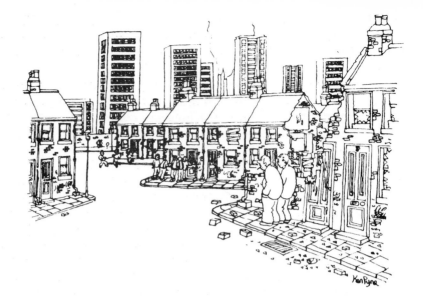

4.1 Government spending on welfare: housing draws the short straw?

Consider the data in Table 4.1 which is taken from John Hills' (1987) examination of changes in pattern of public spending between 1978–79 and 1986–87. Table 4.1 shows clearly that there were winners (such as defence) and losers (such as overseas aid) in changes in public expenditure since 1979. The biggest loser was housing, with the substantial reduction in the construction of council housing through the 1980s (see also Joseph Rowntree Foundation, 1991, p.74, Figure 26).

Table 4.1 UK public expenditure 1978–79 to 1986–87 (£bn, 1986–87 prices)

	1978–79	*1983–84*	*1986–87*	*Percentage growth 1978–79 to 1986–87*
Social Security	34.2	41.8	46.5	+36
Education	17.6	18.0	18.7	+6
Health	15.1	17.6	18.8	+24
Defence	14.6	17.6	18.6	+28
Housing	8.8	5.0	4.0	–55
Personal social services	2.8	3.2	3.5	+28
Overseas aid	1.4	1.2	1.2	–15
Other*	33.7	34.3	34.6	+3
Total	128.0	138.6	145.9	+14
National income	334.8	348.5	380.1	+14

Notes: *Does not include debt interest and does not include privatization as negative spending.

All figures from *The Government's Expenditure Plans 1983–4 to 1985–6* (Cmnd 8789) and *1987–88 to 1989–90* (Cm 56). Adjustment to 1986/7 prices is by reference to GDP (market prices) deflator.

Source: Hills, 1987, Table 1, p.89

These figures, however, hide a shift in government expenditure. The shift to 'real' market-determined rents meant that, despite reductions in the number of those eligible, between 1980–81 and 1995–96 the gross cost of housing benefit paid to council tenants rose from £1.9bn to £5.5bn (at 1995 prices) (Wilcox, 1995). This is reflected in the increase in spending on social security. As Hills (1987, pp.93–4) suggests, this was a case of robbing Peter to pay Paul as government departments attempted to reduce expenditure and a rather ironic and unintended outcome of neo-liberal politics aimed at reducing public expenditure (see Jordan, 1995).

It is thus necessary to look at two categories of public expenditure on housing that are omitted from the government's Housing Public Expenditure chapter of the White Paper on Public Expenditure (see Malpass and Murie, 1994). *First,* there are payments which form part of other government programmes such as housing benefit as part of social security. *Second,* there is the category of payment which is not thought of as public expenditure. The most significant of these expenditures are taxes forgone, such as mortgage interest tax relief (MIRAS). The inclusion of these figures makes the overall picture of public expenditure on housing rather different from that arising from just looking at spending on social housing. Let us focus on MIRAS as an example.

Public spending on mortgage interest tax relief was about one-third of the level of housing public expenditure in 1979–80; by 1984–85 it had exceeded it; and by 1990–91, it was three times as large (Malpass and Murie, 1994, p.108). What this suggests is quite a substantial propping-up, as it were, of the market model for the provision and consumption of housing. Owner-occupation was to be the dominant tenure, regardless of the overall cost. Moreover, there are other types of cost borne by those left out, if not constructed out, of the favoured tenure, owner-occupation. It is the social (and economic) costs that are the outcome of this new market discourse to which we now turn. As we do so, we also explore the nature of housing disadvantage and the shaping of new subjects of welfare in the process of social housing provision.

4.2   Housing tenure and social disadvantage

Housing policy can be seen as one means of implementing social policy objectives. As Clapham *et al.* (1990, p.56) point out, one of the 'most contentious of these aims [is] the alleviation of social disadvantage'. Given this, it is useful to follow Clapham *et al.* (1990, p. 56) and explore issues of social disadvantage in relation to the workings of social housing. Throughout the rest of this section, therefore, you might like to consider the following two questions. First, to what extent is it true to say that patterns of inequality are more or less 'entrenched' in the workings of (social) housing markets? And, second, how might housing policies enacted since the early 1980s have influenced social inequality in and across tenures in the UK?

These questions, and many others you can no doubt think of, raise a bigger, primary question: what is meant by 'disadvantage'? Added to this might be, what form of disadvantage is being referred to when the 'mediation of disadvantage' through certain housing tenures is talked of? What is central to this issue are the ways in which housing is thought about, as a *form of social policy* and the degree to which housing, particularly *social housing*, can be made to link with other areas of social policy and welfare.

We therefore need to arrive at a working definition of disadvantage and to do so with reference to the 'market' and 'social democratic' models introduced in section 3. Under the *market model,* disadvantage is linked to individual action. It can be measured on an absolute scale: disadvantage is viewed as equivalent to poverty. The aims of policy, then, are to raise people over the 'objective poverty-line' and thus help them to participate in society. The *social democratic model,* however, looks at disadvantage from the perspective of how economic and social processes are organized (Clapham *et al.*, 1990, p.57). Disadvantage, in this view, is a relative not an absolute condition and is defined in terms of a society's overall goals, aims and standards. Clapham *et al.* (1990, p.58) conclude that disadvantage can most usefully be 'conceptualized in terms of the varying *combinations* of deprivation and poverty that individuals experience' (emphasis added). If disadvantage is relative rather than viewed as being an absolute, measurable figure, then this 'portrays disadvantage as a *process* rather than as a product of individual or group behaviour, and as a consequence of the differential apportionment of a range of citizenship rights rather than as an outcome of individuals' failure to compete in the economy' (Clapham *et al.*, 1990, p.60).

So, how does all of this relate to the housing system, and to the legislation passed between 1979 and 1997 that has impacted on and around the operation of social housing in the UK? Well, for one thing it pushes us along lines of argument that express inequality produced through housing tenure as being *structured* and helps us to view disadvantage played out through housing tenure as being a *process*. In both these instances tenure, and their associated systems of provision and subsidy, suddenly move from *passive* categories – isolated containers, labelled owner-occupation and so on, as used in section 2 – to now being understood as *active* 'shapers of social disadvantage' (see Clapham *et al.*, 1990, pp.60–62). This is not to claim that there is something particular about housing. Rather it is to say that, just as in education or the labour market, inequality and social disadvantage work through and can be reinforced by housing tenure.

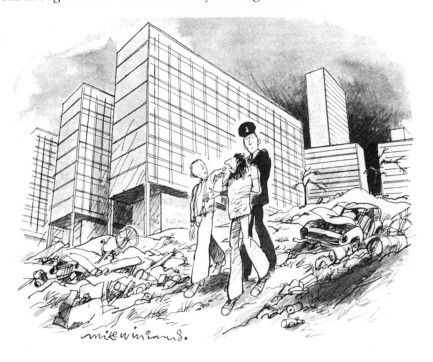

'Personally, I blame it all on Le Corbusier'

Reflect for a moment on the degree to which housing policy enacted between the beginning of the 1980s and the late 1990s has influenced the *process* of disadvantage in and around housing tenures, either directly or indirectly.

Another, in many ways inseparable, question you might like to consider is the issue of how certain groups have been disadvantaged more than others, again as the *direct* result of housing policies, or *indirectly* as a result of the ways in which housing tenure and housing policy intersect with other areas of welfare policy (such as social security payments and housing benefit).

These issues point to an examination of how social policy initiatives have set in train the reconstruction of council housing as a tenure. What we also need to be aware of is how the UK's uneven economic geography influences this reconstruction, in particular the changing geography of employment opportunities. The following subsection takes the issue of the social disadvantages of housing tenure further and concentrates on related processes of residualization and marginalization in the context of privatization and the broader restructuring of the welfare state that has been ongoing since the early 1980s.

4.3 Residualization and marginalization

So far, we have seen the reduction of public expenditure on public housing and the rising importance of market ideology in the delivery of welfare since the early 1980s. Here we want to explore a little further the impact of policy and political decisions through an exploration of social disadvantage and exclusion working through housing tenure. Specifically, the concepts of *residualization* and *marginalization* will be introduced to help us to understand more of what happened within the social housing tenure. In what follows a central aim is to reaffirm how inter- and *intra*-tenure differences align 'with the differential distribution of wealth, resources and life chances in British society' (Clapham *et al.*, 1990, p.66). This (re)alignment followed from the move during the 1980s from subsidizing public sector housing towards financial and ideological support for owner-occupation, leaving public or social housing only for those 'who for reasons of poverty, age or infirmity cannot find suitable accommodation in the private sector' – that is, creating 'a process of residualization' (Malpass and Murie, 1982, p.174). The processes of residualization and marginalization, it should be pointed out, are not new nor peculiar to the years after 1979; they are processes which have always characterized parts of the public housing sector (see Merrett, 1979). For instance, some argue that from 'the 1950s onwards the character of council housing gradually began to change, from a tenure for middle income groups … to a tenure of last resort' (Somerville, 1994, p.165). Nonetheless, the process of residualization *intensified* during the 1980s: in 1980 the income of the average council tenant was 73 per cent of the national average but by 1990 this had fallen to only 48 per cent, while the average for housing association tenants was only 45 per cent of the national average.

residualization

But what exactly are 'residualization' and 'marginalization'? For Forrest and Murie – two leading British social housing researchers who share a left-of-centre approach to social policy analysis – these terms provide helpful conceptual tools for understanding the deeper social welfare implications of the changing role of council housing. However, both terms are helpful, as Forrest and Murie (1994, p.74) note, only if they form part of an approach which lifts analysis out of a one-dimensional, single-tenure-based approach and relocates it within the 'coincidence' of 'longer term and wider trends in the housing market[s]'. In this way, we can avoid the trap of thinking about residualization in terms of single, isolated elements of change, such as the decline in public sector housing stock, or in the role of council housing. If the terms are to prove useful conceptual tools, their use must not be focused only on housing but must embrace, it is argued, wider factors such as ease of entry into (and exit from) particular types of housing and what is happening to social housing within broader processes of economic and social change.

As Forrest and Murie go on to point out, while it is important to understand the process and *direction* of residualization in this way, on its own it says little about *why such a process is possible in the first place*. It is here that the second concept, that of marginalization, is relevant. As they comment, what is important is that, 'The marginal poor, those with least political and economic muscle, have always been in the worst housing. What is new is the close association between this group and state housing' (Forrest and Murie, 1994, p.73). And, as earlier sections and previous chapters have made clear, this process of marginalization is located within a broader restructuring of the welfare state and residualization of public sector housing. Thus what has been ongoing in the British housing markets since the early 1980s is the polarization of forms of provision:

marginalization

> At one extreme, and typically associated with council housing, we have the development of state dependent communities where marginalised groups subsist increasingly on a range of stigmatised and pressurised subsidies. At the other are the highly mobile, high earners extracting the maximum benefit from mortgage interest tax relief, capital gains exemptions and other tax concessions (Forrest and Murie, 1987). What is common and what *cuts across tenures* is a reassertion of the connections between housing opportunities, housing conditions and earning power.
>
> (Forrest and Murie, 1991, p.79; emphasis added)

Both terms, then, in the particular ways they are being employed here, attempt to capture the manner in which what is going on within social housing is shaped by interacting processes of uneven economic change, the reliance on market relationships, the political marginalization of certain groups, as well as the simple reduction in social housing stock. In using these terms in this way, therefore, Forrest and Murie (1991, p.80) '... are concerned with contemporary forms of the reproduction of inequality' through (social) housing. The end-result of these processes of residualization and marginalization, when combined with the sale of council housing stock through the right-to-buy scheme, has left an unprecedented concentration in public sector housing of people who are dependent on benefits and social services (Forrest and Murie, 1986).

This section has sketched out the ways in which social housing has been subjected to substantial government expenditure cutbacks throughout the 1980s and early 1990s, although ironically resulting in greater expenditure on housing benefit. The immediate impact of this has been to limit the provision of new council housing in a broader environment which has seen the promotion of – and through the 1980s, considerable financial support for – owner-occupation. The section then moved on to consider the ways in which the economic policy favouring certain tenures and demoting others, might be viewed as part of a process contributing to social disadvantage.

The ways in which social disadvantage works through (social) housing will be returned to in section 6. Before that we will examine the changes that took place from the early 1980s in the *provision* of social housing. The following

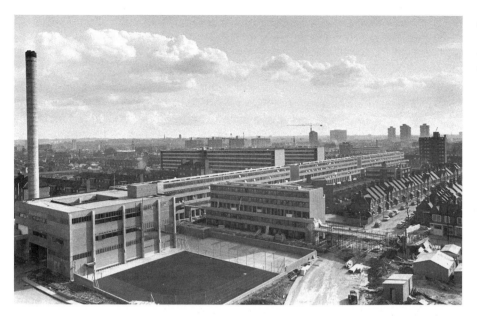

Aylesbury estate in Southwark, London: large-scale social housing

section looks at the way in which government policy has moved housing associations to centre-stage, whilst relegating local authorities to the role of *enabling* – rather than directly providing – the supply of social housing.

5   The (re)emergence of housing associations

We have seen that the move away from local authorities towards housing associations was formulated in the context of privatization of management and control; the other aim was monetary – to replace public with private sector finance. This section summarizes the key elements of this changeover in the 1980s which saw the introduction of two significant pieces of legislation – the Housing Acts of 1985 and 1988. These Acts followed on the back of the right-to-buy policy introduced under the Housing Act 1980, further cutbacks in public expenditure on social housing and the promotion of owner-occupation. As the then Secretary of State for the Environment announced in 1979:

housing associations

> In terms of housing policy, our priority of putting people first must mean more house ownership, greater freedom of choice of home and tenure, greater personal independence, whether as home owner or tenant, and a greater priority of public resources for those with obvious and urgent need.
>
> ...
>
> As for specific policies ... [w]e will be looking at a new subsidy system for public sector housing which will direct help where it is most needed. We certainly intend to ensure that local authorities are able to build homes for those in the greatest need – and I have in mind especially the elderly in need for sheltered accommodation and the handicapped.
>
> (House of Commons, *Official Report*, vol.967, cols 407, 408, quoted in Murie, 1982, pp.38, 39)

As well as conveying the potential for (further) marginalization of council housing, these words suggest the early rethinking of how social housing was to be financed in the 1980s. As Murie wrote in 1982, the combination of these changes heralded 'a new era for council housing in which a concentration on special needs is accompanied by a reduction in the actual size of the council stock, a minimal role of new building, a decline in the quality of new and existing council dwellings and a reduction in subsidy for council housing ... This combination of developments has not occurred before and marks a more thorough shift in policy than has occurred in the past' (Murie, 1982, p.34).

5.1   Why housing associations?

Housing associations are non-profit-making organizations and have a variety of origins. Some associations date back to the almshouses of the Middle Ages, others to philanthropic housing projects from the nineteenth century (see **Mooney, 1998**). Many of the younger housing associations were formed in the 1960s as part of a Shelter-supported, inner-city rehabilitation initiative and reflect the radical views voiced against the old welfare settlement. All associations have been monitored by the Housing Corporation since it came into existence in 1964. In Wales the equivalent body is Tai Cymru and in Scotland it is Scottish Homes, formed in 1989.

Until the Housing Act in 1974 housing associations were negligible providers of social housing; social housing took the form of council housing and was provided by local authorities. But with the Housing Act 1974, introduced by a Labour government, the role of the Housing Corporation grew to include functions of 'primary bank manager' and regulator. Importantly, the Act also introduced the Housing Association Grant (HAG), a form of subsidy that financed associations' expansion into the 1980s (Langstaff, 1992, pp.30–31).

HAG was a capital grant – not a loan – which in effect reduced substantially (at an average of 85 per cent) the cost of housing schemes, and in some cases totally covered the costs of schemes such as those catering for people with special needs (Hills, 1987). All in all, while local authorities were subject to quite savage cuts in capital spending and the target of harsh political attack, the housing association movement suffered little on either front as the subsidy system established in 1974 was allowed to continue into the 1980s. Under this system, it should be added, even cost overruns on an association's development programme would in most cases be met by HAG (see Hills, 1987). Output, however, was running at some 30,000 units a year fewer than in the 1970s (Langstaff, 1992, pp.33–4). A number of things needed to change.

5.2   Housing associations transformed

As the 1980s progressed, the Conservative government began to focus more attention on the ways in which housing associations could not only come to replace local authorities as the main providers of social housing but could do so in a way that fitted with the ideology and practices of the New Right and its market model. To this end the Housing Act 1988, as well as initiatives stemming from the Housing Act of 1985, are important.

The 1985 Act enabled the transfer of local authority stock into the hands of associations newly formed specifically for that purpose, so-called LSVT (Large Scale Voluntary Transfer) associations. (Many LSVTs were initiated by local authority officers to anticipate the perceived effects of the 1988 legislation (see Kleinman, 1996a).) In the period to 1997, 223,000 properties were transferred in 53 rural and suburban transfers. However, of the 27,000 or so associations active in the late 1990s the vast majority were small, managing a stock of under 1,000, concentrated in relatively tiny geographical areas, with only a handful operating at a national level.

By the mid 1980s the HAG system was not viewed as an effective use of public money, nor was a system that allowed cost overruns seen as 'efficient'. Ways were therefore sought to introduce the mechanisms and the thinking of privatization into the housing associations' provision of social housing. To facilitate this move there was a primary need to alter the basis of funding associations, introducing the possibility of using private as well as public finance in the funding of housing associations (Pryke and Whitehead, 1993, 1995). The risk of cost overruns also had to be shifted to the associations, as did the process of establishing rents, so that a closer correlation between the levels of social housing rent and the total costs of producing that housing (to include the cost of private finance) would emerge.

Following several attempts to mix private finance with public grant after the 1985 Act, the Housing Act 1988 established a framework which, amongst other initiatives such as bringing rent determination within the assured rent system (see Whitehead, 1989), set as a requirement the use of private finance in *all* HAG schemes. Moreover, total public funding under the new framework was reduced, with average grant rates lowered initially to 76 per cent and continuing to fall ever since, standing at around 55 per cent in 1997.

The main drive behind the new framework was to reduce public expenditure yet increase the output of social housing – the so-called 'value-for-money' argument. Additionally, the new financial context aimed to make associations more aware of the risks and costs of developing social housing – the so-called 'efficiency' argument. In the process, local authorities were to be sidelined as providers, becoming instead enablers for housing association provision: following the Housing Act 1988 housing associations became the main providers of social housing in the UK. The range and number of associations active in developing and managing social housing was viewed as beneficial as it was a move away from the near monopolistic control of the supply of social housing by local authorities. Additional aims and benefits, the government argued, included increased competition (amongst housing associations) in the provision of social housing in local areas and the establishment of a professional – rather than a political – setting for social housing. This would supposedly enable more efficient and responsive housing management. This was not a view shared by everyone, however. In Scotland, the effect of the Housing (Scotland) Act 1988 meant placing the majority of Scottish social housing under the control of Scottish Homes – an unelected, quasi-government body – thus removing from local councils the means to carry out their housing policies (Glasgow City Housing, 1989, p.5).

Unsurprisingly, while these changes in the funding and rent systems of housing provision were taking place, and as housing associations were pushed into the limelight as the new providers, local authorities faced a further 'campaign of denigration'. In addition to being subject to capital cuts and thus rent increases, and the effect of the right-to-buy policy, they were discredited as housing managers in a number of reports by the Audit Commission and by influential academics (Audit Commission, 1986; Minford *et al.*, 1987; Malpass, 1992, p.15).

While the subject of housing management is vast, the purpose of the following subsection is simply to focus, first, on the criticisms levelled at local authorities as poor managers; second, on trends in housing management; and, third, to outline the way in which housing associations faced up to their 'new' role as providers and managers of a growing stock of social housing.

5.3   A new housing management discourse

What is important to remember in all this is the underlying purpose behind the questioning of the ability of local authorities to manage their housing stock. Just as owner-occupation was promoted using the language of the new market ideology, so local-authority housing management was talked of in terms which influenced public opinion and thus facilitated the implementation of new policy initiatives. Thus, rhetorical formulations such as 'value for money', 'cost-effectiveness' and 'consumer choice' accompanied and eased the effective side-lining of local authorities as providers of social housing and led to the questioning of their role as 'good' housing managers.

What we need to recognize, then, is the way in which a particular ideology and its accompanying discourses have been at work in 'reconstructing' the role of local authorities (see **Clarke and Cochrane, 1998**). In a similar fashion we saw how owner-occupation was constructed as the new 'social norm' – the tenure that any sensible person would want to be in for a number of attendant reasons, not least because other tenures – notably 'social housing' – were portrayed as existing only for 'problem groups'. For example, the Secretary of State for the Environment in 1979 emphasized his view of the limited scope of public provision:

> We propose to create a climate in which those *who are able* can prosper, choose their own priorities and seek the rewards and satisfactions that relate to themselves, their families and their communities. We shall concentrate the resources of the community increasingly on the members of the community *who are not able* to help themselves.
>
> (House of Commons, *Official Report*, vol.967; quoted in Murie, 1982, p.38; emphasis added)

ACTIVITY 4.3

With these emphases in mind, as well as the broad themes that run through the market model outlined in section 3, read through the following quotation. It is taken from a publication from the early 1980s on local government policy published by the Adam Smith Institute, a right-wing think-tank. Can you identify any of the rhetorical devices intended to create the 'acceptance of a new political and economic reality' that would help to establish 'a healthy housing sector' (ASI, 1983, p.49)?

> A key objective is the removal of the barriers which stand in the way of a proper exercise of consumer choice. Arm in arm with this is the need to provide a framework that will facilitate speedy transition to a pattern of tenure that accords with that choice.
>
> ...

Far too much of what is wrong with housing today can be directly attributed to political intervention overriding individual choice and initiative.

…

Price plays a vital role in the private market for housing. It conveys the information about supply and demand … It thus serves to allocate and to increase the available supply. No such price information is available within the public sector, where the tradition has been one of supplying below-cost housing based on perceived needs.

(ASI, 1983, pp.49, 50, 52)

COMMENT

Although this is only a brief extract, there are a number of words and phrases used that echo the sentiments of the New Right and its efforts to have a 'new reality' accepted. For instance, at the very start of the quote emphasis is placed on consumer choice and how efforts must be made to ensure that tenures – particularly owner-occupation – are allowed to develop to meet with that choice. This emphasis made me think about the issue of the social construction of a tenure; about how a particular tenure can be shaped through policy to accord with 'natural' choice.

The rhetoric of the New Right comes through again in the way in which the blame for much of 'what is wrong' with British housing is laid at the feet of interventionist policies. Individual choice, rewards for initiative and so on, should be allowed to express themselves in the housing market just as much as in any other market. And, for this to work, the price mechanism must be allowed to signal preferences. The private rather than the public sector thus comes through as the 'obvious' choice for organizing the production and consumption of housing.

■ ■ ■

Arguably, amidst all of these policy suggestions and claims, there was an ongoing effort to construct a 'welfare consumer' as part of the New Right's attack on the old welfare regime (see, for example, Taylor-Gooby, 1985), an attack that was as much about the promotion of a market discourse as it was about removing the welfare state from 'the social, political and economic landscape'. As Clarke (1996, p.61) has noted, '… the figure of the consumer provided one of the levers with which the Conservatives could dislocate the old welfare regime and its potential as a site for ideological attachments and alliance building.'

It is not surprising to find that the shiny new ideas of 'the consumer' and of 'consumer choice' sat untidily amongst the jaded language of council housing and local authority housing management. The 'customer' and all the other rhetorical baggage of choice and the price mechanism was very much part of the 'business discourse of *managerialism*' (Clarke, 1996, p.65; emphasis added). It was also part and parcel of the 'challenge' to the 'professional paternalism' of the institution of local authorities as providers and housing managers.

Before considering how any of the above influences are filtering through into the way in which housing management is being implemented, it is helpful first to consider the changed context of managing council housing in the 1990s, and, second, to acknowledge that while local authorities have been subject to change in the way they manage their reduced housing stock, housing associations have had to approach the task of managing a different type of social housing.

ACTIVITY 4.4

You should now read Extract 4.1. While you do so, consider what new function the author suggests is being placed on housing associations. Can you see any limitations to the analysis of the process of residualization presented here?

Extract 4.1 Page: 'A new role for housing associations'

The new role which Government has assigned to housing associations is ... one for which most associations are not well prepared: their skill lies in managing a different kind of social housing chiefly provided for those with different categories of need. Managing large estates which house very low income families with children will therefore require new skills and an understanding of how managing an *estate* is something more than the management of a large number of individual dwellings.

Most 'residualised' areas of council housing are large estates of low-income families, with high numbers of children. They may also be associated with poor locations, high building densities, 'utopian' design, a bad state of repair and ineffective housing management. But the common ingredients seem to be scale, poverty, a large number of children and an allocation system which places people where they do not want to be. In the past, this potent combination has rarely applied to housing association property: it seems likely that it could increasingly do so from now on.

Housing associations have chiefly avoided the management problems of local authorities by not producing housing on the same scale or accommodating the same tenants: but there is no intrinsic reason to assume that housing associations are better managers than local authorities. Where associations have had to manage poorly designed or located housing with the same spectrum of tenants as local authorities, the same management problems have tended to arise. But in dealing with these problems, housing associations have certain advantages: they have higher staff-to-tenant ratios; they have a dedicated repairs allowance; they are single-function organisations (whereas local authorities have a multiplicity of functions and a number of departments controlled by separate committees); and they are not subject to direct political control. This means that they have been free to bring greater resources to bear on their own 'problem' estates, but even these efforts have not always been successful.

(Page, 1993, p.5)

COMMENT

Housing associations have had to take on the management of large estates, something which few of them had to do in the past. The author suggests that this produces very different types of problems, compounded by the new type of tenants with whom they are now dealing.

In reading through this extract you, like me, might have been struck by two things: first, by the simple fact that the process of residualization is beginning to emerge within housing association stock; second, by the heavy emphasis placed on both the characteristics of *problem housing* – 'large estates', 'poor locations', 'high building densities' and the like – and the characteristics of those *people* living in them.

It seems to me, recalling the arguments put by Forrest and Murie (1991) outlined in section 4.3 above, that the analysis reported here falls into the trap of a tenure-based approach to the problem of residualization in both council housing and housing association stock. The end-result is that the source of the problem is seen as lying either with the nature of the housing – 'large estates', 'poor locations', 'high building densities' – or with the tenants – 'low income families', 'families with high numbers of children'. The wider *systems of provision* of that housing and changes in its funding and the various subsidies, such as housing benefit, that are attached to it, together with the wider structural changes in both the economy and in the welfare state that go some way to producing 'low-income tenants', never seem to enter the analysis or explanation.

■ ■ ■

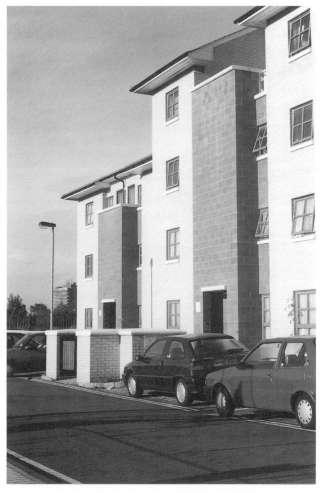

New housing association development, North London

Extract 4.2 is taken from an extensive piece of research which looked at the consequences of housing associations moving 'centre-stage', with a focus on the factors that lead to the residualization of social housing on large estates. Although the majority of associations are not involved in developing or managing such estates, the extract usefully highlights some of the 'new' processes that are leading to the emergence of 'problem' estates within the overall housing association stock; processes, moreover, that almost necessarily are at play within the social housing tenure more generally, although in different combinations.

ACTIVITY 4.5

When reading through Extract 4.2, bear in mind the above points. Try to list the elements highlighted in the analysis of 'residualization' as well as the remedies offered, perhaps set out in a grid. You could then add a third column to the table listing the effects of restructuring in the wider welfare state and in the economy on the problems identified and on the feasibility of the remedies offered.

Extract 4.2 Page: 'Building for communities'

What is the problem?

There is now evidence that the process of rapid decline of large social housing estates which some had thought peculiar to council housing can also apply to the stock of housing associations. There are a number of reasons why this has not been evident in the past:

- housing associations have relatively few large estates;
- associations have generally avoided 'mass housing solutions' like high-rise or deck access forms of building;
- before 1988, only a small number of long-established associations owned very large estates and most of them practised estate-based housing management.

...

Something new is occurring; some newly built estates have shown significant signs of wear and tear after only two years; two of the case study estates had developed problems of vandalism, graffiti, incivilities and drug abuse so serious in only four years that a multi-agency approach was required to deal with them. The problems are not new, but the time-scale is: housing associations are getting there much quicker than local authorities. Run-down council estates are generally the result of two or three decades of decline: housing associations are now meeting similar problems in under 5 years. What is the explanation?

The evidence suggests an explanation in two parts, which are interrelated. One concerns the new estates and the other the populations who live on them: both are now composed differently from when councils last built large estates.

...

There is an assumption that social housing providers cannot go wrong if they provide houses with gardens: but it depends how these houses are let. The suburbs of most towns comprise chiefly family type housing but it is occupied by a diverse range of household types – young and old, families with and without children, single people, couples and extended families. If large new housing association estates were let to a similarly diverse range of households they would meld seamlessly into the communities in which they are set. But that option would require both underletting and letting to households who were not in priority need: in practice the pressure on social housing means that large estates of family housing will be let to those in greatest need and filled to capacity.

...

A different mixture of people

The second thing that has changed is the composition of the population of new estates ... There has been a significant shift since 1979 in the characteristics of the people for whom social housing must provide. This has been caused by changes in both the supply of, and demand for, rented housing.

On the supply side, during the eighties the rented sector as a whole decreased by about one quarter; private renting decreased by one-third and social housing by one-fifth. This amounted to a total supply-side loss of 1.75 million dwellings from the rented sector.

The demand-side changes are less easy to quantify but the pattern is clear. The demand for social rented housing remained strong among low-income households who could not afford to buy their own homes: this pressure was further increased by those (including some of the poorest) who would previously have found a home in private renting, a sector which had decreased by some 600,000 dwellings … Taken together these changes have meant that the people seeking social housing are increasingly the poorest. The selection processes used by local authorities and housing associations give this population a further sift by prioritising according to need.

The excess of the demand for social rented housing over its supply means that tenancy selection processes must be particularly stringent: priority is therefore given to the homeless, the most vulnerable and those least able by virtue of income to compete in the market. Analysis … shows how new housing association tenants compare to the wider community: they have only one-third of the average disposable income; they are less likely to be economically active and those who are active are five times as likely to be unemployed; lone parents are over-represented by five times; and more than half (54%) are wholly dependent on state benefits or pensions. Among new tenants, those who were previously homeless are even more disadvantaged: 64% of those who are economically active are unemployed and 54% of families are headed by a lone parent (95% of whom are eligible for housing benefit).

What this data means in practice can be better understood by considering the effect on a new estate let under fairly typical current allocation arrangements. If we imagine an estate which comprises 80% family houses and 20% one-bed flats where a local authority has nomination rights to all of the family units (i.e. 80% of all) and uses them to re-house homeless families, and we assume that the characteristics of tenants on the estate in each size of dwelling are [typical] …, we could expect the estate's tenants to have the following characteristics: only 21% would be in full-time work; 60% of those who were economically active would be unemployed; 43% of households would be headed by a lone parent; 81% of tenants would be eligible for housing benefit; the average disposable household income would be around £94 per week.

How does this hypothetical case compare to what is actually found on real estates? One of the already stigmatised case study estates has these corresponding characteristics: only 22% of tenants are in full-time employment; 65% of those who are economically active are unemployed; 57% of households are headed by a lone parent; and 85% are in receipt of housing benefit …

Also on some estates, the concentration of disadvantage is further increased by the way that the non-family one-bedroomed accommodation is allocated. Some associations have used this chiefly for those with special needs moving on from hostel-type accommodation or being discharged from institutions under the care in the community programme. These include people with learning difficulties and people with alcohol or drugs problems. The pressure to find accommodation of a good standard for those in greatest need has led to a situation in which, on some estates, almost every tenant is either seriously economically disadvantaged or is vulnerable because of their special needs.

The above comparison … demonstrates that the socio-economic profile of tenants on new estates is not the product of local circumstances nor of perverse decisions by individuals but is instead the likely outcome of current development and allocation practice. Consequently, unless one or other practice is changed, housing associations are likely to produce a number of large new estates, each with a social mix undesirable in itself and similar to existing estates which have become rapidly stigmatised.

How did this happen?
The present situation has arisen as a result of the pursuit of two perfectly legitimate and praiseworthy policy objectives: that publicly funded housing should go to those in the greatest need; and that the best value for money should be obtained by housing associations in building new schemes.

Following the value for money objective, housing associations have been encouraged to achieve economies of scale by entering into bigger value contracts with volume builders … The outcome is the provision of large new estates, chiefly by consortia of housing associations, frequently including some which provide for people with special needs. Local authorities are also encouraged to provide land on which to build new estates in return for nomination rights up to 100%.

The other policy objective, again unimpeachable, is pursued through two main instruments: first, the requirement placed on the Housing Corporation that 50% of its rented programme (this rises to 70% in 1993/94) should be used for housing the homeless; second, through the use of local authority nomination rights under 'Partners' type agreements which require housing associations to allocate a high proportion (around 70% on average) of their family-type accommodation to statutory homeless households (this will often be higher where councils have 100% nomination rights).

When the two policy objectives come together, the result can be a singular concentration of serious disadvantage and vulnerability on a large new estate …

…

There are clearly different ways of providing housing to meet both of the policy objectives set out earlier. If the main objective is to house people in the greatest need, the best way of providing for them is not on large estates, given what is now known about the serious disadvantage and vulnerability of the people to be housed …

Better still, housing associations could again be permitted to buy and rehabilitate street properties using skills they have developed over the last quarter of a century. Both of these alternatives would set disadvantaged and vulnerable people in the wider community in which they are more likely to find support, instead of among other people who are equally disadvantaged and vulnerable on large estates.

(Page, 1993, pp.46–50)

These are just some suggestions to start you off. Draw up your own grid to add further ideas.

The problems	The remedies	Impact of welfare and economic restructuring
large estates	smaller-scale developments	Change in local employment markets leading to pockets of high unemployment
physical structure of the stock, e.g. high-rise blocks	newer low-rise housing	

■ ■ ■

6 Homelessness and marginalization: issues of gender, 'race' and class

This section explores further the issue of social disadvantage and housing tenure, specifically addressing the issue of how inequalities attached to gender, 'race' and class intensify the processes of homelessness and marginalization; in doing so, the effects of the right-to-buy policy will be revisited. The main areas addressed here include:

■ the causes of homelessness – its most immediate reasons, as well as the less visible ones;

■ the 'unintended consequences' of government housing policy on homelessness;

■ the reasons why certain groups of people are more likely to be homeless;

■ the reasons why certain ethnic and racial groups tend to be concentrated in particular tenures;

■ the ways in which gender (as well as 'race', ethnicity and class) 'differences' complicate the supposedly straightforward categories and processes of allocating and consuming housing across tenures.

The emphasis in what follows is almost exclusively on social housing – the public rather than the private sector. The private sector, particularly the rise of owner-occupation, the right-to-buy policy, and the regionally uneven rise and collapse in house prices, nevertheless cannot be ignored, as its changing role affects particularly the most recent reasons for homelessness and the marginalization of council housing. What also needs to be borne in mind is the overall context of change in housing policy that has occurred between the early 1980s and the late 1990s. Most of the 'big changes' in housing policy have been covered in previous sections. Of these it will help to recall the sidelining of local authorities as social housing providers, the rise of housing associations, and the importance placed on choice of housing tenure by successive Conservative governments.

6.1 Gaining and not gaining access to housing

homelessness

In order to understand some of the reasons why homelessness is a continuing and growing problem throughout the UK, it is necessary to consider the different 'access channels' to each tenure. To oversimplify, access to the *private sector* is determined by ability to pay and the 'actions and decisions of "gatekeepers"' (Clapham *et al.*, 1990, p.112). *Private renting* offers a half-way-house, as it were, for those persons or households on low incomes who are unable to gain entry into owner-occupation, nor able to find a way through the procedures involved to qualify for social housing. Although representing only about 10 per cent of the total housing stock, the private rental market has proved to be an important – although in many cases far from desirable – source of shelter.

In the *social sector* it is 'need' rather than ability to pay which determines access (see **Langan, 1998**), but as Clapham *et al.* comment:

> It is important to note that 'need' ... is a social construct. That is to say, rather than being objectively determined and self-evident, need is defined by professionals such as housing managers ... [W]here demand for accommodation is greater than its supply, definitions of need become a bureaucratic rationing device. A particular definition of need can be used to determine which households are to be given priority for accommodation. Those deemed to be in 'greatest need' can then be allowed to join the waiting list or to go to the top of the queue.
>
> (Clapham *et al.*, 1990, p.113)

Once again the price mechanism plays an important part in determining access to tenure, as does the process of socially constructing access to – or socially constructing people out of – a tenure. This is an important point to remember in what follows when, for example, we consider how different ethnic groups and their particular circumstances are confronted by the issue of access to housing: if issues specific to them are not voiced and heard then the social construction of homelessness can easily lead to their exclusion.

The *official* definition of homelessness under Part III of the Housing Act 1985 (an Act that incorporates the Housing (Homeless Persons) Act 1977 which for the first time gave certain groups of 'priority' homeless people the statutory right to be rehoused by their local authority) sets out definitions of those who have such a right. One important criterion is that someone claiming to be homeless must be in priority need: 'i.e., have lost their home through an emergency such as a fire or flood *or* have children *or* be pregnant *or* be sick, elderly or disabled *or* be otherwise "vulnerable"'. As Withers and Randolph write,

> These 'priority need' groups are defined in such a way as to include those who for legal, medical, accidental but not structural reasons, are unable to compete in labour (and therefore housing and welfare) markets ... This identification of 'priority need' carries with it the implicit labelling of different groups as being 'deserving' or 'undeserving' of assistance.
>
> (Withers and Randolph, 1994, p.14, Box A)

As this suggests, such an official definition of homelessness serves to 'define specific areas of responsibility on the part of local authorities' as well as to allow for the supposed quantification of the 'problem' (Watson and Austerberry, 1986, p.12). Local authorities – and now housing associations – can use the Act's definition of homelessness in effect to exclude certain categories of homelessness. For instance, as Burrows and Walentowicz (1992, p.6) report, in 1991 in England 146,290 households – that is roughly 420,000 adults and children – 'were accepted as homeless by local authorities out of roughly double that number who applied'. If one includes Scotland, that figure jumps to 170,000 households. Thus by the end of 1991 there were around one million people *officially* homeless in England and Scotland. Yet, needless to say, official statistics are less than reliable. People who fall outside of 'priority groups' such as the young, or those without children, are simply not registered as homeless. These people may not be 'roofless' but living in private boarding-houses, private tenants with insecure or short-term tenancies, single people, couples and families – the 'concealed homeless', as they are termed, because they may find themselves living in inadequate or unsuitable accommodation, not officially acknowledged as homeless. As this suggests, a complex set of processes lies at the heart of homelessness.

6.2 Causes of homelessness and the characteristics of the homeless

So, what are the main causes of homelessness in the UK? Figure 4.1 suggests the main causes: while looking at it, think about how a succession of government policies – not just those related to housing – and economic trends have affected the patterns and processes of homelessness. These are explored in more detail in the following extract.

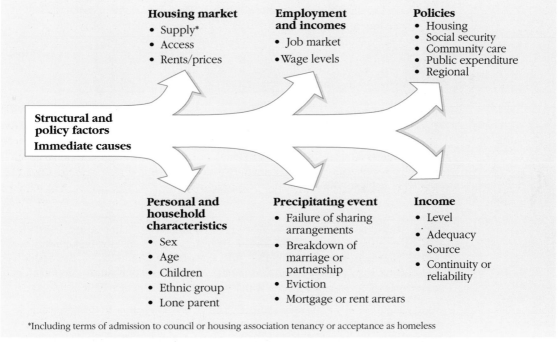

Figure 4.1 Causes of homelessness (Source: Greve with Currie, 1990, Figure 7, p.16)

ACTIVITY 4.6

Now read through Extract 4.3, which is taken from a report by *Shelter*, the pressure group which campaigns for adequate housing provision in the UK. As you read it, consider the differences between 'immediate' and 'underlying' causes of homelessness.

Extract 4.3 Burrows and Walentowicz: 'Causes of homelessness'

Immediate causes

The primary causes of homelessness have changed little in recent years. The most common is the breakdown of previous living arrangements. Around 43 per cent of households become homeless because parents, other relatives or friends are no longer able or willing to accommodate them. Many will have been on a local authority waiting list but without much hope of an offer of a home until a crisis hit them. Many would not have applied as homeless if other housing alternatives had been available to them at a price they could afford [see the figure opposite].

In about 16 per cent of cases, homelessness is caused by the break-up of a settled marriage or relationship. What was originally one household often becomes two households when a family breaks up.

Some people become homeless because they have been evicted. For owner-occupiers it is usually because of mortgage arrears. A tenth of those accepted – about 7,000 households – became homeless because of mortgage arrears in the first six months of 1992. Mortgage arrears as a reason for official homelessness has tripled in a little over ten years. Although mortgage repossessions have fallen slightly from their peak in 1991, they are still historically high. About 36,000 homes were repossessed by mortgage lenders in the first six months of 1992. Those people who do not turn to the local authority or are refused help probably move in with friends or relatives or rent privately.

About 15 per cent of homeless households were previously private tenants. A growing number of officially homeless people is accounted for by private tenants who have lost their assured shorthold tenancy. They now make up around a half of all private tenants who are accepted as homeless. The number of private tenants who could be accepted is limited by the fact that most are single people and ineligible for help. Loss of a social rented home – either a council or housing association letting – is usually caused by serious rent arrears. But only two per cent of homelessness acceptances arise from this cause.

Underlying causes

Government statistics do not explain why a household was unable to find itself an alternative home. Shelter believes the key factor which underlies the increase in homelessness is that insufficient accommodation is available at prices or rents which ordinary people can afford. The main reason for this is the decline in the stock of rented housing – both public and private …

…

At the same time the private rented sector has continued its decline despite legislative and fiscal attempts to stem the tide. The 1988 Housing Act shift to 'market rents' has led to rent increases which have made the private rented sector increasingly inaccessible to most low income households. Many households simply cannot afford to pay market levels of rent, even with housing benefit help (see table).

Most people facing homelessness cannot afford owner-occupation. In 1990, for example, research showed that only 29 per cent of young families were in a position to buy a new home. Despite price falls home ownership remains out of reach of many (see table).

Other government policies, such as high interest rates and the poll tax, have left low income households worse off making it even more difficult to compete in the housing market. Inevitably homelessness has increased.

(Burrows and Walentowicz, 1992, pp.10–13)

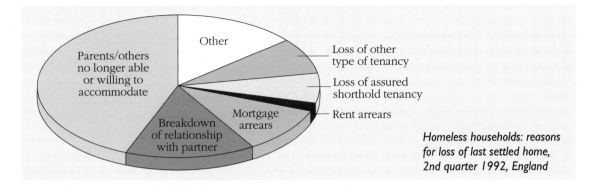

Homeless households: reasons for loss of last settled home, 2nd quarter 1992, England

Can they rent a home from a private landlord?

Description of household	Weekly take home pay	Typical weekly private rent for home of adequate size	Can they afford the rent?
Administrative Officer Couple with child One working, London	£166	£185 (2-bed)	Rent is more than a third of income after housing benefit
Staff nurse Single, Devon	£190	£70 (1-bed)	Rent is more than a third of income – no housing benefit
Kitchen porter Single, South East	£126	£50 (bedsit)	Rent is 40% of income – no housing benefit
Unemployed Single, London	£43.10	£57 (bedsit)	Rent is met by housing benefit. But landlords often do not accept claimants. Many have problems finding deposits and rent in advance

Sources: *Earnings:* Department of Employment, 1992; *London rents:* London Research Centre, 1992; *Elsewhere:* Shelter Housing Aid Centres.

Can they afford to buy a home?

Description of household	Weekly take home pay	Maximum mortgage they could afford	Average price of home	Can they afford to buy?
Administrative officer Couple with child One working, London	£166	£32,167	£69,600 (2-bed flat)	No
Staff nurse Single, Devon	£190	£39,750	£49,000 (Terrace)	No
Kitchen Porter Single, South East	£126	£24,617	£55,800 (1-bed flat)	No
Hairdresser Single, Yorkshire	£110	£20,701	£36,000 (1-bed flat)	No

Note: Maximum mortgage is three times gross income.

Sources: *Earnings*: Department of Employment, 1992; *London house prices and rents*: London Research Centre, 1992; *Elsewhere*: Halifax Building Society, 1992 and Shelter Housing Aid Centres.

The immediate causes of homelessness stem from the break-up of marriages and relationships, from parents no longer willing or able to accommodate their children: that is, broadly as a result of 'changed living arrangements' creating new households. The *underlying* causes identified in this extract are factors such as the inadequate supply of social housing, high real rents, and the lack of affordable accommodation in either the private-rented sector or in owner-occupation. You may have identified more causes than I have.

■ ■ ■

It is important to remember in examining the causes of homelessness that each cause – mortgage arrears, inadequacy of supply of alternative accommodation, the mismatch of local job opportunities to skill base, insecure employment and low wages limiting access to good quality accommodation, and so on – varies spatially; each has a particular geography and when these geographies overlap, so the issue of homelessness intensifies. Figure 4.2 gives some indication of the varying degrees of homelessness as distributed across the local authorities of England in 1991–92. What is interesting about the figure is that it shows that homelessness, though marked in certain metropolitan areas such as London, is by no means an urban phenomenon. Indeed, throughout the 1980s homelessness rose at a faster pace outside London: between 1985 and 1990 average annual increases for Metropolitan districts outside London ran at 14 per cent, compared with 7 per cent for inner London and 9.3 per cent for outer London (Greve with Currie, 1990, Table 2, p.9).

This variation in the rates of homelessness felt by both local authorities and housing associations means that the problem of managing housing association stock and the process of residualization can vary quite substantially within a highly heterogeneous tenure. Faced with these problems, both the government and the Housing Corporation have aided associations in the task of dealing with homelessness. The various 'packages' and 'initiatives' put forward have been financial and include the Rough Sleepers Initiative (targeted at London), the Homelessness Package (targeted at families in London and the South East) and the Housing Market Package which allocated £620m to 27 associations to buy unsold stock in the owner-occupier market with a condition that a proportion of this would be let to the homeless.

The irony is that for many associations the task of tackling homelessness directly – by building new or rehabilitating existing houses – has been complicated and hampered by the new funding regime brought in with the Housing Act 1988. As indicated in section 5.2 above, one of the Act's aims was to shift the risk of cost overruns from the government to housing associations. As a result, certain types of scheme such as renovation, whose final cost is often unknown at the outset, have been cut back severely: 'The effect has been ... [a shift] to more new development away from areas where homelessness has been centred and into green field and suburban locations where pressures to rehouse the homeless have been less acute' (Withers and Randolph, 1994, p.11).

These trends and 'causes' have begun to suggest some of the reasons for homelessness in aggregate, but in order to be able to say something about the

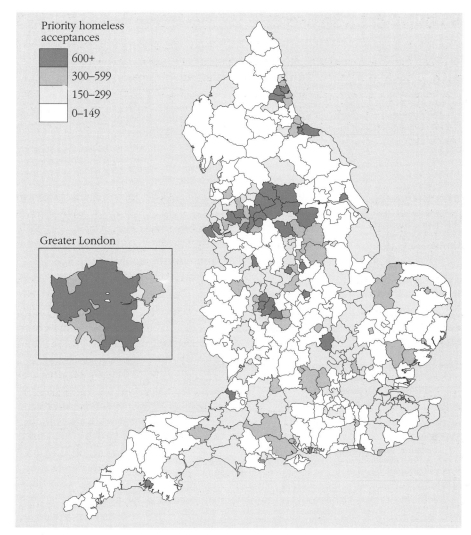

Figure 4.2 The geography of 'official' homelessness: priority homeless acceptances by English local authorities, 1991–92 (Source: Withers and Randolph, 1994, p.5)

social construction of disadvantage in terms of access and – more importantly here – *failure* to gain access to particular tenures, then we also need to look a little more closely at 'the homeless' themselves. Certain groups are more subject to homelessness than others: for example, homelessness and unemployment are very closely linked, particularly amongst young people from African-Caribbean and Pakistani/Bangladeshi ethnic groups. In London in the early 1990s an estimated four in ten households accepted as homeless were from a minority ethnic background (Burrows and Walentowicz, 1992, p.10). The following subsection focuses on the specificity of a couple of these groups that are not reflected in official definitions of homelessness.

6.3 'Race' and gender

It is important to question not just the usefulness of official definitions of homelessness, but also the centrality of certain concepts in the formulation of those definitions. Terms and categories used in housing policy formulation such as 'family household' and 'owner-occupation', as well as categories of broader application such as 'ethnic' but which impinge upon housing in terms like 'social housing for ethnic minorities', are all *constituted positions*: they are the result of defining, of socially constructing, people 'in' or 'out of' housing rights (see Chapter 2 of this volume; **Langan, ed., 1998**). As Watson and Austerberry (1986, p.18) remark, as well as being forever 'ambiguous', definitions of homelessness are *relative* not only to time and culture, but 'between different forms of households and within the household unit itself' (see also Watson, 1986, 1987). The examples of 'race' and gender have been chosen here in order to question the suitability of existing definitions of homelessness and its causes; more broadly, they help us to explore how certain groups are constructed out of tenures and the (mal)functioning of those tenures (see Phillips, 1987; Henderson and Karn, 1984; Peach and Byron, 1994).

In reading through this subsection, keep in mind the way in which housing rights have been reformulated as one consequence of the emergent social settlement informed by the market model.

The reformulation of housing rights is resulting in at least two things: *first,* the emergence of another form of unevenness between different 'categories' of people for whom housing should be a basic right; *second,* the reinforcement of this unevenness for certain groups. So, for some groups – say, those officially constructed and recognized (such as 'ethnic') and those constructed but rarely officially recognized in housing policy (such as 'unemployed, separated women with dependent children' or 'female pensioners') – the problem of obtaining housing may be exacerbated by wider discrimination in the face of a shortage of social housing. For example, racism in the process of housing allocation within the public housing sector did not simply arise out of the process of restructuring, but has been present for a long time (see Commission for Racial Equality, 1988, 1990; Parker and Dugmore, 1977/78; Sarre *et al.*, 1989). However, with a shortage in the availability of public housing – something that has become quite marked since the beginning of the 1980s – the marginalization of racialized groups may have become more acute. As the Chief Executive of a black housing association, Presentation, wrote in 1994, 'It's not difficult to trace the causes of homelessness among black people. When our community is traditionally home to society's lowest paid workers – when our housing is consistently in the poorest condition and when our experience of unemployment is the most marked there can be no surprise that our people find the greatest difficulty in securing and holding onto housing' (Chandran, 1994, p.13).

Particular groups of people and their 'characteristics' produce specific housing needs; they can, moreover, project certain groups along particular tenure paths. For instance, in the UK since 1945, 'Caribbean tenure patterns have evolved in a notably different way from those of the Indian and Pakistani ethnic minorities ... Indian and Pakistani tenures have moved very swiftly in the direction of owner-occupation, while Caribbean tenures moved dramatically towards council housing, although with a substantial presence in owner-occupation' (Peach and Byron, 1993, p.408). Indeed by 1985 while only 39 per cent of African-Caribbean households lived in owner-occupied property, the figures for Indian and Pakistani households were 77 per cent and 74 per cent respectively. At 47 per cent African-Caribbean households were by far the largest group in local authority accommodation; the figures for 'whites', 'Indians' and 'Pakistanis' were 28 per cent, 11 per cent and 16 per cent respectively (Peach and Byron, 1993, p.409, Table 1). And while, as the same authors note, '... class explains much of the tenure pattern of Caribbean *male* heads of household ... the tenure patterns of female heads of household is the product of a much more complex *interplay* of class, gender and racism' (emphasis added).

And once this interplay is recognized and accounted for in the explanation of tenure paths, we can begin to appreciate how these socially constructed groups *and* the social construction of their constituent members, may well compound the problem of access to certain tenures, and may lead to (further) residualization and to unofficial homelessness. For instance, Peach and Byron conclude their analysis of the high concentration of Caribbean tenants in council housing by saying that gender and family structure must be added to class as an explanatory factor:

> Over 40 per cent of Caribbean heads of household are female-headed; 62 per cent of Caribbean female-headed households are in council housing and of this group, more than a quarter (27 per cent) are single parents with dependent children. Lone mothers of any kind (that is, not just single mothers but divorced, widowed, separated and so on) living in council housing, constitute 37 per cent of all Caribbean female-headed households. This is the group with least power in housing decisions.
>
> ... [T]he gender factor is of vital important in an explanation of a Caribbean household tenure structure ... The Caribbean female-headed household category is most likely to encounter racist, gender and class based constraints to tenure options.
>
> (Peach and Byron, 1993, p.422)

Thus, active beneath the surface of the emergent social settlement's badge proclaiming 'customer', is an interplay of practices of categorization('Caribbean minority', 'single mother' and so on) that are filtered through sets of institutional practices which are in themselves not devoid of racism and sexism. All of these result in quite different outcomes for those who should, according to the rhetoric of the new discourse, be treated equally. And it is not that difficult to see, once the interplay of class, gender and 'race' in housing tenure is added to the wider outcomes of welfare change, how the processes of marginalization and residualization would become more extreme, more so when the uneven outcome of council house sales (Forrest and Murie, 1991) and employment opportunities are taken into account.

ACTIVITY 4.7

Read through Extract 4.4, taken from *Black Housing*, a journal concerned with issues of racism and housing from the minority ethnic groups' point of view. Note how the interplay of factors suggested in the article leads to high rates of homelessness and poor housing amongst those groups of people with whom the extract is concerned. How might changes in the structure of the wider welfare state have worsened or lessened the effect of the factors and processes identified?

151

Extract 4.4 Bulgin: 'The sinister arrangement for black homeless people'

A relatively recent report into Tower Hamlets black homeless, *Who's Hiding*, researched and written by the late Carolyn Ye-Myint for the local housing campaign group, No Fixed Abode, is a clear pointer for all who are trying to get to the root of the level of black homelessness in England and Wales.

The report looks at the acute needs of those segments of the Somali, African-Caribbean, Bangladeshi, Irish and Chinese communities regarded by the borough housing department as non-priority homeless.

Among the many findings contained in the report is that 'Existing data about black and ethnic communities in Tower Hamlets is grossly inadequate.' The effect has been a poor service to the black community there. At 35,000, the Bangladeshi represents the largest of the minority communities in the borough followed by the African-Caribbean (10,000), and the Chinese and Vietnamese, 8,000. But there is a sizeable African community approximately 4,800 of which there is no record at the town hall.

Placing non-priority homelessness in context *Who's Hiding* identifies as its primary set of causes racism, poverty, and 'local authorities' policies and practices (which) have exacerbated housing inequalities' and in recent times, 'market forces'. The latter has been a factor in the 'disproportionately high level of unemployment in Tower Hamlets which is '… twice the London average – 20.4% – derived from pre-1983 methods of assessment', with a rate of 'Pakistan/Bangladeshi 21.8%; West Indian/Guyanese 14.4%; Indian 9.4%; all other ethnic groups 7.9%; and white 6%.'

This occurs side by side with a low income problem where 63% of African-Caribbean and 60% of Asian households have an annual income of below £7,800,

Ethnicity and homelessness, Tower Hamlets, 1991

	Approximate % of borough's population	No. of homeless families	% of total homeless
White	68	412	24.5
All minority ethnic groups	32	1061	62.2
Unknown		207	12.3

Source: *Who's Hiding*

Ethnic origin of families registered as homeless, January 1991

Ethnic origin	No. of families	% of total homeless
Bangladeshi	827	49.2
Caribbean/West Indian	27	1.6
Somali	73	4.3
Other African	46	2.7
Chinese	4	0.2
Vietnamese	11	0.6
Other Ethnic	73	4.3
White U.K.	412	24.5
Unknown	207	12.3

Source: *Who's Hiding*

compared with 45% of white households, according to the 1986 Docklands Housing Needs Survey.

The low income–poverty–homelessness continuum weighs heavily on most who experience it, and the ethnicity and homelessness relationship disfavours all black minority ethnic groups. While the combined black population in Tower Hamlets is 32% and the white 68%, the homelessness level is skewed against the black population at nearly 3:1 (63% to 24%), with a 12% unknown number.

The report finds a definite link between the much suffered problems of over-crowding, bad housing and homelessness. Tower Hamlets in a recent report acknowledges that there is over-crowding in the borough, admitting that between 1990–1991, 75% of all applicants were due to heads of black households, throwing out family members or friends living with them because of over-crowding.

Other factors that lead to homelessness include mental illness due to pressure of racism with which a number of people cannot cope, and post-institutional care does not include permanent housing provision. Asylum seekers and refugees also have major problems as all local authorities are free to use their discretion in the way they like and quite often it is in favour of a refusal. Single refugees, who constitute 90% of the total in the United Kingdom, do not qualify for housing.

...

Equally blunt is the authority's 'Intentionally' clause in their housing policy. It complements their 'Sons and Daughters' scheme and keeps a large number of black families off their waiting list. Between November 1991 and May 1992, 48 families were declared intentionally homeless. Four were white, and 37 Bangladeshi.

In the 1980s the London Docklands Development Corporation embarked on a building programme to renew and expand the housing stock in the borough. But in spite of an awareness of the need for larger accommodation for black families, 67% of all units were built with one or two bedrooms only.

Now the building programme in Tower Hamlets, as it is in the rest of England, has come to a near standstill. Public spending in housing fell by £11 billion over the period 1979–1989. In London the building programme has fallen by 50%, and Shelter's estimate at the time was that there were approximately 3 million Britons without a home. Of that figure is the black homeless which is disproportionate to our actual number. Work needs to be done to discover the actual number.

(Bulgin, 1994, pp.10–11)

COMMENT

For me, one of the most striking aspects of this extract is the way in which it highlights the discrepancy between an obvious set of housing needs across quite disparate ethnic groups and what local government policy identifies as the housing needs of those groups. This discrepancy, coupled with racism in the housing allocation process and high rates of unemployment and low incomes amongst ethnic minorities in Tower Hamlets, seems to be one of the major factors producing limited access to good quality housing and to high rates of homelessness amongst members of these groups.

Reduced expenditure on social housing has worsened the situation in Tower Hamlets, as elsewhere: as Extract 4.4 notes, new building by the public sector has more or less dried up. No doubt the impact of the right-to-buy scheme has also worsened the situation.

■ ■ ■

7   Conclusion

This chapter has been concerned to explore the ways in which social policy can be thought into social housing. The analysis of housing and housing policy in terms of tenure was shown to be too static, as the provision and consumption of housing, and the effects of changes in government policy and legislation, is a dynamic process.

This chapter has been concerned with the period after 1980 and the effects on housing policy of the significant shift in ideology which came with the Conservative governments of the 1980s and early 1990s. The introduction of the market model, and the concomitant favouring of owner-occupation as the preferred tenure, took place within a broader restructuring of the welfare state. One consequence of this was shown to be the increased polarization of housing tenures, with the residualization of social housing as the poor became marginalized and concentrated in this tenure. The withdrawal from social housing by the state was achieved through the promotion of housing associations as the main provider, signifying a new housing management discourse of consumerism and commercial financial imperatives. However, housing associations are now facing the same problems as local authorities as they too cope with housing the priority homeless and those unable to compete in the market.

It was shown that the process of marginalization and the incidence of homelessness are not uniformly distributed. Gender, 'race', ethnicity and class are all decisive influences on who is marginalized, on who is made homeless and how they are constructed as the 'new welfare subjects'. Above all, the social processes referred to in the chapter should not be taken as given, but questioned for what they are – social constructions.

Further reading

The People's Home by Michael Harloe (1995) provides a very useful account of the relationship between public sector housing and the welfare state in the UK and in other Western European countries; see also Mark Kleinman's *Housing Welfare and the State in Europe* (1996b). An interesting and alternative account of the growth of owner-occupation in Britain in the 1980s is provided by Peter Saunders (1990) in his book *A Nation of Homeowners*. For one of the best accounts of the issues surrounding the demise of the public sector housing see *The Eclipse of Council Housing* by Cole and Furby (1994). The collection of papers entitled *Directions in Housing Policy,* edited by Williams (1997), provides an extremely useful mix of views on a range of private and public sector housing issues. To find out more about the history and aims of housing associations see *Housing Associations: Policy and Practice* by Cope (1990). Issues relating to housing policy are very well covered in *Implementing Housing Policy*, edited by Malpass and Means (1993).

References

Adam Smith Institute (1983) 'Local government policy', *Omega Report*, London, ASI.

Audit Commission (1986) *Managing the Crisis in Council Housing*, London, HMSO.

Balchin, P. (1995) *Housing Policy* (3rd edn), London, Routledge.

Birchall, J. (ed.) (1992) *Housing Policy in the 1990s*, London, Routledge.

Bulgin, S. (1994) 'The sinister arrangement for black homeless people', *Black Housing*, March/April, pp.10–11.

Burrows, L. and Walentowicz, P. (1992) *Homes Cost Less Than Homelessness*, London, Shelter.

Central Statistical Office (1996) *Social Trends 26*, Government Statistical Service, London, HMSO.

Chandran, K. (1994) 'Homelessness amongst Black people: down and out in Major's Britain', *Black Housing*, March/April, pp.13–14.

Clapham, D., Kemp, P. and Smith, S. (1990) *Housing and Social Policy*, London, Macmillan.

Clarke, J. (1996) 'Capturing the customer', *Self, Agency and Society*, vol.1, no.1, pp.55–73.

Clarke, J. and Cochrane, A. (1998) 'The social construction of social problems' in Saraga, E. (ed.) *Embodying the Social: Constructions of Difference*, London, Routledge in association with The Open University.

Cole, I. and Furby, R. (1994) *The Eclipse of Council Housing*, London, Routledge.

Commission for Racial Equality (1988) *Racial Discrimination in a London Estate Agency*, London, CRE.

Commission for Racial Equality (1990) *Putting Your House in Order*, London, CRE.

Cope, H. (1990) *Housing Associations: Policy and Practice*, London, Macmillan.

Department of Employment (1992) *New Earnings Survey, Part A*, London, HMSO.

Department of the Environment (1987) *Housing: The Government's Proposals*, London, HMSO.

Forrest, R. and Murie, A. (1985) *A Unreasonable Act? Central–local Government Conflict and the Housing Act 1980*, SAUS Study 1, SAUS, Bristol.

Forrest, R. and Murie, A. (1986) 'Marginalization and subsidized individualism', *International Journal of Urban and Regional Research*, vol.10, no.1, pp.46–65.

Forrest, R. and Murie, A. (1987) 'The affluent homeowner', *Sociological Review*, vol.35, no.2, pp.370–403.

Forrest, R. and Murie, A. (1991) *Selling the Welfare State: The Privatisation of Welfare Housing*, London, Routledge.

Forrest, R. and Murie, A. (1994) *Housing Policy and Practice* (4th edn), London, Macmillan.

Gibb, K. (1996) 'Secure foundations? – Scottish house-building in the nineties', *Scottish Housing Monitor*, pp.5–6.

Glasgow City Housing (1989) 'Housing: the Council's proposals for Glasgow', Glasgow, City of Glasgow District Council.

Greve, J. with Currie, E. (1990) *Homelessness in Britain*, York, Joseph Rowntree Foundation.

Halifax Building Society (1992) *House Price Index, 3rd quarter*, No.49, Halifax, Halifax Building Society.

Harloe, M. (1995) *The People's Home*, Oxford, Blackwell.

Henderson, J. and Karn, K. (1984) 'Race, class and the allocation of public housing in Britain', *Urban Studies*, vol.21, pp.115–28.

Hills, J. (1987) 'What happened to spending on the welfare state?' in Walker, A. and Walker, C. (eds) *The Growing Divide: A Social Audit 1979–1987*, London, Child Poverty Action Group, Ch.10.

Housing Review (1995) 'Housing and social exclusion', vol.44, no.6, pp.124–5.

Hughes, G. and Mooney, G. (1998) 'Community' in Hughes, G. (ed.) *Imagining Welfare Futures*, London, Routledge in association with The Open University.

Inquiry into Housing in Glasgow (1986) *Inquiry into Housing in Glasgow*, Professor Sir Robert Grieve (Chair), Glasgow, Glasgow Dstrict Council (Housing).

Jordan, B. (1995) 'Are new right policies sustainable? "Back to basics" and public choice', *Journal of Social Policy*, vol.24, no.3, pp.363–84.

Joseph Rowntree Foundation (1985) *Inquiry into British Housing: Report*, London, National Federation of Housing Associations.

Joseph Rowntree Foundation (1991) *Inquiry into British Housing, Second Report*, York, Joseph Rowntree Foundation.

Kemp, P. (1993) 'Rebuilding the private rented sector?' in Malpass, P. and Means, R. (eds).

Kemp, P. (ed.) (1988) *The Private Provision of Rented Housing*, Aldershot, Avebury.

Kleinman, M. (1996a) 'The Treasury and Mrs T', *Housing Studies*, vol.6, no.1, pp.27–43.

Kleinman, M. (1996b) *Housing Welfare and the State in Europe*, Cheltenham, Edward Elgar.

Langan, M. (1998) 'The contested concept of need' in Langan (ed.).

Langan, M. (ed.) (1998) *Welfare: Needs, Rights and Risks*, London, Routledge in association with The Open University.

Langstaff, M. (1992) 'Housing associations: a move to centre stage' in Birchall (ed.) Ch.2.

London Research Centre (1992) *Survey on the Standards in Bed and Breakfast Hotels used by Local Authorities in London (Bed and Breakfast Information Exchange 1989)*, London, London Research Centre.

Maclennan, D. (1994) *A Competitive UK Economy*, York, Joseph Rowntree Foundation.

Maclennan, D. (1997) 'The UK housing market: up, down and where next' in Williams, P. (ed.) Ch.3.

Malpass, P. (1992) 'Housing policies and the disabling of local authorities' in Birchall (ed.).

Malpass, P. and Means, R. (eds) (1993) *Implementing Housing Policy*, Buckingham, Open University Press.

Malpass, P. and Murie, A. (1982) *Housing Policy and Practice*, London, Macmillan.

Malpass, P. and Murie, A. (1994) *Housing Policy and Practice*, (4th edn) Basingstoke, Macmillan.

Merrett, S. (1979) *State Housing in Britain*, London, Routledge and Kegan Paul.

Mooney, G. (1998) '"Remoralizing the poor?": gender, class and philanthropy in Victorian Britain' in Lewis, G. (ed.) *Forming Nation, Framing Welfare*, London, Routledge in association with The Open University.

Minford, P., Ashton, P. and Peel, M. (1987) *The Housing Morass*, London, IEA Hobart.

Murie, A. (1982) 'A new era for council housing?' in English, J. (ed.) *Social Services in Scotland*, Edinburgh, Scottish Academic Press, Ch.2.

Office for National Statistics (1996) *Regional Trends*, Government Statistical Service, London, HMSO.

Page, D. (1993) *Building for Communities*, York, Joseph Rowntree Foundation.

Parker, J. and Dugmore, K. (1977/78) 'Race and allocation of public housing – a GLC survey', *New Community*, vol.VI, nos 1&2, pp.27–41.

Peach, C. and Byron, M. (1993) 'Caribbean tenants in council housing: "race", class and gender', *New Community*, vol.19, no.3, pp.407–23.

Peach, C. and Byron, M. (1994) 'Council house sales, residualisation and Afro-Caribbean tenants', *Journal of Social Policy*, vol.23, no.3, pp.363–83.

Phillips, D. (1987) 'The institutionalization of racism in housing' in Smith, S. and Mercer, J. (eds) *New Perspectives on Race and Housing in Britain*, Glasgow, Glasgow University Press.

Power, A. (1987) *Property Before People*, London, Allen Unwin.

Pryke, M. and Whitehead, C.M.E. (1993) 'The provision of private finance for social housing', *Housing Studies*, vol.8, no.4, pp.274–91.

Pryke, M. and Whitehead, C.M.E. (1995) 'Private sector criteria and the radical change in provision of social housing in England', *Environment and Planning 'C': Government and Policy*, vol.13, pp.217–52.

Royal Institute of Chartered Surveyors (1997) *The Real Cost of Poor Homes*, Coventry, RICS Business Services Ltd.

Sarre, P., Phillips, D. and Skellington, R. (1989) *Ethnic Minority Housing: Explanations and Policies*, Aldershot, Avebury.

Saunders, P. (1990) *A Nation of Homeowners*, London, Unwin Hyman.

Somerville, P. (1994) 'Homelessness policy in Britain', *Policy and Politics*, vol.22, no.3, pp.163–78.

Sullivan, M. (1992) *The Politics of Social Policy*, London, Harvester Wheatsheaf.

Taylor-Gooby, P. (1985) *Public Opinion, Ideology and State Welfare*, London, Routledge and Kegan Paul.

Watson, S. (1986) 'Housing and the family – the marginalization of non-family households in Britain', *International Journal of Urban and Regional Research*, vol.10, no.1, pp.8–28.

Watson, S. (1987) 'Ideas of the family in the development of housing forms' in Loney, M. *et al.* (eds) *The State or the Market*, London, Sage, Ch.9.

Watson, S. and Austerberry, H. (1986) *Housing and Homelessness: A Feminist Perspective*, London, Routledge and Kegan Paul.

Whitehead, C.M.E. (1984) 'Privatisation and housing' in Le Grand, J. and Robinson, R. (eds) *Privatisation and the Welfare State*, London, Allen and Unwin, pp.116–32.

Whitehead, C.M.E. (1989) 'Rented housing: radical restructuring', *Public Money*, Spring, pp.51–4.

Wilcox, S. (1995) *Housing Finance Review 1995/96*, York, Joseph Rowntree Foundation.

Williams, P. (1997) 'Getting the foundations right' in Williams, P. (ed.) Ch.8.

Williams, P. (ed.) (1997) *Directions in Housing Policy*, London, Paul Chapman Publishing.

Withers, P. and Randolph, B. (1994) *Access, Homelessness and Housing Associations*, Report No.21, London, National Federation of Housing Associations.

CHAPTER 5

Social Work or Social Control? Remaking Probation Work

by Eugene McLaughlin

Contents

1   Introduction

This chapter focuses on the impact that the various attempts to construct criminal justice settlements in the UK in the period since the Second World War has had on probation work. We have chosen probation as a case study because, since its inception, it has been uncomfortably situated in the ill-defined 'social care–social control' borderland between the social welfare and criminal justice systems, and there has been an on-going debate about whether it should be undertaken by a *social work* agency or a *criminal justice* agency.

We will briefly revisit key moments in the post-war development of probation because this contextualization allows us to recognize both the 'natural' ebbs and flows and the real sea-changes that have washed over and shaped probation. However, the central focus of the discussion will be the ambitious attempt, between 1984 and 1992, of the Home Office to assemble a durable criminal justice settlement that could manage:

- the need for Home Secretaries to be seen to be taking a hard line on law and order;
- Treasury requirements that the department make certifiable cost-effective and efficient use of resources;
- the intensifying penal crisis that was paralysing the system and generating international condemnation;
- the policy vacuum that had resulted from the collapse of what was known as the rehabilitative ideal (the supposed basis of the previous criminal justice settlement in the post-war UK);
- the fortress attitudes of the criminal justice agencies which made coherent long-term policy formulation and implementation virtually impossible and encouraged crisis-management or fire-brigade responses.

Although the proposed settlement had implications for *all* the criminal justice agencies, it was the probation service that came under unprecedented pressure to reconstitute its professional ethos, management structures and working practices and to reconstruct the subject of probation work. This relatively small segment of the criminal justice system was given the central role of resolving the prison crisis by providing the courts with credible 'community sentences' which would persuade sentencers to entrust to the probation service large numbers of relatively *serious* offenders who would normally be imprisoned.

When considering the story of criminal justice and probation reform in the 1980s and 1990s it is worth keeping the following points in mind. First, all the criminal justice agencies enjoyed an unprecedented period of growth in overall resourcing. Second, the *organizational* reform process was relatively modest in scope and marked by a considerable degree of consultation, negotiation and compromise, as well as a discursive framing that respected the sensitive constitutional position of the respective criminal justice agencies. In essence, those in charge of the reform process acknowledged that criminal justice was 'different' to the other areas of government activity discussed in this book. Third, any successful criminal justice settlement depends to a large extent on the political will and institutional capacity to organize a broad consensus (see Figure 5.1). And, fourth, when I use the term 'settlement' I do not imply complete harmony, total consensus or a 'common tongue'. The settlement refers to the parameters within which debate and argument take place. So within an organizational setting, for example, there can still be discernible differences of opinion, disputed understandings and conflicting perspectives. In the case of the criminal justice 'system' it is possible for judges, police officers, prison officers and probation officers to hold contrasting, contradictory and often antagonistic constructions of meaning about the role of the system, their function within it, whom they are dealing with and what the others should be doing. Some of these professional and quasi-professional groupings are more powerful and have a higher status and greater agenda-setting capacities than others. Fifth, proposed settlements can, as we shall see in this chapter, be stillborn, short-lived or radically reworked to accommodate new political realities. Finally, proposed settlements play out differently in different jurisdictions.

However, if we are to think through and understand past and present debates, we need first of all to familiarize ourselves with broader aspects of criminal justice discourse in the UK.

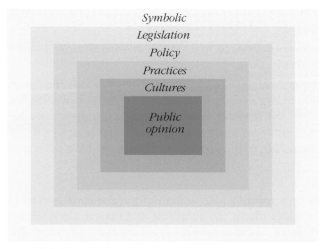

Figure 5.1 The constitutive sources of a criminal justice settlement that must be aligned

2   The official construction of criminal justice difference

We need a base-line knowledge of what the criminal justice system (CJS) is, how it developed, how it works (both in theory and in practice) and what it does. We also need to know how those involved in it make sense of it. This takes us into the realm of organizational discourse. Irrespective of who we are, where we have come from and what we do, I would argue that we need interpretative storylines to make 'common sense' of it all. Elsewhere I have defined storylines as discursive narratives which 'constitute a complex "circuit of meaning" that cannot be treated as either simply true or false, fully imagined or realised, nor as internally consistent. Rather they stand above and outside of rational explanation and critique. What makes particular "storylines" potent is how much the audience and "storytellers" want and/or need to believe them'

interpretative storyline

(McLaughlin and Murji, 1998, p.3). Criminal justice professionals such as police officers, judges, legal representatives, prison officers and probation officers have actively constructed – and have had constructed for them – a very powerful set of storylines that tells them that they are 'different'. At one and the same time these storylines also remind the British public that 'our' criminal justice system is 'different' to every other system.

ACTIVITY 5.1

Think about what is commonly said about the law, the judiciary, the criminal justice system and the police. It is worth noting that these storylines will differ to a degree depending on whether you live in England and Wales, Scotland or Northern Ireland.

COMMENT

Below are some of the key 'ideal typical' storylines that are present in many news reports and official commentaries.

The rule of law

■ The rule of law is *universal* in its remit, offering security and protection from the cradle to the grave.

■ English law is a unique combination of Common Law, Equity and Legislation. This is what distinguishes it from European Roman Law and US Constitutional Law. It is not the result of theorizing, but has evolved from hard experience and trial and error over centuries. It is not the property of any government or even the state, but of the community. This is the basis of its authority.

The judiciary

■ The judiciary is formally independent of governments, and this 'separation of powers' ensures that it can scrutinize and review the actions of parliament. The doctrines of tenure and immunity ensure that each member of the judiciary enjoys freedom in thought and independence in judgement.

■ The judiciary are the guardians of the law and balance justice not only between individual citizens but also between citizens and the state.

■ Judges are and should only be accountable to other judges in a higher appellate court.

The criminal justice system

■ The British criminal justice system is the finest in the world. It is not perfect but it is the nearest that any country has come to producing fair, equal and non-political justice. It has also been remarkably successful in reconciling individual liberties with a high degree of public order.

■ The Home Secretary is responsible for the administration of justice, criminal law, offenders (probation and prisons) and police. He or she does not have the policy powers of a European 'Minister of Justice' because the criminal justice system is not really a coherent, integrated, unified organizational/administrative system, but an amalgam of various agencies with their own distinctive organizational structures, legal powers and statutory responsibilities.

The police

British police forces are unique because:

- Officers are essentially citizens in uniform.

- Every member holds the office of constable and her or his legal authority and powers stem from this.

- Constables are not servants or employees of the state or the police bureaucracy. No-one can tell them to exercise their powers in a particular way. The responsibility for law enforcement lies with them and they are answerable to the law.

- Chief constables are operationally independent of the Executive.

- The police carry out their duties on behalf of the public and enjoy a high measure of public confidence.

■ ■ ■

The discourse of criminal justice 'difference', and the cluster of storylines detailed previously, in many respects constitute *the* overarching ideological settlement on criminal justice. They have a deeply entrenched *symbolic* presence both in public debates about criminal justice and law and order (particularly in debates about possible or proposed reforms) and in media representations. This particular cluster of storylines in turn helps to explain the uneasiness felt by many social policy commentators in discussing the criminal justice system alongside more recognizably public-sector issues such as education and health.

Using the storylines, we can think about what the response might be to those proposing radical reform of the criminal justice system:

- The reforms will infringe upon the *independence* and *autonomy* of the system.

- The reforms will *politicize* the system or are fraught with political consequence – the unintended consequences of radical reform could be a *loss of confidence* in the criminal justice system and a *loss of respect* for the authority of the state.

- Reformers must accept that forms of accountability in the CJS are much more *open textured* and *complicated* than in other spheres of governmental activity.

- Change must be based on a *bipartisan* approach and, ideally, on the deliberations of independent Royal Commissions.

- Changes must be introduced in an *incremental* and *pragmatic* fashion and *not go 'against the grain'* of the organizing principles of the CJS or expose the hidden tensions within it.

This means that all governments have to tread very warily because the criminal justice system deals with fundamental *symbolic* issues of principle – rights, duties, order, equity, justice, punishment – that lie at the heart of a social order that is governed by the rule of law. We may ask ourselves whether any government could successfully overcome the accusation that its proposed reforms would result in: a diminishing of rights; inequities; injustice; or the politicization of law and order or the agencies of the criminal justice system.

3   Probation: the 'jewel in the crown' of the social democratic criminal justice settlement

In the immediate post-war period, commentators applauded and idealized the probation service for providing the first constructive alternative to custodial sentences and ensuring that reformation of offenders had been established as a legitimate goal of criminal justice. Probation officers were told that they should be proud of and never forget their humanitarian origins in the nineteenth century as police court missionaries recruited from charitable organizations whose humane vocation was to persuade magistrates to 'advise, assist and befriend' offenders placed under their supervision:

advise, assist, befriend

> These founder fathers were missionaries in the true sense of the word and they used the methods of missionaries – changing behaviour by changing feeling – through 'conversion'. Their methods were persuasion, exhortation and support. They strengthened weak resolution by administering solemn pledges to renounce drink; they gently admonished the sinner while at the same time they offered him the helping hand of friendship; they advised him for his own good; they assisted him in many ways to improve his social and economic condition; and finally they prayed for guidance for him and for themselves. These men believed in the supreme importance of the individual to God and the parables of the lost sheep and the prodigal son were their casework manuals.
>
> (Newton, 1956, p.123)

As Jordan (1971) has noted, the 1907 Probation of Offenders Act and the Criminal Justice Acts of 1925 and 1948 defined probation as a 'species of liberty rather than a species of imprisonment. The two were as sharply differentiated as they could be, while both being orders of the court.' And Radzinowicz, a leading social democratic criminologist, argued that: 'It contradicts the traditional watchwords of expiation, retribution and deterrence, and though its rules are laced with penal provisions and sanctions, *probation is fundamentally a form of social service preventing further crime*' (Radzinowicz, 1958, p.xii, emphasis added). Penal reform groups and their own representative organizations looked forward to probation officers making the transition from an evangelistic vocation to the leading psychoanalytic social casework profession in the UK:

> … [Seeking] to understand the person in need, not only at that particular moment in time, but in all the major experiences and relationships which have gone into making him the person he is, with conflicts of whose origin he may be unaware, with problems whose solution may lie less in external circumstances than in his own attitudes, with tensions, faulty relationships, inabilities to face reality, hardened into forms which he cannot alter unaided.
>
> (Morris, 1950, p.193)

And its officers, who were organized in 103 local services, under the direction of magistrates' committees, enjoyed a remarkable degree of organizational independence and professional autonomy:

professional autonomy

> Whereas the social work profession generally was characterised by close supervision and control of worker's activities, probation officers were surprisingly free to exercise their own discretion in their work. Once a probation order was made, the probation officer supervised the client as he chose, and his freedom was strengthened by the

fact that he was personally responsible to the court for the conduct of each case. Unlike the local authority social worker, who was supervised by a hierarchy of professional colleagues through whom he was responsible to his employing authority, the probation officer was answerable as an individual to his court. Indeed, he often worked as an individual, as the service was a loose administrative structure with few formal links between the officers serving in different petty sessional divisions. The main limitation on professional autonomy was the fact that officers had to accept the court's decisions over the selection of their cases, but even here their opinions were being increasingly sought and accepted, even by higher courts.

(Jordon, 1971, p.125)

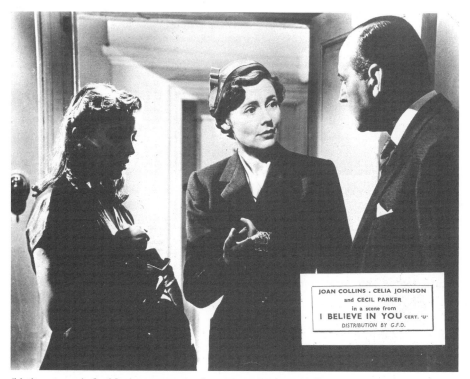

'I believe in you': Cecil Parker represents the post-war probation officer

The final official seal of approval was seemingly produced by the deliberations of the Morison Committee of inquiry into probation work in England, Scotland and Wales. The Committee's report (Home Office, 1962) advocated no significant changes to the functions or administrative structure and affirmed that the probation officer was 'a professional case worker, employing in a specialized field, skill which he holds in common with other social workers. He is also, however, the agent of a system concerned with the protection of society' (para. 54). The focus of probation work should continue to be on the offender's psychological needs and social responsibilities. In terms of the organization of probation work, the Committee acknowledged that the existing structure was 'theoretically insupportable' (para. 171), although it supported the continued existence of a separate generic service, arguing that nationalization or localization (in the form of amalgamation with local government social welfare departments) would interrupt the direct working relationship between probation officers and the courts and threaten the well-developed sense of common purpose. However, it expressed concern that, in Scotland, probation was 'not a court service but a relatively minor local authority service.' It urged probation committees to take a more active role in officers' work and the Home Office to formalize its powers and responsibilities. On the other hand, it also supported the professional autonomy of officers by accepting that probation committees, the Home Office and principal officers could *not* directly interfere with the confidentiality of the officer–client relationship or the conduct of a particular case.

ACTIVITY 5.2

Before leaving this section re-read the quotations and make a list of the key storylines of the probation service and probation work. For example:

1 Where did the probation service originate?
2 Who were probation officers?
3 What was probation work?
4 How was it organized?

COMMENT

Probation's vocational purpose was to 'advise, assist and befriend' offenders, speak for them in court and persuade the judiciary not to impose custodial sentences. Hence, at its core, probation stood in opposition to prison and, indeed, punishment. The unique challenge for the probation officer, as a court social worker, was to balance conflicting *care* (social work) and *control* (criminal justice) responsibilities and identify and resolve, through deep casework, the psychological needs and problems of the subject of probation work – *suitable* clients. Officers enjoyed a significant degree of autonomy and used their discretion to determine the nature, timing, extent and duration of the treatment.

■ ■ ■

The deliberations and recommendations of other governmental committees in the 1960s triggered a period of uncertainty and flux for probation work. However, it was the government's attempt to construct a rehabilitative settlement, represented by the proposals for dealing with young offenders, that triggered an identity crisis in the probation service.

rehabilitative settlement

The government's White Papers *The Child, the Family and the Young Offender* (Home Office, 1965), covering England and Wales, and *Social Work and the Community* (Home Office, 1966), covering Scotland, both pointed to social workers taking over responsibility for young people in need of care, protection *and* control, with probation being absorbed into local authority social services departments. Jordan (1971, p.126) argued that these far-reaching recommendations, which signalled a full-blown social welfare approach to juvenile crime, transformed the probation service 'overnight into a conservative force in the field of delinquency.' The probation service guarded its independent status by taking refuge in a criminal justice discourse arguing that probation work was 'different' to social work because it was a court-based service for offenders.

The next White Paper, *Children in Trouble* (Home Office, 1968), which produced the 1969 Children and Young Persons Act, was a watered-down version which did not pose such a direct threat to the criminal justice model (for a fuller discussion see **Muncie, 1998**). However, the Social Work (Scotland) Act accepted that the functions of the probation service should be undertaken by new generic social work departments and, despite protests by probation officers north and south of the border, this became operative in November 1969. Morris (1974) suggests that Scotland reached a more radical, and what turned out to be a very stable, welfare-oriented settlement than the rest of the UK due to:

- very different judicial traditions and legal system;
- the level of criticism of existing arrangements which ruled out a piecemeal approach;
- the common belief that the Kilbrandon Report (Scottish Home and Health Department, Scottish Education Department, 1964) was an important path-breaking document that did Scotland proud;
- policy-makers in the Scottish Office having the support of the judiciary (in contrast to England and Wales).

Developments in Scotland led the National Association of Probation Officers (NAPO) in England and Wales to resist moves to establish one professional body for social workers and it did not join the British Association of Social Workers. The probation service also successfully campaigned to ensure that probation was not included in the remit of the Seebohm Committee (Department of Health and Social Security, 1968) on personal social services and sighed with relief when the House of Commons Expenditure Committee supported the idea of an independent service in 1971 (see Haxton, 1978; for a discussion of the Seebohm Committee, see Chapter 7 of this volume).

NAPO also resisted the first Home Office attempts to *formalize* the bureaucratic-administrative structure of the probation service and to *enhance* the supervisory role and responsibilities of principal probation officers. It insisted that there was a great degree of uncertainty about the function and role of principal and senior officers in that they could offer support and advice, but they could *not* monitor, inspect or evaluate the work of main grade officers since this would disrupt the professional relationship that existed between probation officers and their clients and the courts (see National Association of Probation Officers, 1966; 1970).

4 Broken dreams and shattered hopes: nothing works

Law and order re-emerged as a potent campaigning issue in the 1970 General Election, when a heated debate broke out between the main political parties and in the media about who and what was responsible for the alarming rise in crime, dwindling detection rates and intractable recidivism, and what should be done about it. With hindsight, we can see that 1970 was a symbolic defining moment because, for the rest of the decade, the UK, as Hall *et al.* (1978) noted, 'edged, bit by bit, towards a "law and order" mood, now advancing, now retreating, moving in a crab-like way.'

As the prison population soared, prisoners demonstrated, and eventually rioted, about serious overcrowding and inadequate facilities. Prison officers, in response, demanded that the government restore 'good order and discipline', eventually taking industrial action for better pay and working conditions. In October 1978 the prison governors sent an open letter to the Home Secretary stating that a 'total breakdown' of the system was imminent (see Fitzgerald and Sim, 1982). Police officers became increasingly vocal in their criticism of the functioning of the criminal justice system and eventually, in an unprecedented move, launched a law and order campaign for increased powers and resources and more pay. Senior members of the judiciary warned that respect for the rule of law was on the verge of collapse and presented the case for stiffer sentences and tougher punishments. The sense of crisis was heightened as it became clear that the Conservative Party intended to centre hard-line law and order policies in future election campaigns.

law and order crisis

The probation service was caught up in the unfolding law and order crisis in a complex manner. First, more officers were appointed, probation areas in England and Wales and funding arrangements were reorganized and training and recruitment procedures were overhauled. Second, the service was allocated new tasks and functions, becoming increasingly involved in statutory after-care of offenders and other forms of compulsory supervision, especially in the aftermath of the 'alternatives to custody' measures produced by the 1972 Criminal Justice Act (see Figure 5.2). A younger generation of probation officers began to protest that they were being drawn ever deeper into the penal system and having to work with more difficult clients in more difficult working environments. They were also concerned that the government was looking to the probation service to solve the prison crisis. Third, the rehabilitation and treatment ethos of the services came under sustained critique from radical left critics (see Cohen, 1979). Probation officers' much vaunted professional discretion and independence was blamed for producing outcomes that were not necessarily in the best interests of these clients but were repressive, controlling and stigmatizing. In addition, the findings of official research in the UK and USA concluded that rehabilitative programmes were having little *meaningful* impact on recidivism rates (Martinson, 1974; Folkard *et al.*, 1976). The following

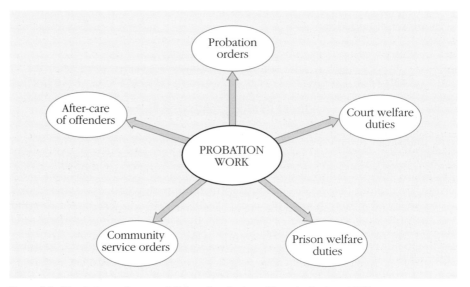

Figure 5.2 The duties and responsibilities of probation officers in the late 1970s

comment sums up the sense of disorientation that many officers experienced: 'How could this incredible situation have come about? The bulk of practitioners in an entire profession appear at worst to be practising in ways that are not helpful or even detrimental to their clients and at best operating without a shred of empirical evidence validating their efforts' (Fisher, 1976, p.63).

The sense of crisis was heightened by repeated attacks from the Right who criticized probation officers for what they saw as their 'touchy-feely' social work platitudes and for refusing to acknowledge that many of their charges posed a serious threat to public safety. A resurgent New Right common-sense 'criminological' discourse reconstructed the criminal subject as a rational, evil, predatory creature who was the product of post-war welfarist policies that had *undermined* the notion of individual culpability and responsibility, *blurred* the distinction between right and wrong, and *incapacitated* the police and judiciary. A consensus took hold within and outside of the service that the status quo was not an option. However, as the following comment from a probation officer makes clear, there was no agreement as to what its future role should be:

> Confused legislation has consistently placed the service in a seemingly impossible position in which it cannot remain true to its compassionate ideals nor retain the empathy or commitment of its political masters for our masters sway with the popular tide of public opinion which largely sanctions the retributive and punitive aspects of punishment whilst ignoring its reformative rehabilitative aspects.
>
> I see the service increasingly offering a beguiling number of roles none of which can be pursued in isolation and most of which offer the transient illusion that we, the officers, can be all things to all people. In future we could exchange our current garb for any number of uniforms, whether it be prison officer, policeman or pin-stripes. We seem to have a foot in many camps and yet constantly need to challenge the assumptions within each.
>
> (Varah, 1976, p.15)

5   From fighting crime to managing crime

If we look at Figures 5.3 and 5.4 overleaf we can see, from rising expenditure and increased staffing, that the Conservative's election pledge of 1979 to provide the necessary resources to crack down on crime was honoured in full. Systemic empowerment was also forthcoming: in the form of a package of measures which tipped the balance towards expiation, retribution and deterrence (Reiner and Cross, 1991). A hard-line law and order discourse equipped the police with contentious new powers; in addition, judicial powers, in determining type and length of custodial sentence (particularly for juveniles), were strengthened and extended. The courts were also encouraged to hand out longer sentences. In tandem, the largest prison building programme of the twentieth century was initiated.

However, as Figures 5.5 and 5.6 indicate, despite the emphasis on deterrence, the crime rate escalated to an unprecedented level and the police clear-up rate remained alarmingly low. British society became painfully aware of the economic costs of the crime wave: legitimate businesses complained about the impact of a flourishing illegal economy in stolen goods; hospitals, general practitioners and employers protested about the costs of supporting victims of crime; local authorities had to divert scarce resources to combating vandalism on public

Figure 5.3 Expenditure on Home Office services in the criminal justice system in real terms, 1978–87 (actual to 1984–85, estimated for 1985–86, plans for 1986–87. Base year 1978–79 = 100): (a) prisons, court services and probation; (b) police (Source: Home Office, 1986, p.45, Table 3)

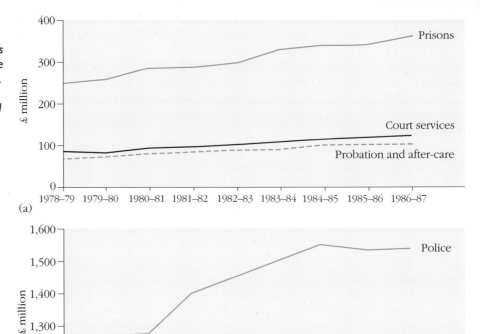

Figure 5.4 Personnel in the criminal justice system (year averages, actual up to 1984–85): (a) police officers; (b) police civilians, prison staff, and probation officers and ancillary staff (Source: Home Office, 1986, p.48, Table 6)

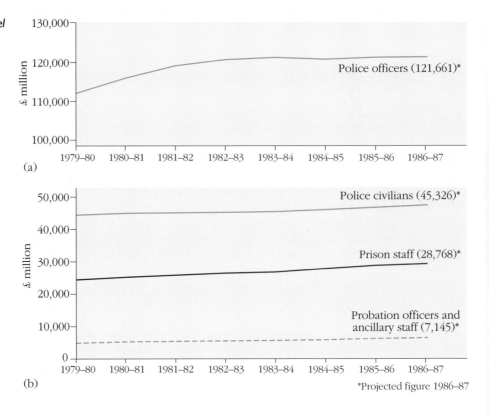

housing estates; and house and car owners were confronted with spiralling insurance premiums to cover escalating theft and burglary. Far from guaranteeing a sense of personal security and giving individuals peace of mind, successive British crime surveys revealed that the public's fear of crime – rational or not – was as great a problem as crime itself. The period also witnessed outbreaks of urban rioting and industrial conflict which, although not unprecedented, underlined the depth of racial and social division in British society.

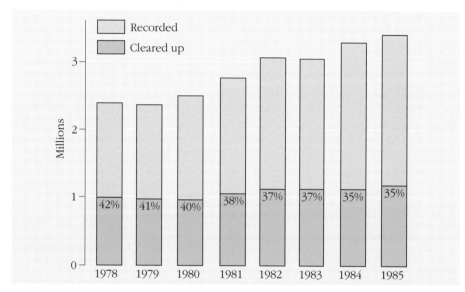

Figure 5.5 Offences recorded and cleared up, 1978–85 (Source: Home Office, 1986, p.4, Table A)

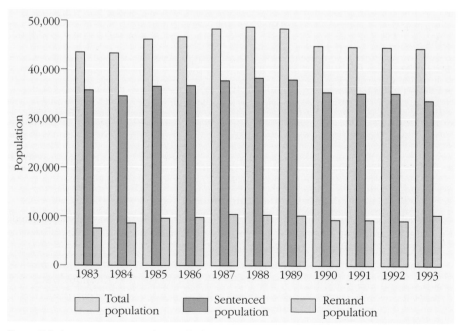

Figure 5.6 Average prison population, England and Wales (Source: Barclay, 1995, p.42, Figure 2)

The political reverberations of this ignominious political 'failure to deliver' compelled a radical rethink of law and order policies and the uncritical support traditionally given to the *deterrent* potential of the criminal justice agencies. In this moment, the discourse on law and order was challenged by one which demanded the formulation of policies which would re-establish public confidence, maximize the *effectiveness* of the various criminal justice agencies and make the most *efficient* use of *available* resources. Home Office officials and eventually ministers, under pressure from the Treasury to account for the dramatically increased law and order budget, began to make headway in persuading key members of the 'policy community' that a self-generated crisis was engulfing the criminal justice system. The sheer number of non-violent offenders entering and re-entering the criminal justice system was threatening to paralyse the functioning of the courts. The knock-on effects were overcrowding and disturbances in the prisons, and prison service demands for more resources. The experience of imprisonment was entrenching patterns of offending and increasing the likelihood of more serious offending upon release. Spiralling levels of re-offending were increasing levels of victimization, the public's fear of crime, and intolerance which resulted in demands for more police officers, tougher policing and harsher sentences, which in turn propelled even more people into the system. As the then Home Secretary, Douglas Hurd, made clear in his speech to the Conservative Party conference in 1988: 'If we doubled the police, doubled the penalties, doubled the prisons – say, until all three reached American levels – we might still find ourselves with American levels of crime and violence' (quoted in *The Times*, 18 October 1988). As far as Home Office officials were concerned, a new interlocking political and organizational settlement had to be pieced together if the vicious circle set in motion by the hard-line law and order model was to be broken.

Part of the official response was a gradual withdrawal from moralistic debates about the causes of crime. Home Office officials tutored the public that extreme caution was needed in 'reading' crime statistics because, despite media representations, most crime was petty in nature and the UK remained a relatively crime-free society. Certain statements even suggested that certain levels of crime were normal and inevitable and that it was therefore unrealistic to expect any set of policies to eradicate crime. All that governments could do, according to this new situational crime-prevention orthodoxy, was to work with and in the community in order to lessen the opportunistic crime rate and the fear of crime to manageable and acceptable levels (see Clarke and Mayhew, 1980; Heal and Laycock, 1985).

The public was told that it must recognize that the sources of crime and victimization and their prevention and reduction lay, first and foremost, in the actions of individual citizens and communities. Stress was placed on shared responsibility and individual self-discipline which were encouraged through the 'target-hardening' of homes and businesses and the presumed greater security offered by membership of Neighbourhood Watch.

Private self-help efforts were also to be supplemented and augmented by multi-agency approaches to crime prevention. The Home Office redoubled its efforts to create partnerships between local authorities, local businesses, voluntary organizations and statutory agencies which would prepare effective policies and localized strategies to design out crime and reduce the fear of crime (Locke, 1990).

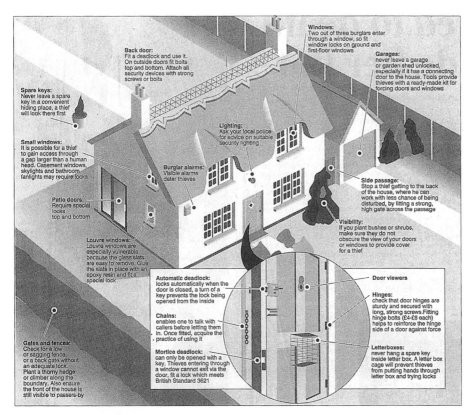

Fortress UK: target-hardened house. By the late 1980s householders were being told by the Home Office that they should take the necessary steps to target harden their homes

5.1 Managerial reform of criminal justice

A series of overlapping managerial reviews and directives signalled the government's commitment to addressing the problems of the criminal justice services. The recommendations emanating from these sector-by-sector reviews, as we shall see in the following sections, acted as a stimulus for further inquiries because they uncovered the need for ever deeper and broader change if a clearly defined, co-ordinated criminal justice *system* was to be realized. Reform was to be achieved, as in the rest of the public sector, within an overall framework of organizational restructuring, transformation of organizational culture and rationalization of tasks. The different agencies would in future have to justify their existence and restructure themselves in terms of core tasks, market competitiveness, resource control and certifiable cost-effectiveness. As a consequence, certain activities and *responsibilities* were centralized, others devolved and yet others were contracted out or privatized (see Fowles, 1990; Jones, 1993; McLaughlin and Muncie, 1994).

The attempt to inject modern managerial ideas and construct a 'mixed economy' of criminal justice provoked considerable organizational opposition as criminal justice professionals and their representative bodies found their professional expertise and judgement effectively excluded from the reform process. Their 'special pleading' and claims to 'difference' were redefined as self-interest and seen as being part of the problem. However, the government faced particular difficulty in attempting to structure the discretion, and curb the autonomy, of criminal justice workers for three reasons. First, the rank and file had traditionally enjoyed a remarkable degree of autonomy and had been empowered during the first half of the 1980s. Second, as we saw earlier, they had a set of powerful discursive storylines which stressed criminal justice difference. And, third, there was the difficulty of devising adequate processes and mechanisms to measure performance for organizations pursuing a multitude of instrumental *and* symbolic objectives.

6   Unsettling probation work

In the early 1980s, the probation service was a beneficiary of the Conservative's law and order policies, enjoying an unprecedented increase in resources (see Figure 5.7). The professional standing of probation officers was also enhanced by the establishment of a new university-based social work course. However, it was also concerned about what the government might demand of a service that the tabloids viewed as 'soft on crime' and 'the criminal's friend'. NAPO orchestrated opposition to the 1982 Criminal Justice Act which empowered the courts to impose specific restrictions and conditions on offenders as part of a probation or a supervision order. Probation officers argued that the act would transform them into 'screws on wheels', monitoring and controlling rather than helping offenders. Concerns were heightened when it became clear that the plans to re-establish the troubled Northern Ireland probation service on the Scottish model had been rejected. The head of the new centrally funded *criminal justice* service did not help matters when he spoke of offender management, the importance of corporate plans, measuring cost-effectiveness, concentrating on core responsibilities, and purchasing services (see Griffiths, 1982).

Probation officers were also aware of developments in other parts of the world. In New Zealand, it was being proposed that the probation service be renamed the 'Offender Supervisory Service' to stress its crime-control role. And in the USA pressure was mounting on probation to switch from 'client rehabilitation' to 'offender control': what became known as the 'trail 'em, nail 'em and jail 'em' approach with the primary emphasis on enhancing public safety.

6.1   Opening up the debate: SNOP, SLOP and FMIS

In this uncertain context, the publication of the Home Office's *Statement of National Objectives and Priorities* (SNOP) in April 1984 rocked the service (Home Office, 1984a). The text was a Home Office response to the 1983 Financial Management Initiative that demanded that central government departments take steps to ensure that resources were being deployed and managed in an *efficient*, *effective* and *economical* manner (Treasury, 1983).

ACTIVITY 5.3

Read Extract 5.1, which is taken from the Home Office's *Statement of National Objectives and Priorities*, and, as you do so, work through why the probation service was so alarmed by its tone and content. It would be worth referring back to the probation storylines summarized in Activity 5.2.

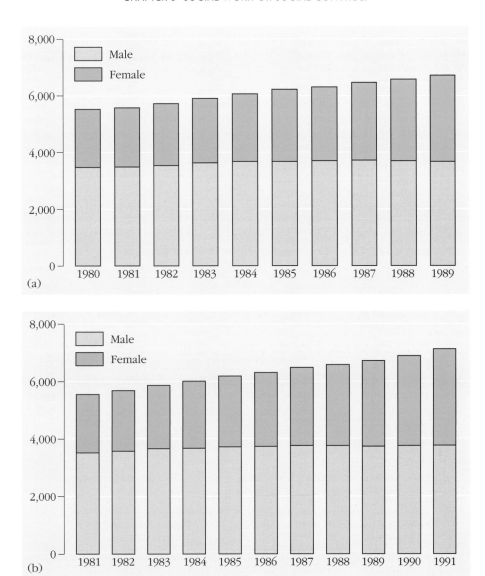

Figure 5.7 Number of probation officers: (a) all grades; (b) in post on 31 December
(Source: (a) Barclay, 1991, p.68; (b) Barclay, 1993, p.71)

Extract 5.1 Home Office: 'Statement of national objectives and priorities'

6. At a time when recorded crime and public concern about crime have been
    increasing, the Probation Service has constantly to ensure that its work is
    effective, that it is relevant to the needs of the community which it serves and
    that it has the confidence both of the courts and of the public at large. There
    must be a continual process of interaction with other agencies and other
    interests – locally between probation committees, the management and staff
    of area services, the courts, the police, the prison service, local authorities,
    local government services, educational institutions and a variety of voluntary
    organisations; and centrally between the representative organisations and
    central Government, especially the Home Office. New opportunities and
    demands are opening up in the fields of preventive work, mediation and

reparation, where the Service is already involved to some extent and where its experience, knowledge and skill should enable it to make a significant contribution.

7. New activities and new interests of this kind inevitably raise questions of resources. The provision by the Government is intended to allow the Probation Service to grow by rather more than three per cent in 1984–85 as compared with 1983–84. But the response to changing needs and circumstances cannot always be the provision of extra resources. The first task must be to check that existing resources are being deployed in a cost-effective way. It can then be seen how far any new requirements can be met by adjusting priorities or adopting new methods of working with the resources that are already available. The following paragraphs are intended to provide the context in which such an examination should take place.

Purpose, objectives and priorities of the Probation Service

I   The Probation Service, together with others involved in the criminal justice system, is concerned with preparing and giving effect to a planned and co-ordinated response to crime. It must maintain the community's confidence in its work, and contribute to the community's wider confidence that it is receiving proper protection and that the law is enforced.

II   The main purpose of the Service within the criminal justice system is to provide means for the supervision in the community of those offenders for whom the courts decide that it is necessary and appropriate.

III In pursuance of this purpose, the Service has the following principal tasks:

(i)   the provision of reports to the courts which may include reasoned advice on sentencing;

(ii) supervising offenders subject to probation, supervision and community service orders;

(iii) providing through-care for offenders sentenced to custody, and exercising supervision after release in cases where required by law.

IV   The Service has other statutory tasks arising from the civil work of the courts in relation to matrimonial disputes and the welfare of children.

V   In fulfilment of these purposes, and in the discharge of its statutory responsibilities, the Service should seek to attain the following specific objectives.

A   Working with the courts

(i)   concentrating the provision of social inquiry reports on cases where a report is statutorily required, where a probation order is likely to be considered, and where the court may be prepared to divert an offender from what would otherwise be a custodial sentence;

(ii) maintaining the confidence of the courts in the ability of non-custodial measures to cope with a wide range of offenders.

B   Supervision in the community

(iii) ensuring that each area probation service is able to accept and put into effect as many orders as the courts decide to make, especially in cases where custodial sentences would otherwise be imposed;

(iv) maintaining a range of facilities which, used in conjunction with probation and supervision orders in suitable cases, will increase their effectiveness and thereby the Service's capacity to cope with the widest possible range of offenders;

(v)   ensuring by clear planning and follow-up action that the supervision, support, advice and guidance available to offenders under probation or supervision orders, through the exercise of social work skills and use of available facilities, are applied as efficiently and effectively as possible in each case so that the risk of offending is reduced, to the benefit of the offender and of the community.

C   Through-care

(vi)   assisting prisoners while in custody, and in preparation for and following release;

(vii) ensuring that offenders under statutory supervision comply with the requirements of their licences, and assisting them so far as possible to make a successful and law-abiding adjustment to ordinary life.

D   Other work in the community

(viii) encouraging the local community in the widest practicable approach to offending and offenders, taking account of the influences of family, schools and other social factors and of the potential contributions of other agencies;

(ix)   developing the service to the wider public by contributing to initiatives concerned with the prevention of crime and the support of victims, and playing a part in the activities of local statutory and voluntary organisations;

(x)   civil work: providing services to courts in accordance with statutory requirements.

VI   In the allocation of resources towards these objectives, the following broad order of priorities should be followed:

(a)   The first priority should be to ensure that, wherever possible, offenders can be dealt with by non-custodial measures and that standards of supervision are set and maintained at the level required for this purpose.

(b)   Resources should be allocated to the preparation of social inquiry reports on the basis that standards will be similarly set and maintained, but that reports will be prepared selectively in accordance with the objective set out above.

(c)   Sufficient resources should be allocated to through-care to enable the Service's statutory obligations to be discharged (including the reduction in the minimum qualifying period for parole). Beyond that, social work for offenders released from custody, though important in itself, can only command the priority which is consistent with the main objective of implementing non-custodial measures for offenders who might otherwise receive custodial sentences.

(d)   The Service should allocate sufficient management effort and other resources if necessary to ensure that each area probation service is making an appropriate and effective contribution to wider work in the community (objective D). The scale and pace of development will depend on local needs and the opportunities available.

(e)   The proportion of resources allocated to civil work should be contained at a level consistent with local circumstances and the foregoing priorities.

(Home Office, 1984a, pp.2–5)

COMMENT

As probation officers read SNOP, alien and hostile words, phrases and directives stood out with alarming clarity:

- concentrating on criminal justice work;
- supervising offenders in the community;
- effectiveness and efficiency;
- prioritizing the needs of the community, the courts and victims;
- management responsibilities in resource allocation;
- new evidence-based working methods.

There was no mention of 'clients', 'assisting, advising and befriending' or professional autonomy and a very clear downplaying of social welfare; that is, care tasks. And as Smith (1996, p.233) has noted, 'the explosive character' of the text came 'from the fact that it existed at all: it announced that the Home Office was going to take a much closer interest in the doings of the probation service than the service had been used to.'

■ ■ ■

A Home Office working paper entitled *Criminal Justice* (Home Office, 1984b) was released the following month reiterating that existing resources must be used in a cost-effective way, and not dissipated into activities which were peripheral to the main functions of the service. And in July 1984, David Faulkner, then Under Secretary of State at the Home Office, informed a NAPO conference on the future of the service that SNOP signified that the 'old ways' of doing things – including ignoring Home Office circulars – were no longer an option:

> it is meant to be taken seriously, and we do expect the managers of the probation service to start applying the statement to their own areas' services, testing its practical implications, measuring and evaluating what is happening, and making those adjustments in the organization or deployment of the service which they believe to be needed. It is not a theoretical exercise which the probation service can set aside while more discussion takes place.

(Faulkner, 1984, p.3)

Conference delegates attacked SNOP as a 'soulless' and inappropriate document that stressed management over working relationships between colleagues, policy over professional practice, control over care, central over local; denied the needs of the offender; and failed to recognize the distinctive values of the service.

The 56 probation areas were obliged to produce their own local statements (SLOPs) and participate in developing a Financial Management Information System (FMIS) which would facilitate objective setting, performance measurement, delegated resource management responsibilities and critical scrutiny (Mair, 1989). The response suggested that, despite Faulkner's warning, probation officers were circumventing, undermining and/or ignoring these central initiatives. Those areas that bothered to respond produced SLOPs that bore little resemblance to each other. Some fundamentally disagreed with SNOP, especially its proposed prioritization, whereas others were not sure what it meant. Some SLOPs were drafted by chief probation officers, some by probation teams, others by probation committees, and many of the responses asserted the non-negotiability of the service's social work ethos (Lloyd, 1986; Parry-Khan, 1988).

The resistance to FMIS was just as notable. The private management consultants who were appointed to carry the work forward seem to have been bewildered by the wide variations in staff activities, primitive information-gathering 'systems', lack of agreement over what might constitute 'good practice', a refusal to prioritize activities or cost the various activities, and non-existent or underdeveloped managerial processes and controls (see Humphrey, 1991). Two things were obvious from reading the responses to SNOP and FMIS. First, England and Wales did not have a probation *service* but a diversity of eclectic practices and activities with little sense of organizational direction. Second, the points of unity were (i) a distancing from criminal justice discourses and a commitment to a social work ethos, and (ii) a determination to resist all attempts to encroach upon professional discretion.

However, some probation areas were developing practices that were in line with or, indeed, in advance of Home Office thinking. Examples included:

- day centres with intensive group work rather than traditional one-to-one social casework with a focus on changing offending behaviour of relatively serious offenders;

- developing 'risk-of-custody' scales to estimate the outcome of sentencing decisions. This again represented a move away from depending on an officer's professional judgement, intuition and 'practice wisdom' to a more formalized, focused system which would enhance the monitoring and evaluation of practices;

- responsibility for bail/remand decisions which drew probation officers deeper into the penal realm and produced more systemic working practices;

- involvement with crime prevention schemes and 'moving out' into the wider community;

- thinking about the interest of victims – for example, mediation, reparation and conciliation initiatives which brought offenders closer to the consequences of their actions.

Parts of the service in England and Wales began to confront the critically important questions of 'race' and gender in relation to criminal justice and probation practice. Probation officers in certain urban localities were drawn, in the early 1980s, into the debate about whether the dramatic increase in the number of black people in custody was a result of their criminal activities or of racist criminal justice agencies. A Commission of Racial Equality report (Taylor, 1981) and a Central Council of Probation Committees (CCPC) report (1983) concluded that there was evidence to suggest that the traditional social casework approach was not relevant to the needs of black clients and that the inappropriate, highly racialized content of social enquiry reports was partly responsible for the number of young black men receiving custodial sentences. Both reports signalled the need for probation areas to think seriously about why there were so few black officers and how black offenders were 'constructed' in and produced by probation work. Areas were also advised to develop practices tailored to the needs and concerns of black clients and to prioritize *community-based* programmes which would divert black people from the criminal justice system. Of great significance was the fact that the service also agreed to the setting up of a working party on the establishment of a *national* system of ethnic monitoring of clients and employment practices (see Holdaway and Allaker, 1990).

In the same moment, feminist criminological research suggested that the patriarchal and paternalistic discourses present in social enquiry reports and court discussions were constructing female offenders as suitable for supervision by the probation service. However, probation programmes were not capable of addressing the roots and nature of female offending. The result? Female offenders were not responding in a positive manner and were in danger of being drawn into the deep end of the criminal justice system. For the rest of the decade certain probation teams attempted to construct innovative practices and policies that were geared towards identifying and meeting the specific needs of female offenders (see Eaton, 1985; Worrall, 1990; 1995).

6.2   Towards a shared vision?

In 1987 two texts appeared that attempted to use a form of words with which both the Home Office and the probation service could possibly constitute a framework for a new organizational relationship. Both texts attempted to gloss over the fundamental differences that existed. A Home Office brochure for prospective probation officers explicitly acknowledged:

- that 'it shall be the duty of probation officers to supervise the probationers and other persons placed under their supervision and to assist, advise and befriend them';
- the importance of the social casework approach: 'direct personal relationships are the foundation for everything that follows during the supervision of offenders … The moment you move into other people's problems, you are tackling problems within yourself'.

However, it also stressed the need for probation officers to:

- 'inspire the confidence of the courts and the general public' by guaranteeing effective supervision of offenders which in many ways would be 'tougher than imprisonment' and recognize the need to protect the public;
- work to nationally agreed objectives and priorities;
- 'show offenders, through the legal requirements and sanctions of a court order, that whatever their misfortunes, they are still responsible for their actions'.

(quotations from Home Office, 1987, pp.17, 18)

A briefing statement, entitled *Probation: The Next Five Years,* the first issued by all ranks of the service, attempted to make common cause with the Home Office and government by stating that it was willing to play a prominent and full role in 'improving the overall effectiveness of the criminal justice system'. The service would 'adopt initiatives which encourage courts to make greater use of existing non-custodial sentences, and thus reduce the pressures on the prison system' (Association of Chief Officers of Probation, Central Council of Probation Committees and National Association of Probation Officers, 1987, p.3). However, the text reiterated the service's opposition to SNOP's demand that it only prioritize the 'controlling offenders' part of its work and laid out an alternative list of priorities:

- increased community involvement;
- increased use of non-custodial option;
- improved service to the courts;
- improved service to civil courts;
- improved through-care with prisoners.

Moreover, it reasserted the 'traditional' value base of the service:

> It is important that developments build upon the *established strengths* of the probation service, utilise the skills of its professional and other fieldwork staff and *work with the grain of the service.* Any other approach risks *disorientation, dislocation* and *inefficiency.* New developments should therefore be *consistent with the main values underlying probation work* – a respect for the worth of each individual; a belief in the freedom of the individual and the capacity for individuals to change for the better; a belief that lasting change can only be developed from within, not imposed from without; a commitment to the minimum necessary intervention and to constructive humanitarian approaches.
>
> (Association of Chief Officers of Probation, Central Council of Probation Committees and National Association of Probation Officers, 1987, p.3, emphasis added)

In the same moment, however, new voices joined the debate and added to the destabilization of the probation service. In April 1987, a House of Commons Home Affairs Committee recommended that the Home Office investigate whether electronic tagging should be introduced for non-violent petty offenders (Home Affairs Committee, 1987). Experiments in the USA suggested that such schemes could reduce the prison population and allow offenders to continue to work and support families who would have to be looked after by the state, as well as pay fines and offer compensation to their victims. The Association of Chief Officers of Probation attacked the idea as 'repellent', while NAPO stated that it would refuse to co-operate with such an initiative (*The Times*, 24 April 1987). This was followed, later in the year, by press reports that Home Office ministers were concerned that many members of the judiciary did not trust or have confidence in the outcomes of probation work or the attitudes and practices of probation officers. Officers in many parts of the country, it was claimed, continued to 'over-identify' with offenders; were seemingly incapable of mentioning the words 'custody', 'guilt', 'responsibility' or 'punishment'; were producing inadequate, poorly prepared or irrelevant social enquiry reports; and not providing satisfactory information on the progress or outcome of court orders. Home Office sources informed the press that 'alternatives to custody' would have to be turned into a 'gruelling' experience and 'genuine hardship' for offenders because, as they stood: 'a convicted felon is given a bucket of whitewash and told to go away and paint an old lady's wall. It is not much of a task or a deterrent to reoffending and there's little chance of the offender being shamed into misbehaving himself in the future' (Home Office minister, quoted in *The Times*, 13 October 1987, p.3).

The Home Office also pointed out that ministers were contemplating taking their 'business' elsewhere. There were plenty of *voluntary-* or *private-*sector organizations working in the field which did not have the same philosophical or political difficulties in devising rigorous schemes for supervising juvenile offenders and managing ex-offenders. As can be seen from Table 5.1 overleaf, an alternative organizational model of probation work was emerging.

Table 5.1 The past and future shape of probation

	WELFARE *Old model*	*CRIMINAL JUSTICE* *New model*
Probation subject	Client, with complex of needs and problems like other human beings	Offender, the criminal 'Other' who has broken the law
Probation officer	Individual practitioner	Devising and supervising programmes
Probation philosophy and values	Social work within criminal justice setting	Specialist criminal justice agency
Probation work	Care, assistance, facilitation, guidance	Control, supervision, punishment, discipline
Purpose of probation intervention	Rehabilitation, diversion from custody; resettlement	Reduce re-offending: complying with requirements
Organizational culture	Bureau-professional	Managerial
Interests served	Needs of client	Needs of public, courts, victims, offenders, government
Relationship with Home Office	Relative autonomy	Tighter control, monitoring and evaluation
Relationship with courts	Advocate for client	Impartial advisers to the court on appropriate sentence for offenders
Control of work situation	Maingrade officers	Chief officers
Basis of relationship between probation officer and client/offender	Consent, trust, confidentiality	Compulsion, surveillance, control, confrontation

6.3 A new settlement: punishment in the community

Between 1988 and 1991, the government published legislative proposals which it claimed would pave the way for a new long-term settlement on criminal justice. The resultant Criminal Justice Act 1991 was described by its supporters as the most radical and far-reaching piece of criminal justice legislation in the UK in the twentieth century.

ACTIVITY 5.4

Read Extracts 5.2 and 5.3, which are taken from the words of a Home Office official and John Patten, then Minister of State at the Home Office, respectively. As you do so, note down the key features of the new approach to sentencing as outlined in both extracts.

Extract 5.2 Home Office: 'The rationale of the 1991 Criminal Justice Act, 1'

The act can be seen as a first attempt to construct a truly comprehensive piece of legislation governing sentencing. It covers the whole process: virtually the whole range of disposals available; the reasoning to be applied when reaching decisions; the methods by which sentences can be calculated and implemented; and in the case of custody, the whole process from reception, right through to the expiry of the term imposed. The sheer scale of the attempt, taken as a whole, is probably unprecedented. Previous reforms have tended to be more piecemeal.

(Home Office official, quoted in Gibson *et al.*, 1994, p.33)

Extract 5.3 Patten: 'The rationale of the 1991 Criminal Justice Act, 2'

Sentencing will not be effective until we are clear about its purpose. The first aim of sentencing should be to punish the offender. The sentence of the court denounces criminal behaviour and exacts retribution for it in proportion to its gravity. If that fact is going to be clear to the offender, to the victim and to the public, the offender must be punished justly and proportionately according to the seriousness of his offences. …

The Act makes it clear that a court should not sentence an offender on the basis of his record. It is unfair to punish offenders twice for an offence for which they have already been convicted and punished. Experience and commonsense suggest that little can be gained by sentencing persistent petty offenders to custody. Prison tends to erode an offender's sense of personal responsibility. It deprives him of the ties in the community – both family responsibilities and opportunities for employment – which might encourage him to turn away from crime. We seem more likely to get offenders to learn to exercise self control and to resist the temptation to commit petty offences if they stay in the community where the temptations exist.

Minor offenders who have a history of offending show that they are unlikely to be deterred by the sentence which they receive. It is unrealistic to construct sentencing arrangements on the basis that most offenders will weigh up the possible consequence of their actions in advance. Evidence and experience shows that often they do not. Most offenders are opportunistic and impulsive; they see an opportunity and they seize it.

(Patten, 1992, p.29)

COMMENT

The proposals sought to establish a rational sentencing framework in line with the 'just deserts' theory that would ensure that punishment was commensurate with the seriousness of the offence rather than the offender's past record. This bifurcatory approach, which made a sharp distinction between violent and non-violent offenders, accorded with the managerial cost-effective calculus. Custodial sentences would be reserved for the most serious, violent offences. The majority of petty opportunistic offenders who were clogging up the criminal justice system would be dealt with at a considerably lower cost and just as constructively in the community (see Figure 5.8 overleaf). The Home Office hoped that the new measured approach would reduce the prison population by 3,000 by 1995 (Gibson et al., 1994). It is also worth noting how the extract from the article by John Patten attempts to reconcile the Conservatives' traditional emphasis on punishment and retribution with the principles of situational crime prevention.

■ ■ ■

The probation service was allocated the role of making the proposed 'twin-track' settlement work by persuading the judiciary to make use not of 'alternatives to custody' but 'punishments in the community'. Community *punishments* were to be strengthened, clearly structured and cleansed of ideas of 'treatment', 'rehabilitation' and 'clients' and become an integral and credible part of the structure of punishment which included:

'twin-track' settlement

■ probation orders becoming a *sentence of the court*;

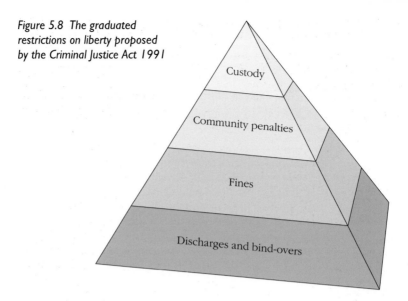

Figure 5.8 The graduated restrictions on liberty proposed by the Criminal Justice Act 1991

- a new combination order (which already existed in Scotland) under which elements of probation supervision and community service work could be combined in a single order;

- a curfew order which would require an offender to be at home for a specified time period. Such orders could be enforced with the assistance of electronic monitoring systems;

- national standards for supervision in day centres which were to be renamed probation centres;

- the service having to keep the courts informed of the outcome of the orders it supervised;

- national standards for parole supervision;

- social enquiry reports becoming pre-sentence reports assisting the courts to determine the most suitable sentence.

A comparable shift in emphasis took place in Scotland. In what McIvor (1996) describes as a 'landmark' address, the then Secretary of State for Scotland, Malcolm Rifkind, detailed the government's commitment to follow a bifurcated policy on sentencing to tackle the overcrowding crisis in Scottish prisons. However, unlike England and Wales:

> our main objective is *not* widening further the range of non-custodial sentences – for we have sufficient number and sufficient flexibility within those to cover our needs – but on strengthening the non-custodial disposals already available to the courts so that they, and the public also, can have confidence in their suitability for a significant number of offenders guilty of non-violent crimes who are at present imprisoned.
>
> (Rifkind, 1989, p.88)

Community service was to be used in future in a much more focused manner – 'for those offenders whose offences genuinely warrant a custodial sentence, except where the court considers that other factors, such as the protection of the public, require a period of detention or imprisonment' (Social Work Services

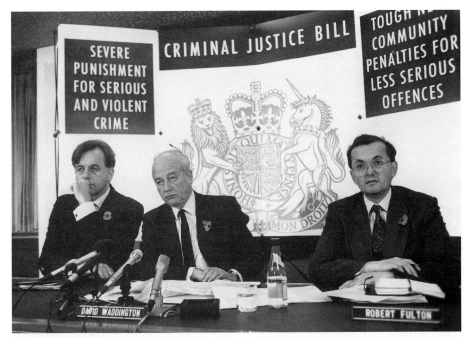

David Waddington, then Home Secretary, at the launch of a twin-track approach to sentencing offenders

Group, 1989, para. 1.2.2). And probation orders were to be revitalized to persuade courts to make more use of them. Ditton and Ford (1994) and McIvor (1996) suggested that probation fell into disuse in Scotland because of the absorption of probation work by social services departments.

The probation service in England and Wales faced an acute dilemma. All levels of the organization could wholeheartedly support the general objective of working to reduce the prison population to manageable proportions. It became clear that many senior officers viewed the 'punishment in the community' proposals and the extra resources as an opportunity to extend probation's social casework methods under cover of punitive rhetoric. However, NAPO (1988) was much more cautious, arguing that the proposals were 'an elaborate confidence trick' that disguised ministers' refusal to fetter the sentencing freedom of judges and magistrates. There was no guarantee, according to NAPO, that providing sentencers with a broader range of tough non-custodial options would persuade them to curb the use of imprisonment. Only mandatory and tightly defined sentencing guidelines; abolishing custody for certain offences; cutting maximum sentences; and tackling the underlying socio-economic causes of crime, and providing 'ladders of opportunity', would reduce the prison population. NAPO also argued that there was no evidence that the new non-custodial options enjoyed public confidence and that, if there was a backlash, the probation service would be scapegoated. NAPO was concerned that the punitive rhetoric of punishment, control, protecting the public, seriousness of the offence, etc., would colonize and eventually define out the social work aspects of probation work:

NAPO is absolutely clear that the transformation of community supervision into a system of 'punishment in the community' represents a major shift in the role of the probation service which will have far-reaching effects. It involves a shift from 'dealing constructively with the problems arising from crime and social breakdown' (*Face to Face*, Home Office, 1987) to a narrower policing role …

We see this proposed transformation as one of fundamental importance. It would mark a clear break with the established role and values of the probation service and would severely damage the ability of the service to maintain its current successful contribution to the criminal justice system. …

Probation supervision has always involved a set of obligations on offenders and placed constraints upon them. However, the purpose of those requirements has been clear – to provide a framework for supervision, within which the emphasis will be on constructive engagement with offenders' problems based on co-operation and positive influence. The imposition and monitoring of punitive restrictions would destroy the balance built by the probation service over many years. Offenders cannot be expected to place trust in, or work co-operatively with, a service which is perceived as policing their punishment.

(National Association of Probation Officers, 1988, p.11)

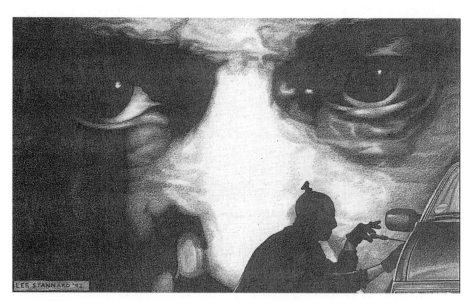

Was probation's new role 'watching' to make sure that offenders did not return to their old habits?

However, the service was informed that it was living on borrowed time. David Faulkner (1989), the Home Office civil servant responsible at that time for piecing together the new criminal justice settlement, told probation officers that the pressures on the service to make 'the transformation from a social work agency to a criminal justice agency with a social base' would increase because such a move was crucial if the new legislation was to work. He warned that the determination of some sections of the service to define themselves as social workers would mean that they were viewed as part of the problem:

an exclusive commitment to the interests of the so-called 'client'; an assumption that the individual social worker/offender relationship is so much at the centre of things that everything else is secondary to it; or worst of all a belief that probation officers are somehow the 'nice guys' of the system, balancing or even correcting the repressive work of other agencies.

(Faulkner, 1989, p.2)

But as the following quotation from Mike Worthington, then Chief Probation Officer of the Northumbria Probation Service, indicates, the service was torn between the old ways and the new demands:

> On Friday last I attended a celebration of the career of a long serving probation officer in this area. At the celebration, the Clerk to the Justices, speaking on behalf of a range of other agencies in the town and representing the local community, spoke movingly of the officer's dedication, helpfulness, integrity and concern for others, throughout a career spanning over thirty years.
>
> We in the probation service have long recognized that in caring for those offenders placed under our supervision, it is also our duty to exercise control on behalf of our community. Over a long period of uncertainty, we are also adjusting to the new central government language of efficiency, cost effectiveness and punishment in the community. As a chief probation officer, I believe that I and my colleagues have a responsibility to do so.
>
> However, Friday reminded me that we carry a far greater responsibility than that of engaging with the current political agenda. It is to ensure that values such as compassion for individuals and service to the community continue to be upheld, even though they may be unfashionable at the present time.
>
> (Mike Worthington, in a letter to *The Independent*, 27 January 1990)

7 Towards a new model probation service

During the formulation and passage of the new legislation a series of official reports was published signalling the government's determination to ensure that the probation service could deliver 'punishment in the community'. The Audit Commission (1989; 1991), as part of its intensifying review of the economy, efficiency and effectiveness of local authority activities, released the most systematic evaluation that had ever been compiled on the organization of probation work in the UK.

The 1989 report provided an unusually clear window on the workload, work span, resourcing, expenditure practices and structures. It told the service that the government had marked out a new path which it must follow and concluded that the managerial processes were not in place to (i) determine and evaluate effectiveness; (ii) disseminate and introduce best practices; (iii) establish national standards; and (iv) ensure consistency. A hard-hitting National Audit Office report (1989) was critical of the Home Office for relying on near-petrified information systems and having no control over expenditure or effective powers over direction of policy; and for inadequate monitoring practices to determine whether policies were being implemented or were successful. The inspectorate was criticized for not providing adequate oversight and being unclear about its purpose; and for wide and unacceptable variations in inspection methods and inadequate dissemination of report findings. Both audits concluded that reform was necessary *at all levels of the service* if it was to iron out divergent practices and processes and meet its new responsibilities.

Read Extracts 5.4 and 5.5 which are taken from Audit Commission and National Audit Office reports respectively. As you do so, concentrate on the key reforms that are being proposed and note the managerialist *tone* and *framing* of the analysis that they present.

Extract 5.4   Audit Commission: 'The probation service: promoting value for money'

The probation service's role has expanded considerably over the years and it is now involved in some way at every stage of the criminal justice system. Its key functions are to *provide information to decision makers (particularly the courts)*, to *supervise offenders on court orders in the community,* and to *work with offenders in custody and on release.* It also undertakes various duties for the civil courts.

It consists of 56 separate autonomous probation areas of very mixed size, with the 12 largest making up over half of the service. Expenditure levels are also very variable, ranging between £230 and £870 per indictable offence. *This variety is more the result of history than present need.*

Probation practice itself has changed over the years, from a social casework approach aimed at providing an understanding of the individual's development, to *a more pragmatic approach which directly addresses the offender's problems.* The process of change continues. But *the emphasis remains on rehabilitating the offender, albeit by confronting him with the consequences of his offending.* This creates some tension between probation and the rest of the criminal justice system. Some regard probation as a 'soft option' which does not mete out to criminals their just deserts. The Green Paper argues that 'the restriction on the offender's freedom of action is a punishment' and that restrictions inevitably occur during a probation order. Thus the *process* [original emphasis] of probation may satisfy the just deserts requirement, even while the *outcome* [original emphasis] should still be the rehabilitation of the offender.

The probation service is in any event moving its focus of activity, reducing involvement with people who commit minor offences and increasing activities with people at risk of going to custody. *To do this effectively and give value for money* the service must *target* its activities, co-ordinating them with other agencies within the criminal justice system, and it must develop and apply new ways of working with more difficult offenders. These changes in turn require it to be *managed differently.*

The way the service *currently targets its activities* gives cause for concern. Increasing probation activity has coincided not with a reduction in the proportion of offenders receiving custody, but with a reduction in the proportion receiving fines. Various monitoring procedures are being introduced with some success to refocus probation activities. But change ultimately must depend on the actions and policies of others. In particular, the service must influence sentencers; *improving performance* requires a partnership between the probation service and the courts. Such a partnership must take account of the separation of powers, and a careful balance must be struck so that sentencers become better informed without compromising their constitutional independence. *Where partnerships have been developed, improved value for money can follow.*

At present there is *considerable variation across the country* in sentencing and cautioning practices, making consistency and co-operation difficult. However, in the field of juvenile justice inter-agency co-operation has progressed considerably, with many examples of close inter-agency working resulting in major changes to the way young people and children are dealt with. There is a marked contrast with the treatment of adults, with 17-year olds being three times less likely to be cautioned and twice as likely to be given a custodial sentence as 16-year olds (without any parallel change in record or nature of offence).

Probation skills and methods of working have also been developing and examples abound of creative and imaginative initiatives for dealing with offenders. But if these skills are to be put to best use, and if inter-agency co-operation and the targeting of probation activity are to be improved, *better management systems* are required. The Home Office has given a lead with a Statement of National Objectives and Priorities, and all services now have equivalent local statements, but the extent to which these statements have changed the actual operations of the service is mixed. Further progress is required in six important areas:

Demonstrating effectiveness While there is a striking variety of probation schemes in operation involving much vision, creativity and imagination, these schemes must be *evaluated*, and their impact on offending behaviour *assessed*. It is unsatisfactory that, at present, *considerable sums are spent with relatively little understanding of the effects achieved*.

Spreading good practice Successful schemes and practices should be disseminated. The distribution of such schemes is currently very uneven, and strategies are needed which promote *greater consistency* between services, taking account of *'best practice' identified through evaluation*. There is a clear role for HM Probation Inspectorate in assisting this process.

Developing management systems Such developments depend on *adequate monitoring*, and each service should have an appropriate system. It is unnecessary to develop large complex systems; a better approach is to develop a flexible system tuned to local targets and objectives. Improvements in cost controls are also necessary.

Clarifying lines of accountability Current arrangements for financing the service (both revenue and capital) are under review and care must be taken that new proposals give *clear lines of accountability*. Probation committees should be required to provide annual reports to improve accountability.

Developing skills in a multi-disciplinary service As probation objectives change, it is important that staff skills keep pace. The trend towards a *multi-skilled workforce* should continue. Furthermore it should be made possible for services to grant-aid independent agencies and local community initiatives, allowing the funding or contracting-out of services where appropriate.

Working with other agencies If the role proposed in the Green Paper and Action Plan is to be fulfilled successfully, the service will need more *effective working relationships* with other agencies in the criminal justice system.

In current circumstances it is hard to assess the value for money provided by the probation service. But there can be no doubt about the need to seek more effective non-custodial options. The probation service is the logical place to look. A carefully *managed programme of action* on the above lines could allow the service to validate its own belief in the value of probation work and to play a much more significant role within the criminal justice system.

(Audit Commission, 1989, pp.22–3, all emphasis added except where indicated)

Extract 5.5 National Audit Office: 'Home Office: control and management of probation services in England and Wales'

Overall conclusion

5. Improving the *economy, efficiency and effectiveness* of the probation services, and securing their full contribution to the tasks facing the criminal justice system, involve responsibilities of both the Home Office and the probation services. Primary responsibility for *management and delivery* of probation work on the ground has rested with local probation committees and probation officers; and local autonomy in these matters has encouraged flexibility and initiative in adapting probation work and methods to local circumstances. Professional judgement has had an important part to play.

6. On the other hand, *increasing demands, finite resources*, and the need to harness probation work more closely to central policy objectives mean that Home office oversight and monitoring will inevitably assume greater prominence. The development of *common standards*, more *consistency of approach* and greater selectively and direction are already under way.

7. In pursuing these various goals, and thereby seeking to improve the contribution of probation work to the operation of the criminal justice system, it will be important to establish and sustain an appropriate constitutional and operational balance between the central role of the Home Office and the level of autonomy exercised by the local probation services. The natural role for the Home Office is to provide *strategic direction* and an *overview of performance* whilst encouraging the *drive and initiative shown by local probation services in day to day management.*

8. There will consequently be a need at both Home Office and local level for more and better information and analysis about which aspects of the probation service work well and which do not and why; about how *resources* are being deployed and to what effect; about *comparative costs and performance against targets*; and above all how far *achievements match up to agreed objectives*, at both *operational and strategic level.* At present information on all these matters is incomplete and of variable quality, and this stands in the way of *effective management.*

9. More generally, the National Audit Office consider that there is scope within the present constitutional framework for improving liaison and the exchange of information between the probation service and other elements of the criminal justice system: the police, the Crown Prosecution Service, the courts and the prisons. Obviously in this area there are sensitive relationships which derive from the essential nature of the checks and balances within the British constitution. Nevertheless it is evident from the work of the National Audit Office and Audit Commission that the full *potential of the probation service is not yet fulfilled* so that *economy and efficiency suffer* and ultimately the *effectiveness of the effort is diminished.*

10. In the National Audit Office's view the Home Office have a vital central role and considerable opportunity to foster greater co-operation and understanding, the importance of which is underlined by the proposals in the recent Green Paper. The improved *relationships and partnerships* that could thereby be secured would facilitate the development and implementation of agreed, common objectives, within clear priorities for the probation service as a whole.

(National Audit Office, 1989, p.6, emphasis added)

COMMENT

Notice how both extracts centre the managerialization of all aspects of probation work. Managerialization does not refer just to the appointment of managers, but also to the application of managerial principles to all aspects of the organization and its work. Both extracts acknowledge that there were established ways of doing things, *but* that only managerialization is deemed capable of meeting the government's objectives and priorities, improving performance and effectiveness, ensuring value for money and generating new working practices (see Figure 5.9). Professional judgement and discretion will have to be reworked within a managerial framework of accountability and the social work ethos within the punishment-in-the-community discourse. These broad parameters were intended to constitute the new organizational settlement for probation.

managerial-ization

■ ■ ■

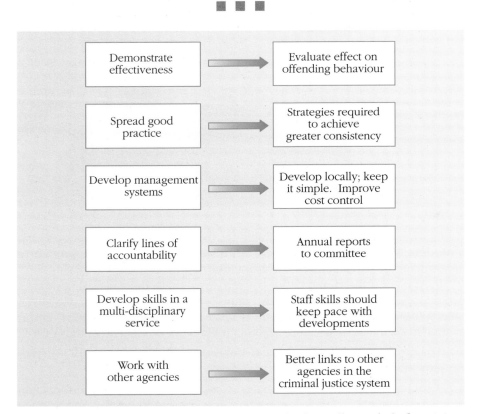

Figure 5.9 The Audit Commission's six recommendations for change (Source: Audit Commission, 1991, p.3)

In February 1990, the Home Office, drawing upon the analysis presented in the two texts (Audit Commission, 1989; National Audit Office, 1989), released *Supervision and Punishment in the Community*. This Green Paper made it clear that a radical root-and-branch reorganization of structure, funding, accountability, personnel policies and relations with the private and voluntary sector was necessary if the service was to take responsibility for supervising and controlling offenders sentenced to community-based punishments. A follow-up discussion document signalled the government's desire for the private and

In April 1990 serious disorder engulfed Strangeways Prison in Manchester and quickly spread to other penal institutions. The intensity and costs of the rioting lent weight to the view that the prison crisis could only be resolved through greater use of non-custodial sentences

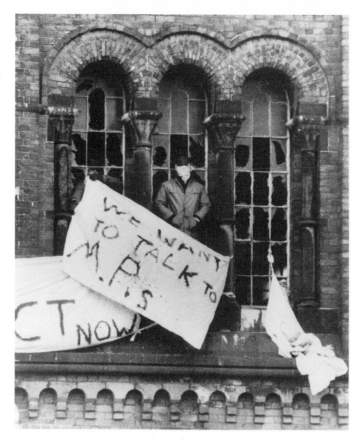

voluntary sectors to take responsibility for the welfare aspects of supervising offenders in the community. This would allow the probation service to concentrate on its core criminal justice tasks.

In April 1991 the Home Office backed down on its most radical option – a national agency funded and directly controlled by the Home Office. However, other reforms were forthcoming in the decision document (Home Office, 1992a) to strengthen the local structure within a framework of greater central control:

- The probation grant was cash limited to control probation service expenditure more effectively.

- A national resource planning process was put in place, with the introduction of a statement of purpose and rolling three-year plans (replacing SNOP) to enable the setting of local objectives, deployment of resources and assessment of progress towards the achievement of objectives.

- The structure of probation committees was to be overhauled.

- There was to be strategic liaison with the judiciary, prison service and Crown Prosecution Service.

- Probation areas were to be amalgamated to make them coterminous with police force areas.

- The calibre of senior management staff was to be improved and performance-related pay introduced.

- The probation inspectorate was to be placed on a statutory footing.

■ The government was to be provided with a default power to enable the Home Secretary to intervene in a seriously or persistently under-performing area.

In 1992, to coincide with the coming into force of the Criminal Justice Act 1991, the Home Office released a handbook of *National Standards for the Supervision of Offenders in the Community* (Home Office, 1992b).

ACTIVITY 5.6

Read Extract 5.6 which is taken from the *National Standards* handbook. As you do so, notice how much more prescriptive it is than SNOP.

Extract 5.6 Home Office: 'National standards'

National standards are intended to achieve several purposes:

• **Quality assurance** As well as setting requirements for probation and social services work, and criteria for the return to court of offenders under supervision, the national standards provide for *monitoring* to ensure that standards are met (and if not, for sentencers to be advised). They are backed by *independent review*, through internal monitoring and inspection and through external inspection by HM Inspectorate of Probation and, where appropriate, the social services inspectorates;

• **Accountability** The standards establish a clear and consistent framework, within which work can be viewed and decisions justified. The standards support and encourage local discretion and initiative. Where an officer finds it necessary to depart from a normal expectation in the standards, the case file should note the departure and explain why it was necessary. The standards provide a basis of accountability for individual cases, and for services as a whole;

• **Consistency** No two offenders are identical. It is essential that supervision takes adequate account of the individual needs and circumstances of each person. Nevertheless, some degree of consistency, particularly of general approach, is important to ensure fairness to the individual and to give assurance to the courts and others;

• **Equal opportunities** The work of probation services and social services departments must be free of discrimination on the ground of race, gender, age, disability, language ability, literacy, religion, sexual orientation or any other improper ground. All services must have a stated *equal opportunities policy* and ensure that this is effectively implemented, monitored and reviewed. Effective action to prevent discrimination (*anti-discriminatory practice*) requires significantly more than a willingness to accept all offenders equally or to invest an equal amount of time and effort in different cases. The origin, nature and extent of differences in circumstances and need must be properly understood and actively addressed *by all concerned* – for example, by staff training, by monitoring and review and by making extra effort to understand and work most effectively with an offender from a different cultural background. This is in keeping with the duty not to discriminate confirmed in section 95 of the Criminal Justice Act 1991, and is reinforced, in context, in each of the national standards. This is not simply a matter of fairness in what is provided to others: in the context of the firm requirements in the standards and the consequent risk of breach, effective anti-discriminatory practice is essential to avoid further disadvantaging those already most disillusioned and disadvantaged in society;

- **Good practice** The framework of the standards leaves, as it should, much of the application of probation and social services work with offenders to the exercise of skill, imagination, discretion and judgement on the part of individual practitioners and services; it also provides a consistent basis for developing and promulgating good practice;

- **Good management** Management has a key role in formulating policy and ensuring that it is delivered effectively and consistently in individual cases, in accordance with these standards. The standards contain important guidance for management at all levels in achieving the required standards, for example, through planning, training, practice guidance, efficient use of resources, liaison and monitoring. Good management involves clear, deliberate choice over strategy; effective leadership of staff; and consistent promotion to all concerned of the value and credibility of work undertaken;

- **Targeting of community orders** All the standards relating to the supervision of community orders (probation, supervision, CS [community service] and combination orders) contain guidance on when that order may or may not be the most suitable for a particular offender, and the need to relate restriction of liberty to the seriousness of the offence, linking to the section on assessment in the PSR [pre-sentence reports] standard;

- **Management of risk** Some offenders and defendants coming to the attention of social and probation services present a significant potential risk to the public. While guarantees cannot be given about offenders' future behaviour, the standards give consistent support to positive management of risk: through advice to courts (eg in PSRs and on breach) and careful assessment of individual offenders to devise suitable programmes of supervision.

(Home Office, 1992b, pp.3–5)

COMMENT

Even though commentators such as Smith (1996, p.238) argue that its content 'more or less reflected the best of existing practice', if we look closely at the text we can see a much more prescriptive Home Office perspective on all aspects of probation work. Harry Fletcher, then Chair of NAPO, seemed to be only too aware of what was happening: 'Just as with the National Curriculum into schools, the government is laying down national standards in an attempt to control the probation service. There are now set standards for report writing, day centres, hostels, probation supervision and discharged prisoners, which take away much of the discretion probation officers once had' (quoted in *The Guardian*, 3 March 1992).

The real problem for opponents was that criticisms could be interpreted as supporting (i) unaccountability, (ii) inconsistencies and (iii) discriminatory practices. It is also worth noting how probation's responsibility for more high-risk offenders is also used as a justification for national standards.

■ ■ ■

Managerialism also cast its shadow over Scotland. National standards and objectives for community service, probation orders, social enquiry reports and through-care were introduced:

> The Government's objective in refunding to local authorities the full approved cost of providing social work services for the criminal justice system is to ensure that the services which the courts require for dealing with offenders in the community are

available in the right quantity and at the right quality ... the provision of community disposals of sufficient quality and quantity will enable sentencers to use them in cases where otherwise they might have imposed a custodial sentence. The overall aim is to create a situation in which it is practicable to use prisons as sparingly as possible through providing community based disposals which contain and reduce offending behaviour, assist social integration, have the confidence of the courts and the wider public, and make efficient and effective use of existing resources.

(Social Work Services Group, 1991, paras 4, 5)

Social work departments had to restructure the delivery of offender services on specialist lines to facilitate strategic planning and funding processes. The work of voluntary agencies was also formalized through the introduction of full central funding. And as in England and Wales, an Inspectorate was established to oversee social work in the criminal justice system. It also resulted in the appointment of senior officers who had direct responsibility for the management of criminal justice services.

However, there was not a comparable ideological assault on the working ethos or occupational identity of criminal justice social workers in Scotland. Smith (1996, p.19) notes how the national standards and objectives were not framed within an overtly punitive discourse and were 'less preoccupied with procedures for enforcement, and more hospitable to the aims of providing help and support.' He also argues that the changes provoked considerably less conflict and opposition.

We can put forward a number of reasons for the difference in the Scottish approach:

- The proposals were less radical and less antagonistically framed.

- Law and order issues were less prominent in public debates in Scotland and not seen as vote winners.

- It is easier to create a policy consensus in a smaller country where policy-makers, practitioners and personnel are more likely to meet on a routine basis.

- There was a common consensus that Scotland's prisons were a national disgrace and that something must be done.

- The Scottish settlement of the late 1960s was still in place and had not been subject to the ideological assaults and organizational crises that had taken place south of the border.

8   Coming apart at the seams

Even before the new criminal justice settlement came into force, senior members of the judiciary, police officers and the members of the Magistrate's Association voiced grave misgivings about the underlying anti-custodial philosophy of the 1991 Criminal Justice Act. Two parts of the Act were identified as the source of judicial misgivings: first, the system of means-related fines, which magistrates argued were producing perverse outcomes; and, second, Section 29 which limited the judiciary's ability to take previous convictions into account when sentencing. Ironically, it was left to the Association of Chief Probation Officers, NAPO and penal reform groups to defend the new legislation and plead with the judiciary to work with the grain of the proposals.

It is possible that the Home Office could have negotiated a new compromise which did not undermine the general principles of the Act. However, the nature of the law and order debate in England and Wales shifted dramatically in the year from 1992 to 1993. There was heightened political and media concern about a seemingly relentless surge in crime, persistent young offenders, 'bail bandits' and joy riders and ram raiders who were in open defiance of the law (see **Muncie, 1998**). However, it was the murder of James Bulger in February 1993 that triggered an anguished and polarized public debate about evil, wickedness and the 'devil children' of a morally depraved 'underclass', with the main political parties seeking to prove that they were tough on crime. In a headline-grabbing speech, the then Shadow Home Secretary, Tony Blair, fired the first salvo by signalling a sea-change in Labour's policy on crime and punishment. He effectively side-lined the party's traditional emphasis on the social and economic causes of crime in favour of a new 'tough on crime, tough on the causes of crime' stress on moral values and the importance of individual responsibilities and duties. He demanded that children be taught 'the value of what is right and what is wrong' (*The Guardian*, 20 February 1993). John Major, then Prime Minister, immediately responded with a highly emotive call for a new public attitude towards criminals: 'I would like the public to have a crusade against crime and change from being forgiving of crime to being considerate to the victim. Society needs to condemn a little more and understand a little less' (*Daily Mail*, 21 February 1993, p.1).

In October 1993, Michael Howard, then Home Secretary, led what *The Times* (7 October 1993) described as 'a right wing policy charge' at the Conservative's annual conference. In an attempt to wrestle back the law and order debate from New Labour, he resurrected the debate about the underlying causes of crime. He blamed Britain's crime wave on the collapse of individual responsibility, the decline of the two-parent family and growing dependency on the welfare state. He subsequently announced that legislation would be passed to 'correct the thirty year inbuilt bias in favour of the criminal and against the protection of the public', acknowledging that this would mean sending more offenders to prison:

'prison works'

> I do not flinch from that. We shall no longer judge the success of our system of justice by a fall in our prison population. Let us be clear. Prison works. It ensures that we are protected from murderers, muggers, and rapists and it makes many who are tempted to commit crime think twice. Today I make this announcement. We shall build six new prisons. And I can tell you one thing. Butlins won't be bidding for the contracts.
>
> (Michael Howard, quotation from his Conservative conference speech as broadcast on BBC Radio 4, 12 October 1993, emphasis added)

New prisons, privately run secure offending institutions and harsher regimes for persistent juvenile offenders were promised to ensure that felons finally got their just deserts.

Howard's speech puzzled and confused political commentators, criminal justice professionals and criminologists. Some argued that the Home Secretary, like all Conservative Home Secretaries, was having to employ tough rhetoric to appease the law and order lobby within the Conservative Party, public opinion and sections of the media. The 'bark is worse than its bite' theory believed that the moral panic surrounding the Bulger case would not undermine the legislative and organizational settlement that had been painstakingly pieced together over the previous decade. It was felt that no Conservative government committed to

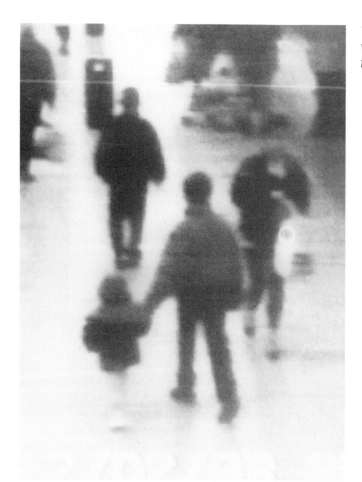

This closed circuit television image associated with the murder of James Bulger came to personify the crime crisis in the UK in the 1990s

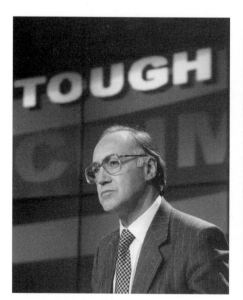
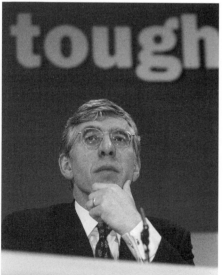

In the countdown to the 1997 General Election, both the Conservative and Labour Parties sought to reassure voters that, on the issue of crime, tough words would be matched with tough deeds

197

'economy, efficiency and effectiveness' would sanction throwing away billions of pounds of taxpayers' money on a knee-jerk imprisonment strategy that patently did not work. At least the 'value-for-money' principles of 'new managerialism' would hold any attempted law and order u-turn in check. Other commentators suspected that Howard's speech sounded the death knell for the settlement heralded by the Criminal Justice Act 1991. Finally, a Conservative Home Secretary was willing to synchronize words and deeds. The Prime Minister at the time, John Major, supported the new approach on the populist grounds that 'People want us to go back to basics in our attitudes towards crime.' He also attacked those commentators who argued that 'deterrence and public protection' policies did not work: 'Those who make such points must not miss two simple facts. First, while criminals are in prison they cannot commit crimes; and second, the existence of prison as a sanction against crime deters many others from committing crimes. In short, prison works' (John Major, all quotations from *The Independent,* 14 October 1993).

A battery of controversial legislation was produced to prove that the Conservatives' words were no idle threat. The Criminal Justice Act 1993 allowed, among other things, courts to be permitted to take account of an offender's past criminal record. It also abolished the unit fines system. The Criminal Justice and Public Order Act 1994 curtailed the right of a defendant to remain silent during police questioning and in court. Police 'stop and search' powers were extended, as was their right to ban public demonstrations. This was followed by a Crime (Sentences) Act which sought to introduce *mandatory* life sentences for a second serious sexual or violent offence, *mandatory* minimum sentences for repeat drug traffickers and burglars and the end to automatic early release. Critics of the new 'prison works' approach warned that the government would have to build 40 new prisons, each costing between £70 million and £100 million each, to house the thousands of extra prisoners who would cost £30,000 per prisoner a year to feed, clothe and accommodate.

The effects of Michael Howard's rewriting of the criminal justice script were immediate, with a dramatic increase in the number of offenders receiving custodial sentences. A prison service already rocked by the sacking of its head in October 1994 in the aftermath of two high-profile breakouts, protested that the government's policies conflicted with the operational realities facing an overcrowded and extremely volatile penal system where discipline and morale were at breaking-point. Prison governors in conjunction with penal reform groups and the probation service demanded a return to the bifurcation principles of the Criminal Justice Act 1991.

The crime debate intensified in the aftermath of the Dunblane massacre, the Frederick and Rose West case and the murder of head teacher Phillip Lawrence. And in the run-up to the 1997 General Election both political parties vied with each other to come up with populist soundbites to prove who was the toughest on crime. Jack Straw, then shadow Home Secretary, claimed that the Conservatives were soft on crime and promised action to reclaim the streets from beggars, squeegee merchants, noisy neighbours, vandals, under-age drinkers and threatening children. In a desperate attempt to seize back the initiative on law and order, Michael Howard promised voters that a re-elected Conservative government would intensify its crusade against crime by implementing minimum jail sentences, toughening up community punishments, building more private prisons, extending closed circuit television, introducing

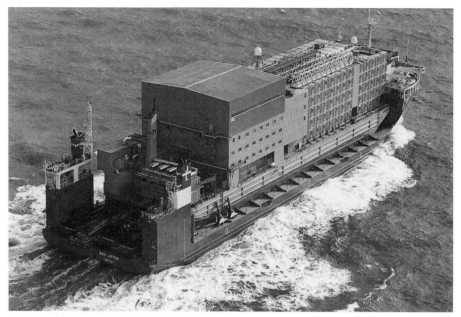

By March 1997 the prison population had reached 59,000 with numbers forecast to rise at 300 per week. The Home Office response was to authorize another prison-building programme and to acquire floating accommodation as a short-term measure

identity cards and supporting 'zero tolerance' policing. Commentators such as Rod Morgan, a penal expert, warned that the political parties had 'entered into a sort of arms race on law and order' predicated upon the need for ever tougher denunciations of crime, aggressive policing, harsher sentencing and stricter prison regimes (quoted in *New Statesman*, 22 November 1996, p.6).

9 A new model probation officer

The 'prison works' philosophy and law and order atmosphere had serious implications for the probation service: first, resources were redirected to the prison system; and, second, ministers launched a fresh assault on the service, arguing that authoritative research findings indicated that prison was just as effective as probation and community service in reducing offending. The probation service came under yet more pressure to show that it had changed. The first annual report of the revamped Probation Inspectorate acknowledged that the service had made considerable progress in a short time period and had proven that community sentences represented 'real value for money'. However, it was the Inspectorate's criticisms on which the media focused. These included:

- the failure of certain probation areas to produce rigorous and demanding schemes for *serious* offenders that were credible with sentencers, protected the public and reduced re-offending;
- the service's persistence in clinging to its social work ethic and resisting efforts to integrate 'punishment in the community' into its work;
- the persistence of wide and unjustifiable variations in practice.

The service was subsequently informed by the Home Secretary that the Inspectorate reports would evaluate service delivery and effectiveness, and that national standards for community penalties would be tightened and made more prescriptive in nature.

In March 1995, the Home Office presented a new framework for community sentences which placed more curbs on the discretion and autonomy of probation officers. A single 'community sentence' (incorporating the existing orders) would be introduced to simplify matters; the power to specify the content and purpose of these sentences would be transferred from the probation service to the courts; and courts would receive more feedback on the effects of their sentencing decisions as well as on the progress and outcome of sentences. Finally, the requirement for offenders to consent to community sentences was to be ended (see Home Office, 1995).

Official attempts to reform probation work in England and Wales took a dramatic, if not unexpected, turn in February 1995 when a shake-up of recruitment and training procedures was announced to replace, once and for all, its 'liberal do-gooding ethos' with a 'tougher, disciplinarian' organizational culture. A highly critical Home Office report (1989) on the quality and nature of the statutory two-year social work based training courses accused them of not being able, or refusing, to meet the specific needs of trainee probation officers. Criticism was aimed at curricula for paying too much attention to generic social work issues and not recognizing that probation officers were different to social workers, and highlighted the lack of attention paid to:

- offence-centred treatment and behaviour modification programmes;
- philosophical debates about punishment (for example, retribution versus deterrence) and rehabilitation;
- victimology;
- assessment of effectiveness both at the level of outcomes of probation work and officer performance;
- the specifics of criminal justice legislation;
- the core criminal justice duties and responsibilities of probation officers.

> It is right for any academic course, or its individual staff members, to take their own view on the appropriate role and location of probation work and the methods and approaches suitable for it. But it must also be right for public bodies to expect a basic sympathy with their aims from vocational courses which receive tax payers' money specifically for training recruits to become public employees ...

> It is important to look beyond the Probation Service for consumer views. In many respects the Probation Service is a deliverer rather than a consumer. Furthermore, most senior management have now been recruited through the generic social work training route, which may tend to keep their comments bounded within the assumptions and values of that system.

> The ultimate consumers are the courts of which they are officers, the community they serve, the Home Office which pays 80% of their salaries, the Probation Committees which employ them and the offenders whom they supervise.

> ... it is vital for probation officers to be left in no doubt during their training that they are involved in the punitive process and are cast to play an important role in the control of offenders in the community ...'

(Home Office, 1989, pp.7, 9)

The report also commented on the dramatic over-representation of students from minority ethnic backgrounds on certain courses and it posed questions about:

- the recruitment practices of universities and colleges;

- the 'undue priority' given by social work tutors to issues of anti-racist and anti-sexist practice which bordered on 'consciousness raising and indoctrination';

- the unprofessional and unjustifiable belief that social work practices could abolish racism in British society.

As we can see from Table 5.2, higher education institutions, in conjunction with the probation service, reformulated certain aspects of the Diploma in Social Work (DipSW) to make it more skills based and relevant for probation officers in the light of these criticisms.

Table 5.2 Core elements of probation training

Assessment :	of risk to the public
	of offender need in relation to reducing offending
	of resources/programmes available
	of the efficiency and effectiveness of a planned intervention
Negotiating contracts:	with courts
	with offenders
	with victims
	with potential providers and beneficiaries (e.g. community service)
Managing contracts:	continuing risk assessment
	maintaining motivation and compliance enforcement
	evaluating outcomes for court and offender
	providing direct work with offenders

Source: Central Probation Council, Association of Chief Officers of Probation, Joint Universities Council – Social Work Education Committee, 1991

However, in 1994, in the aftermath of another highly critical and controversial report (Dews and Watts, 1994), the Home Secretary stated:

> The present arrangements for recruitment and training have some great strengths, but the work of probation officers and social workers is different, and there is no longer a good reason for a common training qualification. I propose to sweep away the barriers to the recruitment of people who have relevant skills and experience to offer but who lack the social work qualification required by law.
>
> (quoted in *The Guardian*, 23 February 1995)

This decision to remove control of probation training from higher education institutions and repeal the legal requirement that probation officers hold a social work qualification inaugurated another bitter struggle between the service and the Home Secretary. The Home Office stressed that the reforms would enhance the *criminal justice* role of officers:

There are 150,000 offenders serving their sentences in the community. On present trends, too many of them will re-offend. Those offenders are supervised by the probation service. The service's role in the criminal justice system cannot be overstated. ...

Although the work of probation officers includes a social work dimension, it is very distinct from that of social workers. The probation service is an important part of the criminal justice system and plays a critical role in the corrective punishment of offenders. ...

For criminals serving community-based sentences of the court, we have introduced tougher, more rigorous national standards. Both the Government and the public expect community sentences to be a punishment – and that needs probation officers to implement those standards. We also want fewer offenders to return to their criminal ways. That means probation officers, along with others, working hard to prevent re-offending.

(Lady Blatch, then Home Office Minister of State responsible for the probation service, 1995, p.7)

The service stressed the importance of broad *social work* training:

Often, the offending is a symptom of another problem which should be addressed. Drugs or alcohol misuse, mental ill-health, education or lack of it, dysfunctional relationships, poverty, homelessness and unemployment can all contribute.

Most adult offenders stopped listening to their parents long ago – if they ever did. To encourage them to toe the line, a probation officer needs to use many tactics including encouragement and positive reinforcement. A probation officer needs knowledge of human behaviour, developmental psychology, counselling, sociology, law and social history and a working knowledge of legislation and how to apply it. This must include an understanding of how the system works to uphold that legislation.

(Walter Henry, probation officer, 1995, p.5)

After taking office in 1997, Jack Straw, the Labour Home Secretary, announced that he supported the move away from social work training on the grounds that it no longer reflected the core tasks of probation officers (see Figures 5.10 and 5.11). In future, local probation services would be expected to recruit trainees and arrange for them to obtain a relevant qualification. He also indicated that the service should think of renaming itself to make it clear to the public that it was not a 'soft' social welfare service for offenders (*The Times*, 28 December 1997).

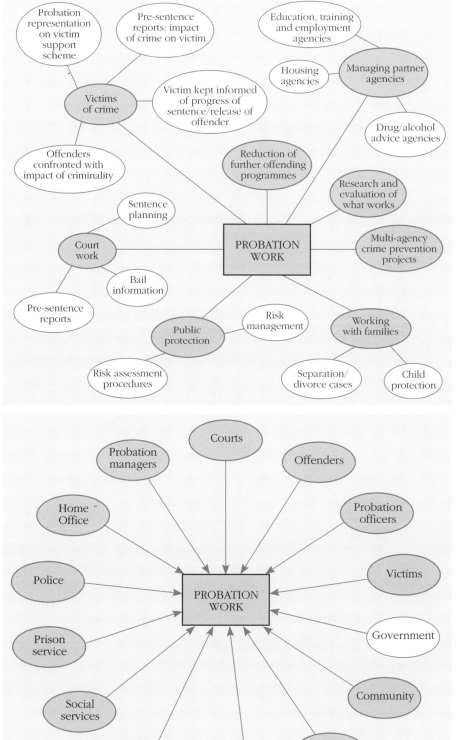

*Figure 5.10
The 'New Probation
Work', governed by
national standards
covering objectives
and priorities and
cost effectiveness*

*Figure 5.11
National and local
stakeholders in the
'New Probation
Work'*

10   Conclusion: the same only different?

This case study has illustrated just how difficult it is to establish the groundwork for, never mind realize, criminal justice settlements in England and Wales. Why? First, criminal justice professionals and quasi-professionals have the necessary organizational and legal discretion to rework policy initiatives to dovetail with their own preferences and interests and they also have the power to resist and subvert policies they do not support. Second, questions of law and order have come to saturate the media and the public mood and fear of crime; moral panics and social anxiety can determine the outcome of political elections. This means that settlements will be sacrificed for short-term political advantage. Third, there are no neatly arranged plans, 'magic bullet' policies or rounded formulas that will reduce the complex of criminality and fear of crime and disorder that afflicts contemporary UK society. Indeed, it could be argued that the traces of each 'deserted settlement' seem to have *deepened* rather than *resolved* the endless crises of law and order. And we must always keep in mind that, even though settlements in Scotland and Northern Ireland seem to be more durable and meaningful, this has not produced 'crisis-free' or indeed laudable criminal justice systems.

The probation service, because of its distinctive position – 'facing both ways' – on the borders of criminal justice (control) and social welfare (care), was deeply affected by the attempted criminal justice settlements following the Second World War and actively responsible for their abandonment. The proposed social democratic 'rehabilitative' moment of the 1960s should have signalled the end of a separate probation service, but, because of a successful campaign of resistance, quasi-welfarization only happened in Scotland. The proposed managerial-based settlement of the late 1980s and early 1990s had equally far-reaching implications for probation work. In order to move 'centre stage' as a *criminal justice agency*, the probation service in England and Wales came under unprecedented scrutiny and pressure to restructure its work practices, organizational structure and professional culture. Not surprisingly, given the radical and relentless roller-coaster nature of the reforms, the service split between those who argued that they should take the extra resources on offer and work with or 'soften' the proposals, and those who maintained that the punitive reframing of probation work and organizational changes had to be resisted as a matter of principle because they represented a direct assault on the 'traditional' social work ethos, operational purpose and identity of probation officers. What has been particularly difficult for many officers to accept is the very public 'naming and shaming' that has accompanied each new set of reforms. In many respects the service has been treated by certain Home Office officials and ministers as a persistent offender to be threatened with harsher and harsher punishment to modify his or her behaviour.

However, the changes wrought by the 1980s and 1990s have not been as damaging to probation work as many commentators prophesied. It must always be kept in mind that successive Conservative governments, as part of their patronage of the criminal justice system, allocated unprecedented resources to the service, and probation work has been strengthened considerably in Northern Ireland and Scotland. The Conservative government was also forced in England and Wales to drop its most radical proposals – that is, outright nationalization and or privatization/voluntarization of many of its activities. Nevertheless, many organizational reforms and rationalities are in place and it is likely that they will be deepened by New Labour's criminal justice programme. Probation has been repositioned as a core criminal justice agency whose primary duties are reducing the risk of further offending, servicing the courts and protecting the public. *Local* work with offenders is framed by *national* objectives and priorities and cash limits. Management is attempting to continue to develop and implement processes and systems that will drive highly structured, cost-effective 'what works' working practices and ensure that professional discretion and field work culture are *aligned with* the strategic purposes of the criminal justice system. The work of main grade officers is tested, and the outcomes are evaluated and appraised by both their immediate managers and the Inspectorate. And so long as probation is willing to forget its old 'storylines' and is able to 'talk up' the toughness and effectiveness of non-custodial measures, take on new risk-management and community crime-prevention responsibilities, and ensure that the gap between *promise* and *performance* is not publicly exposed, what is left of its reworked 'care and control' discourse will be respected. If, however, probation officers fail to deliver – and this is a distinct possibility given the volatile law and order climate in which they are working – we can expect to see headlines announcing yet another fundamental review of the service.

Further reading

Worrall (1997) provides a valuable overview of the issues that have engulfed the probation service in the 1990s. The emerging policy and practice agenda for probation is discussed in a collection edited by Burnett (1997). Williams (1995) provides a succinct overview of the debate about the values that should underpin and direct probation work, and an important overview of the development of probation work from 1945 to the late 1970s is provided by Haxton (1978).

References

Association of Chief Officers of Probation, Central Council of Probation Committees and National Association of Probation Officers (1987) *Probation: The Next Five Years*, London, Central Council of Probation Committees.

Audit Commission (1989) 'The probation service: promoting value for money', Appendix 1 in National Audit Office (1989).

Audit Commission (1991) *Going Straight: Developing Good Practice in the Probation Service*, Occasional Papers No.1, London, HMSO.

Barclay, G.C. (ed.) (1991) *A Digest of Information on the Criminal Justice System. Crime and Justice in England and Wales*, Home Office Research and Statistics Department, London, HMSO.

Barclay, G.C. (ed.) (1993) *Digest 2: Information on the Criminal Justice System in England and Wales*, Home Office Research and Statistics Department, London, Home Office.

Barclay, G.C. (ed.) (1995) *The Criminal Justice System in England and Wales*, Home Office Research and Statistics Department, London, Home Office.

Blatch, Lady (1995) 'Quality recruitment', *The Guardian*, 18 October, p.7.

Burnett, R. (1997) *The Probation Service: Responding to Change*, Oxford, Centre for Criminological Research.

Central Council of Probation Committees (1983) *Probation: A Multi-Racial Approach*, London, Central Council of Probation Committees.

Central Probation Council, Association of Chief Officers of Probation, Joint Universities Council – Social Work Education Committee (1991) 'Joint statement on probation training', in Dews and Watts (1994).

Clarke, R.V.G. and Mayhew, P. (1980) *Designing Out Crime*, London, HMSO.

Cohen, S. (1979) *Crime and Punishment: Some Thoughts on Theories and Policies*, London, Routledge and Kegan Paul.

Department of Health and Social Security (1968) *Report of the Committee on Local Authority and Allied Personal Social Services* (The Seebohm Report), Cmnd 3703, London, HMSO.

Dews, V. and Watts, J. (1994) *Review of Probation Officer Recruitment and Qualifying Training*, London, Home Office.

Ditton, J. and Ford, R. (1994) *The Reality of Probation*, Aldershot, Avebury.

Eaton, M. (1985) 'Documenting the defendant: placing women in social inquiry reports', in Brophy, J. and Smart, C. (eds) *Women in Law*, London, Routledge.

Faulkner, D. (1984) 'The future of the probation service', in National Association of Probation Officers (ed.) *Probation: Direction, Innovation and Change*, London, National Association of Probation Officers.

Faulkner, D. (1989) 'The future of the probation service: a view from government', in Shaw, R. and Haines, K. (eds) *The Criminal Justice System: A Central Role for the Probation Service*, Cambridge, Institute of Criminology.

Fisher, J. (1976) *The Effectiveness of Social Casework*, London, Charles C. Thomas.

Fitzgerald, M. and Sim, J. (1982) *The Prison Crisis*, Oxford, Blackwell.

Folkard, M.S. *et al.* (1976) *IMPACT: VOLUME II*, London, HMSO.

Fowles, A. (1990) 'Monitoring expenditure in the criminal justice system', *The Howard Journal*, vol.29, no.2, pp.82–100.

Gibson, B., Cavadino, P., Rutherford, A., Ashworth, A. and Harding, J. (1994) *Criminal Justice in Transition*, London, Waterside Press.

Griffiths, W.A. (1982) 'A new probation service', *Probation Journal*, vol.29, no.3, pp.98–9.

Hall, S., Critcher, C., Jefferson, T., Clarke, J. and Roberts, B. (1978) *Policing the Crisis*, London, Macmillan.

Haxton, D. (1978) *Probation: A Changing Service*, London, Constable.

Heal, K. and Laycock, G. (1985) *Situational Crime Prevention*, London, HMSO.

Henry, W. (1995) 'Criminal cuts that will increase crime', *The Guardian*, 22 November, p.5.

Holdaway, S. and Allaker, J. (1990) *Race Issues in the Probation Service: A Review of Policy*, London, Association of Chief Officers of Probation.

Home Affairs Committee (1987) *The State and Use of Prisons: Vol. 1 Session 1986–1987*, London, House of Commons.

Home Office (1962) *Report of the Departmental Committee on the Probation Service*, Cmnd 1650, London, HMSO.

Home Office (1965) *The Child, the Family and the Young Offender*, Cmnd 2742, London, HMSO.

Home Office (1966) *Social Work and the Community*, Cmnd 3065, London, HMSO.

Home Office (1968) *Children in Trouble*, Cmnd 3601, London, HMSO.

Home Office (1984a) *Probation Service in England and Wales: Statement of National Objectives and Priorities*, London, HMSO.

Home Office (1984b) *Criminal Justice: A Working Paper*, London, Home Office.

Home Office (1986) *Criminal Justice: A Working Party*, London, Home Office.

Home Office (1987) *Face to Face with the Probation Service*, London, Home Office.

Home Office (1989) *Probation Training: Review of Home Office Sponsorship Scheme*, London, Home Office.

Home Office (1990) *Supervision and Punishment in the Community*, Cmnd 966, London, HMSO.

Home Office (1992a) *Partnership in Dealing with Offenders in the Community: A Decision Document*, London, HMSO.

Home Office (1992b) *National Standards for the Supervision of Offenders in the Community*, London, Home Office.

Home Office (1995) *National Standards for the Supervision of Offenders in the Community*, London, Home Office.

Humphrey, C. (1991) 'Calling on the experts', *The Howard Journal*, vol.30, no.1, pp.1–18.

Jones, C. (1993) 'Auditing criminal justice', *British Journal of Criminology*, vol.33, no.2, pp.187–302.

Jordon, W. (1971) 'The probation service in the sixties', *Social and Economic Administration*, vol.5, no.2, pp.125–37.

Lloyd, C. (1986) *Response to SNOP*, Cambridge, Institute of Criminology.

Locke, T. (1990) *New Approaches to Crime in the 1990s*, London, Longman.

Mair, G. (1989) *Some Developments in Probation in the 1980s*, Home Office Research Bulletin No.27, London, HMSO.

Martinson, R. (1974) 'What works? Questions and answers about penal reform', *The Public Interest*, vol.35, pp.1–47.

McIvor, G. (1996) 'Recent developments in Scotland', in McIvor, G. (ed.) *Working with Offenders*, London, Jessica Kingsley Publications.

McLaughlin, E. and Muncie, J. (1994) 'Managing criminal justice', in Clarke, J., Cochrane, A. and McLaughlin, E. (eds) *Managing Social Policy*, London, Sage.

McLaughlin, E. and Murji, K. (1998) 'Resistance through representation: storylines, advertising and Police Federation campaigns', *Policing and Society*, forthcoming.

Morris, A. (1974) 'Scottish juvenile justice: a critique', in Hood, R. (ed.) *Crime, Criminology and Public Policy*, London, Heinemann.

Morris, C. (ed.) (1950) *Social Case-work in Great Britain*, London, Faber and Faber.

Muncie, J. (1998) '"Give 'em what they deserve": the young offender and youth justice policy', in Langan, M. (ed.) *Welfare: Needs, Rights and Risks*, London, Routledge in association with The Open University.

National Association of Probation Officers (1966) *Seniority in the Probation Service* (Probation Papers No.4), London, National Association of Probation Officers.

National Association of Probation Officers (1970) *Future Development of the Probation and After Care Service*, London, National Association of Probation Officers.

National Association of Probation Officers (1988) *Punishment and Custody in the Community: A Response*, London, National Association of Probation Officers.

National Audit Office (1989) *Home Office: Control and Management of Probation Services in England and Wales*, London, HMSO.

Newton, G. (1956) 'Trends in probation training', *British Journal of Delinquency*, vol.VII, no.2, pp.123–35.

Parry-Khan, L. (1988) *Management by Objectives in Probation*, Social Work Monographs No.63, UEA/Social Work Today.

Patten, J. (1992) 'The underlying philosophy', *The Magistrate*, vol.48, no.2, pp.29–30.

Radzinowicz, L. (1958) 'Preface', in Cambridge Department of Criminal Science, *The Results of Probation*, London, Macmillan.

Reiner, R. and Cross, M. (eds) (1991) *Beyond Law and Order*, London, Macmillan.

Rifkind, M. (1989) 'Penal policy: the way ahead', *The Howard Journal*, vol.28, pp.81–90.

Scottish Home and Health Department, Scottish Education Department (1964) *Report of Committee on Children and Young Persons* (The Kilbrandon Report), Cmnd 2306, Edinburgh, HMSO.

Smith, D. (1996) 'Reforming the probation service', in May, M., Brunsdon, E. and Craig, G. (eds) *Social Policy Review 8*, London, Social Policy Association.

Social Work Services Group (1989) *National Objectives and Standards for the Operation of Community Service by Offenders Schemes in Scotland*, Edinburgh, Scottish Education Department.

Social Work Services Group (1991) *National Objectives and Standards for Social Work Services in the Criminal Justice System*, Edinburgh, Scottish Office.

Taylor, W. (1981) *Probation and Aftercare in a Multi-Racial Society*, London, Commission for Racial Equality.

Treasury (1983) *Financial Management in Government Departments*, Cmnd 9058, London, HMSO.

Varah, M. (1976) 'Probation problems: why time is running out', *The Sunday Times*, 14 November, p.15.

Williams, B. (ed.) (1995) *Probation Values*, Birmingham, Venture Press.

Worrall, A. (1990) *Offending Women: Female Law-Breakers and the Criminal Justice System*, London, Routledge.

Worrall, A. (1995) 'Equal opportunity or equal disillusion? The probation service and anti-discriminatory practice', in Williams (ed.) (1995).

Worrall, A. (1997) *Punishment in the Community*, London, Longman.

CHAPTER 6

Choice, Selection and the Social Construction of Difference: Restructuring Schooling

by Ross Fergusson

Contents

1 Introduction

Education is the only area of welfare in which participation is a legal requirement. Almost everyone attends school for at least eleven years of their life. Much longer educational careers are common. In most of our minds the education system, along with the National Health Service (NHS), symbolizes state welfare provision, and, after social security, it vies with the NHS for consuming the second largest share of government spending. However, in the context of this book the education system has a very particular significance for understanding the purposes and processes of restructuring welfare. As Chapter 2 argued, the crisis of welfare and the emergence of newly structured welfare sites entailed the construction of new welfare subjects, positioned in a quite different set of relations to the welfare state from that established under the old settlements. Education is a critical site for the social construction of subjects, and subject positions. Its structural importance to the welfare state and its cultural contribution to the construction of subjects combine to make it a key institution for understanding welfare restructuring.

It takes only a moment's reflection to conceptualize the structural prominence of the education system. Its institutions and structures are evident everywhere. The school term and school day shape many adults' days and years. A huge industry services the movement, maintenance and equipping of its subjects. But what of its cultural influence?

ACTIVITY 6.1

Look back to Chapter 2 section 7.1. Note down as many ways as you can in which the person you are has been 'made up' as a subject. These might include ways in which you understand and present yourself as racialized, as able-bodied or disabled, as masculine or feminine, as a person with certain abilities or limitations, as someone who relates to others in a particular way, as someone whose identity relates to their occupation (paid or not), and so on.

Now consider what aspects of this 'making up' you associate with your own experiences in education. How did the early experience of being a pupil 'make' you? Which school did you go to, and what did that seem to tell you and others about who you were? How did you respond to being one member of a large class? Can you remember special moments – of achievement, failure, anguish, satisfaction and so on – which might have helped define the person you are? How did you react to the culture of school – its regimes, its authority patterns, its rituals, its social values?

In answering these questions, try to concentrate on how your education as a whole helped to 'make' you objectively, in a way which might have shaped the course of your life (rather than on your feelings and the more intimate aspects of your personal identity).

COMMENT

You probably have a 'story' you tell yourself and others about your experiences in education, and about how they contributed to the person you are now. Asked to describe how you became that person, it is quite likely that a good part of your account would touch on school experience – especially if you were trying to give a really in-depth description to a close friend. You are probably aware of how you were identified by others in school, in what ways you were similar to others, and in what ways different. Most of us learned in school which differences were important, and which not, and in whose eyes. We might have learned, for example, that our Irishness seemed to matter more than our friend's Welshness, if we went to school in England. We might have learned that some of our interests did not 'fit' our gender well, according to our friends, our teacher, or other pupils. Or we might have picked up a sense that some people were drawn to us or kept distant from us because of where we lived. Few people leave school without a strong sense of whether they are bright, average or stupid, good at this kind of thing and hopeless at that. There are defining moments: which class you are put into, whether you got into this secondary school or that one, how your teacher dealt with a racist comment directed at you, when you felt you were being criticized for who you were, not what you had done or failed to do.

In making these kinds of connections, you have begun to describe the influence of education in the processes by which you have become constructed as a subject. Of course, social constructionism views these as continuing processes in which people are constantly made up as subjects throughout their lives. But it is probably clear to you that your schooling had a marked influence – and perhaps a greater one than you can now piece together in a few minutes.

■ ■ ■

In constructing subjects, schools, along with other areas of welfare, also construct subject positions in a social world in which distributions of power and resources are highly differentiated and embedded within particular sets of social relations. So this chapter's exploration of the place of schools in the restructuring of welfare emphasizes how schools contribute to the allocation of subjects to differentiated positions, principally through the mechanisms of selection and the construction of difference.

This chapter looks at the restructuring of education over the last 50 years in three closely related ways.

1   First, it looks specifically at the ways in which schooling and the allocation of children to places in the state system has been structured, and at the social, political and economic context in which changes to the structure have been made. Here we trace some key developments from the structures which predated the post-Second World War settlements, through the period of consensus to its breakdown, following some of the main ideas from Chapters 1 and 2. The chapter then goes on to explore the impact of the New Right on the structure of school provision, and the possibilities for resettlement after the 1997 General Election.

2   Second, much of this exploration is drawn together around the question of how schools are organized socially, whether as selective, comprehensive, the product of a market, or an amalgam of what powerful groups think best in any locality. Historical changes in the organization of schooling were frequently driven by the desire to re-form social differentiation. But their social organization is also of fundamental importance to an understanding of how particular welfare regimes construct and treat difference.

3   This focus on the social construction of subjects and subject positions is the third way of looking at restructuring. One important aspect of this is the use

of the idea of ability to structure schools and allocate places. Another is the contribution of the cultures and curricula of schools to the construction of differentiated subjects. Yet another is the part taken by schools in constructing national belonging, social citizenship, and inclusion within a moral order.

The chapter presents a very brief and particular account of the recent development of education. It is confined to secondary schooling, and concerned only with specific features of restructuring and selection. Tracing the links, correspondences and gaps between the development of the education system and its social, political and economic context in one chapter has meant compressing coverage of many areas and neglecting others. The differences between the development of state education in Scotland, Northern Ireland and England and Wales are so great as to mean that any serious consideration of them here has not been possible. Similarly, there has not been space to take more than passing account of the large and important private sector. Which features are included is determined by whether they contribute to a wider understanding of the restructuring of the post-war welfare state, and of how restructuring differs in different areas of welfare. Also important has been whether particular features illuminate the construction of differentiated and unequal welfare subjects.

The terms 'education', 'schools', and 'schooling' are used throughout. As **McCoy (1998)** points out, they are not synonymous. Much of this chapter will be concerned with the processes of social construction, and 'schooling' will be used to denote the experiences of participation in the culture and curriculum of schools. 'Education' is used mainly to refer to the system and its structures, and 'school' to refer to specific sites or an institutional framework.

2   Choosing a school

This section is organized around three activities all concerned with the issue of choosing a school. The first two activities ask you to use your own views and/or experiences of choosing schools. The third activity then asks you to compare and contrast your initial thoughts with your responses to two extracts taken from guides to choosing a school. You should now work your way through this section.

ACTIVITY 6.2

What is your idea of a good school? What would you regard as important issues in deciding? What would you look for? Without too much pause for reflection, make a quick note of what comes to mind.

You will return to your responses to Activities 6.2 and 6.3 later in the chapter (section 7), so it is important that you keep notes.

COMMENT

You might have set out some general ideas about what makes a good school: for example, an experienced and enthusiastic staff, good relations with parents, a respected headteacher, students whom people living locally regard as well behaved, suitable buildings, adequate resources and so on.

Or you might have been more concerned about what the school produces: its examination results, how it ranks in the local league tables, the breadth of its curriculum, its capacity to stretch bright students, the successes of its ex-pupils.

You could have focused on whether the school engenders responsible attitudes in students, how it regards bullying, how effective are its policies on racism and sexism, whether it is producing socially well-balanced young people, whether it represents a mix of social backgrounds and tries to meet the range of needs they generate.

Perhaps you thought about the school's stated philosophies: its approach to teaching, its arrangements for taking into account children with differing abilities, whether the governors are people whose views match your own, how receptive the school is to new ideas.

■ ■ ■

ACTIVITY 6.3

In your response to Activity 6.2 you probably included a mixture of the criteria listed above, as well as some others. Pause now to make a note of your reference points. In what capacity were you making judgements? Whose benefit did you have in mind? What were the grounds on which some things seemed important and others unimportant? Were there whole aspects which you completely overlooked? If so, what can you deduce about your own stance?

Whether or not you were considering the idea of what makes a good school from the point of view of a parent probably influenced your response. If you were, you may have re-interpreted 'what is a good school' to mean 'is this a school I would be (or would have been) happy to send my daughter or son to?' From whatever standpoint you answered, think now about how many other identities you have which might provide other perspectives on what makes a good school. Make a short list.

Most of us have at least two and perhaps several of the following kinds of identities, all of which could be said to have a direct or indirect interest in the quality of education:

■ close relative or friend of someone who has children in school

■ employer

■ black teacher

■ member of a household which pays taxes

■ shopper who is served by teenagers

■ organizer of a local women's refuge

■ supervisor of young part-time or full-time workers.

Choose one of these and note any additions to your list of criteria. Does this alter your approach?

Make a note of the criteria you would want to add to your list if you adopted the subject position of **social citizen**. The premise of the concept of social citizenship is that there is formal equality among all social citizens.

social citizen

We will return to your responses to this activity in Activity 6.10.

ACTIVITY 6.4

Read Extracts 6.1 and 6.2 which are taken from two guides to choosing a state school, both written before the election of the Labour government in 1997. Make notes in response to these questions:

1   How well do the concerns in these extracts match with the issues which concerned you?

2   Are they closer to one of the four sets of factors listed in the comment that follows Activity 6.1?

3   What assumptions do the extracts make about children, parents and education?

4   In what ways do they construct the reader's position in relation to education?

Extract 6.1   Cox et al.: 'Choosing a state school'

The school that your child attends for the next few years will play an important part in shaping the rest of his or her life. There will be a number of schools to choose from in your area, but how do you go about finding the best one amongst them for your son or daughter?

The world of education is specialized and complicated and most parents have had little experience of it since the day they left school themselves. How can you tell if a school is the best one and the one most likely to provide the kind of education which will be the basis for a good career?

Many factors make up a good school. We mention most of them in the following pages but, of course, not every school can excel at everything. Research shows, however, that there are significant differences among schools, even those in the same neighbourhoods and especially in the big cities. The aim of this book is to help you identify these differences. It describes the kinds of education which you may find locally and your legal rights as a parent to information about schools. It indicates what you should look for when you visit a school, and shows you how to appeal if your child is not awarded a place at the school of your first choice.

The results of external examinations, such as GCSE, are very valuable objective indicators of the standards of a secondary school. They are one amongst a number of criteria on which a school's success can be judged, and we offer others. We believe, however, that it is extremely important to bear examination results in mind when you are choosing a school.

This book is unique in providing parents, for the first time, with a simple and trustworthy method of comparing examination results. Using it, a parent can compare the local school's figures, not just with those of neighbouring schools, but also with the national benchmarks for that type of school. National benchmarks are the national average number of passes per fifth-year pupil for all schools of a particular type. They are given subject by subject and from them you can easily see how, for instance, a school's mathematics department measures up to those in similar schools elsewhere …

Another result of the 1980 Education Act was to give parents a far greater measure of choice among state schools than ever before and to oblige all schools to publish prospectuses containing useful information on which parents can base that choice. Before the Act, parents were often directed to use a particular school or had to plump for a school without knowing very much about it.

Remember that it is now government policy that parents should have much greater say in the education of their children; in effect, as ratepayers and taxpayers, parents are 'customers' of the education service.

We hope that you will find help and advice in this book and with it you will be able to make an informed choice among the schools in your locality. It is worth making the effort; after all, schooldays, once gone, cannot be repeated and you will want to ensure that your child receives the best possible education from them.

(Cox *et al.*, 1989, pp.9–10)

Extract 6.2   Atha and Drummond: 'The good schools guide'

Introduction
Here we are with the fourth edition, by popular request.

Since we first appeared in 1986 there have been a flattering number of guides like ours, some in misleadingly similar form. However, as far as we know we are the only guide to fee-paying and state schools which is completely independent. Most other books are funded by schools to some extent, either directly, by charging money for including the school in the book, or indirectly, e.g. by advertising. Our guide dares tell you what it's *really* like – does the headmaster have a limp handshake, is the wallpaper peeling, does the place smell of cabbage, is the Geography master out of control, are the results cooked up?

This time round we have observed an amoeba-like shifting as schools struggle to find their identity and niche in the current climate …

We detect distinct signs of strain as heads endlessly have to project a positive successful public face at odds with the facts. Economy with the truth is everywhere – over numbers in total, numbers in the Sixth Form: 'one or two leave at Sixth Form' is headspeak for eighteen at last count and still leaving. Numbers to Oxbridge. Numbers of subjects (and 'options') genuinely on offer. League tables can be accidentally on purpose filled in so A–D reads A–B …

How to read this book
Read between the lines. For obvious reasons we have had to be mealy-mouthed at times. For example, 'keen' could mean just that, or it may mean enthusiastic but not actually very good. 'Lots of' may mean heaps of whatever it is, or that we are reserving judgement. The curate's egg is still with us. 'Sport not worshipped' could mean they don't play games when it's wet – and couldn't care less when they lose. 'Competitive' might imply precisely the opposite. 'Traditional' has to be seen in context. Could mean just that; or it may be time-warped.

Numbers of pupils are approximate throughout – some Heads appear to give us 'projected' figures (i.e., wishful thinking). In any case, numbers change daily, particularly in today's climate …

What the league tables don't tell you
League tables have caused a lot of agony and misunderstanding. As raw statistics, they are more or less meaningless. You will observe, for a start, that results swing wildly according to which newspaper you happen to look at. Among other things they don't tell you:

1. The pupils' I.Q: two Ds for some pupils is a triumph of wonderful teaching.

2. The pupils' background: how much help/support are they getting at home?

3. The school's background: is it academically selective or mixed ability? How many are on Assisted Places/scholarships? Size of class and ratio of staff to pupils – and the whole question of teaching facilities, resources, funding (books, labs, space, etc.).

(Atha and Drummond, 1994, pp.vii–viii, xi, xiv)

Extract 6.1 is obviously very close to the concerns in the comment that follows Activity 6.2. My subject position as reader is constructed as that of a parent who is a consumer of education. My responsibility in that subject position is to take this critical opportunity to do the best for my child, and I am assured that this means sending him or her to a school with a good published examination performance.

Extract 6.2 takes a broader view, is cautious about examination league tables and is ready to include opinionated judgements in its assessment of schools. But its construction of the reader as subject is similar: a consumer of education who is a parent and who is acting in the best interests of his or her child.

■ ■ ■

Using your own views and experiences in this way may have helped you to deepen your understanding of the ways in which our views and experiences are themselves socially constructed; that is, they are produced in a wider social and cultural context. Comparison and contrast with the views and assumptions contained in the two extracts also illustrated that our individual views and experiences are only *partial*; that is, they emerge within the context of the specific social positions we occupy and the identities we adopt. This is why **Clarke and Cochrane (1998)** stress that a social scientific approach to questions of social policy requires adopting the stance of a 'sceptical stranger'. Becoming a 'sceptical stranger' enables us to both question and challenge our own assumptions and those of others, including assumptions found in academic and social policy texts. It also makes us more able to discern the processes by which we are 'made into' subjects.

The issue of choice of schools, and the related matter of selection, are themselves processes by which we are 'made into' subjects, but this raises two important questions:

1 Who are the subjects of education?

2 How has it come about that parents are constructed as consumers of education?

The rest of this chapter tries to answer these questions by describing the restructuring of secondary schooling from 1944 to the present day, and the contested conceptions of whom and what education is for.

3 The education settlement and the collapse of consensus

Education was a keystone of the four post-Second World War settlements. The term 'education settlement' is not being used here to imply a distinct, fifth settlement, but to refer to the realization of the four settlements in the area of education. The introduction of free secondary education for all, provided by the state, was a critical moment in the formation of a welfare state. As Chapter 1 noted, connections drawn between education, social citizenship, equality of opportunity and social mobility were prominent and powerful. Ignorance was one of Beveridge's five giant evils. In fact the consensus which emerged on the importance of free secondary education for all had a number of quite different sources. For Beveridge, ignorance was an evil 'which no democracy can afford among its citizens' (1942, p.59). The development of human capital in pursuit of international competitive advantage was another driving force. For others, the promise of open access to plentiful jobs, with equal opportunity for occupational and social mobility based on merit, was central. In other quarters, securing social order and a sense of nationhood were vital if deference, hierarchy and class barriers were to accede to merit and mobility. As we shall see, all these priorities were at times visible in negotiating how schooling should develop, and were often in some tension with one another.

3.1 Settling for bipartism

This section looks at the three aspects of restructuring introduced in Section 1: the structures of education, the social organization of schooling, and the construction of educational subjects.

Extract 6.3 is taken from a report which heavily influenced the social organization of schooling. The introduction of compulsory free secondary education and the duty placed on the state to make provision was the greatest single innovation of the 1944 Education Act. But, significantly, the form it should take was left unspecified. In practice, state provision was already extensive but incomplete, and based on a bipartite system of grammar and secondary schools. The Norwood Committee had been set up to consider the secondary curriculum and examinations, but commented more extensively on school organization.

ACTIVITY 6.5

Read Extract 6.3, which is taken from the Norwood Report published in 1943. Pay particular attention to:

■ how Norwood views educational subjects;

■ the conception of ability with which the report is working;

■ the implications of this approach for the construction of subjects.

Extract 6.3 Norwood: 'Curriculum and examinations in secondary schools'

The evolution of education has in fact thrown up certain groups, each of which can and must be treated in a way appropriate to itself. Whether such groupings are distinct on strictly psychological grounds, whether they represent types of mind, whether the differences are differences in kind or in degree, these are questions which it is not necessary to pursue. Our point is that rough groupings, whatever may be their ground, have in fact established themselves in general educational experience, and the recognition of such groupings in educational practice has been justified both during the period of education and in the after-careers of the pupils.

For example, English education has in practice recognized the pupil who is interested in learning for its own sake, who can grasp an argument or follow a piece of connected reasoning, who is interested in causes, whether on the level of human volition or in the material world, who cares to know how things came to be as well as how they are, who is sensitive to language as expression of thought, to a proof as a precise demonstration, to a series of experiments justifying a principle: he is interested in the relatedness of related things, in development, in structure, in a coherent body of knowledge. He can take a long view and hold his mind in suspense; this may be revealed in his work or in his attitude to his career. He will have some capacity to enjoy, from an aesthetic point of view, the aptness of a phrase or the neatness of a proof. He may be good with his hands or he may not; he may or may not be a good 'mixer' or a leader or a prominent figure in activities, athletic or other.

Such pupils, educated by the curriculum commonly associated with the Grammar School, have entered the learned professions or have taken up higher administrative or business posts …

Again, the history of technical education has demonstrated the importance of recognizing the needs of the pupil whose interests and abilities lie markedly in the field of applied science or applied art …

The various kinds of technical school were not instituted to satisfy the intellectual needs of an arbitrarily assumed group of children, but to prepare boys and girls for taking up certain crafts – engineering, agriculture and the like. Nevertheless it is usual to think of the engineer or other craftsman as possessing a particular set of interests or aptitudes by virtue of which he becomes a successful engineer or whatever he may become.

Again, there has of late years been recognition, expressed in the framing of curricula and otherwise, of still another grouping of pupils, and another grouping of occupations. The pupil in this group deals more easily with concrete things than with ideas. He may have much ability, but it will be in the realm of facts …

The time has come, we believe, when the real meaning of secondary education, the significance of child-centred education, the value of the Grammar School tradition, the difficulties of the present Secondary Schools should all be recognized and admitted. This means that within a framework of secondary education the needs of the three broad groups of pupils which we discussed earlier should be met within three broad types of secondary education, each type containing the possibility of variation and each school offering alternative courses which would yet keep the school true to type. Accordingly we would advocate that there should be three types of education, which we think of as the secondary Grammar, the secondary Technical, the secondary Modern, that each type should have such parity as amenities and conditions can bestow; parity of esteem in our view cannot be conferred by administrative decree nor by equality of cost per pupil; it can only be won by the school itself.

(Norwood quoted in McLure, 1968, pp.201–3)

COMMENT

The Norwood Report views educational subjects as highly differentiated. It avoids explicitly attributing difference to biology, but views it as inevitable and so by implication as naturally rather than socially created. This follows principles established much earlier in state provision (see **McCoy, 1998**). Differences are portrayed as explicit, falling into quite rigidly bounded and hierarchical categories. The Report begins from an essentialist view of the individual (see **Saraga, 1998b**), a view that sees people as born with fixed abilities and unlikely to vary or develop significantly beyond them. According to the Norwood Report there are just three broad categories of individuals. Within this conceptual framework pupils would be constructed as principally of academic, technical or 'general' ability. The Report argues that a tripartite social organization of schooling, consisting of grammar, technical and secondary modern schools, will meet the needs of the three broad categories of individuals. There is a discourse of ability running through this extract from the Norwood Report; that is, a distinctive set of linked and deeply embedded ideas and meanings about what ability is, how it is to be understood, and what follows from these meanings. This discourse shapes the Norwood Report's ideas about how schooling should be organized socially and the way in which it conceptualizes the purposes and possibilities of schooling. In practice, tripartism was never effectively realized. Technical schools were rare, and the key division remained between grammar and secondary modern schools – in effect, a bipartite system.

tripartite

discourse of ability

bipartite

■ ■ ■

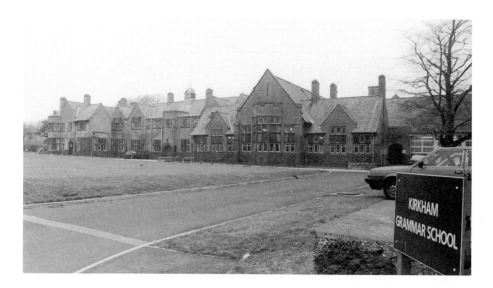

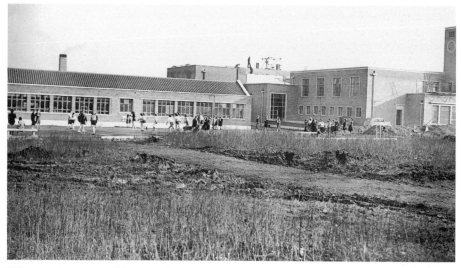

What are the recognizable signs of secondary modern schools and grammar schools? What do they signify?

219

Bipartism closed off children from particular backgrounds from highly valued and resourced schools. The effect of the Norwood Report was to differentiate and exclude, at a time when expansion allowed for greater inclusion. The 1944 Act, celebrated for its inclusiveness, allowed these exclusions to proliferate by making no recommendations on social organization. By building on existing class divisions underpinning the old bipartite system, the guarantee of secondary education for all actively masked the new forms of inequality it was institutionalizing. The architect of the Act was R.A. Butler, Conservative minister in the wartime coalition. That a Labour and Conservative coalition could agree on a selective system is characteristic of the political settlement. Education was embedded within a political settlement based on compromise and alliance. The social democratic consensus was at its earliest stages, and the advance of universal secondary education was a sufficient cause for unity. The forces in the alliance were delicately balanced, and it is far from clear that the Labour Party of the time was hostile to tripartism (see Lawson and Silver, 1985). As Carr and Hartnett (1996) point out, successive ministers of education well into the 1950s actively supported the selective system as a means of providing differentiated educated labour, and securing economic advantage.

3.2 The evolution of the education settlement: comprehensivization

The events surrounding the 1944 Act, and the tensions and paradoxes they embodied, illustrate the complex interplay between the social, political, economic and organizational aspects of the settlement. The origins of Norwood and of the Act were as much political and economic as they were social. Competition and the concern for nation-building were powerful influences. The pursuit of a skilled workforce and a sense of nationhood were driving forces, as they had been for earlier reforms (see **McCoy, 1998**). The expectation that universal education might promote social equality became prominent later, as the consensus evolved. Extract 6.4, from an academic history of democracy and education, describes an important turn in that evolution.

Extract 6.4 Carr and Hartnett: 'Education and the struggle for democracy'

By the middle of the 1950s, the tripartite system was beginning to lose credibility for a number of reasons. One was the growing complaints of primary school teachers that the eleven-plus examination, by forcing them to 'coach for the test', was having a disastrous effect on the primary curriculum. Another was the increasing doubts about the validity of intelligence testing as a basis for selection. Psychologists began to question whether the tests could measure general intelligence in a way which avoided cultural bias or remained divorced from social influences. By 1957, the British Psychological Society had to concede that it was not possible to predict accurately the educational potential of pupils by measuring their intelligence at the age of 11. In their view 'intelligence' was not static and fixed, but could develop through education. Intelligence tests reflected previous educational experience rather than innate intellectual endowment ...

These psychological criticisms were reinforced by a series of sociological studies which brought to light the extent to which the tripartite system was itself enmeshed in social factors and had done less than was thought to promote more equal educational opportunities for working-class pupils in it. For example, *Early Leaving*, published in 1954, found that there was an over-representation of middle-class children in grammar schools and of unskilled working-class children in secondary modern schools. In the grammar school sample examined by the *Early Leaving* inquiry, there should have been 927 unskilled working-class pupils. In fact there were only 436 and, of these, two-thirds left with less than three O-level passes ... These findings were reinforced and extended by other influential studies: *Social Class and Educational Opportunity*, conducted by Floud, Halsey and Martin (1957); Hoggart's *The Uses of Literacy* (1957); Bernstein's work on language and class (1958); Jackson and Marsden's *Education and the Working Class* (1962); and Douglas's *The Home and the School* (1964) ... These studies not only demonstrated the failure of grammar schools to benefit children from working-class backgrounds, but also began to raise questions about the complexity of the interaction between home culture and school culture and the ways in which educational achievement was still mediated through the 'grammar school tradition' that derived from the nineteenth-century class-based educational system. The Floud study, for example, revealed that opportunities for working-class boys were not 'strikingly different from what they were before 1945'. Douglas's work, which demonstrated 'the effects of a variety of domestic influences upon children's school performance' ... was used by Crosland in his book *The Future of Socialism* (1956), and influenced his policy when he became Minister for Education in the 1964 Labour government ...

By the end of the 1950s the scientific 'objectivity' of intelligence tests could no longer be seriously defended and the political legitimacy of the tripartite system of secondary education began to crumble. What had, in 1944, been a relatively unquestioned way for furthering the democratizing trend towards 'secondary education for all' had itself become highly questionable, and it was no longer self-evident that a meritocratic system of education was any more democratic than the class-based aristocratic system that it had replaced. In this climate, the movement to do away with all forms of 'separatism' and 'differentiation' and to reorganize secondary schools in accordance with the 'comprehensive' principle of single **comprehensive** non-selective schools offering a common educational experience to all pupils began to gather force. In the 1960s the Labour Party, and then the Labour government, announced plans to end selection at age 11, and in July 1965 it set this policy in motion by issuing the famous Circular 10/65 which requested all local authorities to submit plans for reorganizing secondary schools on comprehensive lines. Despite the fact that it had no direct legal force, the impact of the Circular was considerable, and a large number of local authorities of all political persuasions and from all regions of England and Wales adopted and implemented comprehensive plans.

References

Bernstein, B. (1958) 'Some sociological determinants of perception', *British Journal of Sociology*, vol.IX, pp.159–74.

Central Advisory Council for Education (1954) *Early Leaving*, London, HMSO.

Crosland, C.A.R. (1956) *The Future of Socialism*, London, Cape.

Douglas, J.W.B. (1964) *The Home and the School*, London, MacGibbon and Kee.

Floud, J., Halsey, A.H. and Martin, F.M. (1957) *Social Class and Educational Opportunity*, London, Heinemann.

Hoggart, R. (1957) *The Uses of Literacy*, Harmondsworth, Penguin.

Jackson, B. and Marsden, D. (1966) *Education and the Working Class*, Harmondsworth, Penguin.

(Carr and Hartnett, 1996, pp.104–5)

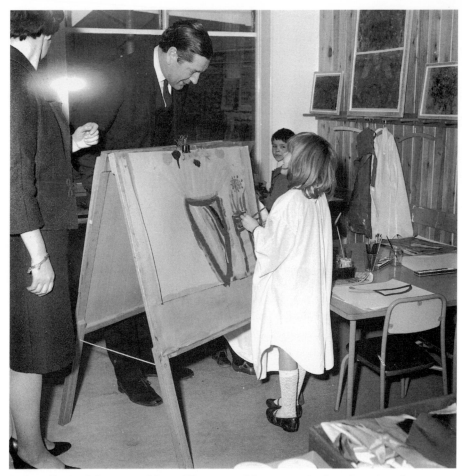

Anthony Crosland, Secretary of State, Education and Science, at the formal opening of a new open-plan primary school in 1967

Carr and Hartnett's account conveys a sense of why the post-war period is referred to as one of consensus. There is a strong impression of an evolving rational debate. It is as though the principles of universalism enshrined in the 1944 Act are steadily being taken a stage further in response to well-founded realizations that they did not produce the advancements intended. Debate amongst social scientists directly influenced policy development. 'Scientific' research refined understandings about intelligence and demonstrated under-representation of particular categories of children in élite schools. This is the classical model of reformist social democracy at work: progressive, consensual social engineering based on hard evidence. Much of the rationale for comprehensivization was based on wastage of talent, unfair bias against 'bright' working-class children (especially boys), and the potential benefits of the new system to the skills needs of the economy, and maintaining the UK's international competitive edge. Once again the requirements of nationhood are integrally entwined with social organization and the way schools construct subjects.

Extract 6.4 suggests that discourses of ability were superseded by discourses **meritocracy** of meritocracy, that is, advancement on the basis of achievement. These saw intelligence as changing, not fixed, and recognized the possibilities of cultural bias in assessing merit. Despite this significant shift, the major turn from selective to comprehensive schooling was achieved within the terms of the political settlement: no legislation was needed, and the vast majority of Conservative local authorities complied. One interpretation of this is that the discourses of ability were untouched by the research findings. The academic underpinnings of the shift may have questioned the predictive value of intelligence testing, or its cultural neutrality, but they did not abandon the essentialist tenets that made individual performance and measurable ability touchstones of meritocracy. As a result, the pro-comprehensive lobby turned out to be a very broad church which included traditionalists who saw it as little more than a fairer and more efficient version of bipartism under the roof of one school. Hence the consensus on education continued into the early years of the comprehensive era without challenge to its premises about the social order. Just as the original motivations and purposes of universalism were ambiguous, so too were the steps towards greater social equity. As such, they were conceived in different ways by actors with significantly differing priorities. Contestation began only when the struggles of one set of interests began to impact upon the priorities of another.

3.3 The beginnings of unsettlement: the attack on comprehensives and progressivism

By the early 1970s most of the state selective system had been dismantled. Comprehensive schools were in place in almost all local authorities. But struggles over education had not been confined to selective schooling. There had long been an awareness that ending selection was not sufficient to alter the construction of unequal subject positions. The conceptions of inequality which occupied reformers were principally those of class and social mobility. The construction of gendered and racialized subject positions had not begun to be tackled. There was also a growing awareness that the culture of schools, the forms of knowledge schools transmitted, and the assumptions about curricula, reproduced unequal subject positions. Some kinds of curricula and some modes of teaching were increasingly recognized to correspond closely to the knowledge and expectations of some social groups. Progressivism sought to redress this balance by developing curricula and teaching methods which were more familiar and of greater interest to groups which traditional approaches tended to disadvantage. These movements had gained sufficient influence by the late 1960s to prompt a strong reaction. Extract 6.5 is taken from one of the Black Papers in Education, an extensive series of short articles published between 1969 and 1977 by groups of right wing academics, educationalists and others opposed to comprehensivism and progressivism.

progressivism

ACTIVITY 6.6

Read Extract 6.5, 'Why comprehensives fail', which is taken from *Black Paper 1975: The Fight for Education*. As you read it, make notes on the following questions:

1   How does the author conceptualize educational subjects?

2   What is his interpretation of the principles of comprehensivization?

3   In what ways do the ideas in this extract reflect the collapse of the consensus?

4   In what ways are ideas of ability and differentiation part of its argument?

Extract 6.5 Green: 'Why comprehensives fail'

In 1956 when I moved to teach in a newly opened, purpose-built comprehensive school, we were all, I believe, inspired and informed by the need to establish real equality of opportunity in education. Most of us saw the lack of this as an area of concern which was not being satisfied by the tripartite system, because we were unable to ignore the increasing evidence of high academic and creative potential in the secondary modern and technical schools. We believed that the comprehensive school could go some way to help to avoid the creation of a divided society; not that we could by a different pattern of organization create the ideal of Christian brotherliness, but we expected that, at least, a real and mutual appreciation between the different strata of the social system might result. In academic and social terms we hoped that the traditions of excellence, integrity, altruism, and sense of service established by the grammar schools could inform the day-by-day school life of all children, as we thought these ideals were at the very root of quality in education …

Equality of opportunity – a realizable and common-sense objective – has over the past decade been replaced by the objective of *equality*, at the same time a political and biological absurdity. The reorganized school system has been seen as a way of achieving this aim, with disastrous effects on curricula, and standards of achievement in every respect. Is it now acceptable that the overall academic achievement in Manchester schools as measured by the C.S.E. and by G.C.E. 'O' and 'A' levels should be much lower in the reorganized situation? All men should be equal in the eyes of the law and are so in the eyes of God, but any schoolmaster of even limited experience will tell you that the great joy of his work lies in the differences – academic, social, creative, emotional – between children. It is right that compensatory programmes should be implemented and used to redress social deprivation, but we make a grave mistake, as many amateur educationists have done, if we imagine that any system of programmes will eliminate intrinsic natural differences between children – some children are better at some activities than others. This is an inescapable fact:

> To be given equality of opportunity is the right of every child: to expect equal capacity to make use of this opportunity runs counter to common sense and experience. In fact, it has harmful consequences because such expectation is bound to engender a sense of failure.
>
> (M. Kellmer Pringle, *Able Misfits*)

The comprehensive school, like any school, should recognize this fact and work with it, ensuring that the uniqueness of the individual is preserved as far as is possible, and ensuring that all children are made to feel that justice is being done to them and everyone else, and that they are valued for what they are and for what they have to offer, whatever it be. Regrettably, comprehensive schools, because many of them have no recognizable academic goal, have a distorted picture of enrichment/compensatory programmes and much of our education over the past decade has been steered away from the able towards the average and less than average. We are, and have been, exchanging excellence for mediocrity and in the process are beginning to create a pool of frustration and deprivation among able children:

> In spite of popular prejudice there is, or there should be, no insuperable conflict between equality as a principle of justice and inequality as a fact of genetics. In education equal opportunity means equal opportunity to make the most of differences that are innate. The ideal is a free and fair chance to each individual not to rise to the same rank in life as everyone else, but to

develop the peculiar gifts and virtues with which he is endowed – high ability if he possesses it, if not, whatever qualities of body, mind and character are latent within him.

(Sir Cyril Burt, 1962)

The supporters of the notion of equality have been reinforced by a persistent, vociferous anti-intellectual faction most evident in comprehensive schools, some universities and among politically motivated educationists. 'Academic', 'intellectual', have become almost pejorative terms; 'formal', 'traditional', words of abuse; 'progressive', 'forward-looking', words of divine revelation. Teachers as a group have been brainwashed into thinking that there must be something wrong with them if they are interested in the needs of the able, of preserving standards of learning and attainment, of believing that things were not always badly done thirty years ago. However, the writing is on the wall for all to see; the flight from the reorganized, maintained sector has not only begun, it is becoming a flood. Instead of introducing doctrinal legislation in a panic-stricken way, our administrators need to examine very closely the reasons which are impelling so many parents to choose to spend quite considerable sums of money, in addition to their taxes, to send their children to schools out of the maintained system. The root causes are a profound disquiet about academic and social standards; about learning and discipline; about culture and anarchy. There is evidence in London and elsewhere of increasing consumer resistance to 'progressive', 'do-your-own-thing' secondary schools, be they never so well endowed with buildings and equipment. Parents are preferring neighbouring schools where the physical conditions are perhaps less prepossessing but where the atmosphere is one of discipline and where learning takes place. It is a sad fact that many parents have to endure for their children 'educational' practices of which they do not approve, being fobbed off with comments about 'learning readiness', 'self-awareness', 'self-development' as substitutes for the fundamental securities of teaching and learning. Parents in this situation, who can afford to, choose the private school.

(Green, 1975, pp.24–5)

COMMENT

Green was a comprehensive school headteacher who had rejected the old tripartite system because it sometimes allocated pupils to inappropriate schools for their abilities and repressed the full development of talent. He also valued the mixing of the 'different strata of the social system' which comprehensive schools brought. But neither of these diminished his essentialist belief in innate differences, and in the legitimacy of schools reproducing differentiated, stratified subjects. He attacks progressivism, utilizing the discourses of individualism, the pursuit of excellence, the power of parents as consumers, and the exercise of choice. These ideas were later critical in restructuring education.

Extract 6.5 epitomizes the shift from consensus to contestation in education. The consensus which produced first a selective system, then a largely comprehensive one, was not sufficiently resilient and flexible to accommodate some of the challenges posed to education during the late 1960s and early 1970s. Progressivism, as it was labelled, and some other challenges from the so-called 'radical' educationalists, were not content with what they interpreted to be the unstated social purposes of education. In particular, they fundamentally questioned the ways in which the processes of schooling (that is, being educated in institutions which had specific values and methods) constructed highly differentiated educational subjects. Deep rifts began to open up over social purposes, which had been concealed during a period of consensus. Much of the growing call for a return to traditionalism went much further than Green's essay, demanding outright rejection of comprehensive schools. On morality, a central claim of the Black Paper authors was that progressivism and comprehensivization had resulted in a deterioration of behavioural standards. Similarly, the introduction of modern 'relevant' curricula was viewed as diluting knowledge of tradition and culture. Part of the collapse of consensus turned on the Right's reassertion of traditionalist conceptions of morality which were largely grounded in Christian doctrine. Taken together, these criticisms make explicit the important role of the curriculum and culture of schools in the construction of subjects.

■ ■ ■

These attacks on comprehensive organization also show some of the early signs of profound divisions within the Conservative Party, many of which were to become significant tensions in the development of its education policies. Green's advocacy of parental choice signals the emergence of neo-liberal thinking in policy-making (see Chapter 2). On the other hand, his and others' pursuit of traditional values represents the conservative strand which continued alongside neo-liberalism in Conservative policy.

4   The discourse of markets and choice

The history of the social organization of schooling repeatedly finds political parties taking unexpected positions. The 1940s' Labour Party accepted the selective plans of a Conservative minister. In the 1960s Conservative local education authorities followed Labour directives to adopt comprehensive schools. During the 1970s Margaret Thatcher presided over the largest number of grammar school closures in any period of office. These are precisely the kinds of paradoxes which 'settlements', as provisional balances of powers, produce. As Chapter 1 argued, they are not unified, consistent or monolithic. And settlements cannot contain contradictions indefinitely, nor do they have clearly finite ends. Labour's 1976 Act requiring resistant local education authorities to adopt comprehensive arrangements, and its repeal in 1979 by the Conservative administration, were probably the most significant moments in ending the education consensus, but they were prefigured by struggle, and they were followed by uncertainty and retrospection (see Chitty, 1992; Jones, 1989). Both debate and policy moves were relatively sterile and did little to alter a hybrid system which was obviously the product of past compromises. The crude binary oppositions of comprehensive/selective, equality/quality, universal/élite governed much of the thinking.

The turning point was the New Right neo-liberal thinking described in Chapter 2. Commitments to 'rolling back the state', reducing public expenditure, and promoting free choice in a competitive environment began to have their impact. In the early 1980s these ideas were applied to education, mainly through the work of a number of think-tanks, including that of the Adam Smith Institute.

ACTIVITY 6.7

Read Extract 6.6, which is taken from an influential document produced by the Adam Smith Institute. As you read consider the following questions:

1   In what ways is the power of professionals portrayed?

2   In what ways are subjects constructed in relation to education?

3   What clues are there to a 'discourse of the market' at work here?

4   What is the social organization of schooling implied by this extract?

Extract 6.6 Adam Smith Institute: 'The omega file'

Producer capture

The problems which beset state education share a common origin with those that incapacitate the other nationalized service industries: the phenomenon of producer capture. When any service is put under political direction and control, the satisfaction of political objectives becomes more important than the satisfaction of consumer interests. Whether the administration is done directly by legislators or through a quango, consumers have little opportunity to express their views, and almost none if the service is a virtual state monopoly ...

Yet without this source of consumer pressure, it is impossible for a service to be run in the interests of customers, even by the most public-spirited administration. An assured income leads to complacency about existing practices and a failure to innovate. Political fears about strikes or unemployment generate lax labour relations and overmanning. Political generosity in wage settlements leads to the (less obvious) trimming of capital replacement. Administrative overheads grow while services often decline.

Those who work in such an industry represent a very concentrated and united interest group, and so they have much more power in the political processes that decide the organization of state industries than do ordinary members of the public who pay for and consume their services. Producer capture – whereby the service comes to be organized more to suit the interests of producers than consumers – is therefore a common and perhaps inevitable feature of state concerns.

Producer capture in education

Education has proved easier for the producers (teachers and administrators) to capture than other industries, partly because its shortcomings can be disguised by jargon. The school with poor examination results can claim that knowledgeable educationalists nowadays hold 'school spirit' or 'awareness' more important. Although the consumers (parents and children) demand examination passes and other measurable achievements from their schools, education producers are able to argue that they, as 'professionals', know better; and they are able to substitute completely new values for those of their 'unqualified' parental customers ...

Unlike private schools, which operate on their own as business units, state schools are enmeshed in a suffocating web of bureaucracy which greatly curtails the flexibility and freedom of action of each school. Local education bureaucracies determine many of the details of how schools should be run, provide the ancillary services (often at very high cost), help plan the curriculum, and generally take many of the decisions about allocation of time and resources within each individual school. Teachers' salaries, grades, conditions, and hours, and many other important decisions are taken centrally.

The result of this centralization of decision-making is that schools in any education area – and indeed nationally – tend to become more similar as time goes on, denying parents any escape from the system at all. If schools retained more independence, then parents would be able to express their preferences by rejecting some schools and sending their children to one whose methods they prefer ... At least there would be *some* prospect of assessing consumer preferences if each school were more of an autonomous unit; but today there is none.

Parental control through school boards

They key to successful reform of the state school system is for parents to be given more power and responsibility. There is a need for increased accountability of teachers and schools to the parents, increased parental involvement in the schools themselves, and more diversity in the education system. Increased parental responsibility, involvement, and choice will encourage improvements in educational standards, since all parents want their children to receive a good education that will qualify them for good jobs. Our school system must be accountable to them if they are to ensure that this happens ...

Choice between schools

Even if parents had no choice on the question of which school their children must attend, the new school board concept would undoubtedly bring rewards in terms of better management and accountability of education producers. But the greatest benefits would be seen only if parents were given the choice in deciding between different schools. Only then would a successful and innovative school board receive its just reward in terms of lengthening application lists; while falling rolls would signify to other boards that there was something wrong with their management and with the appeal of the school. In other words, for good management incentives to prevail, there must be no fixed catchment for each school from which parents cannot escape.

(Adam Smith Institute, 1984/5, pp.269, 271, 274)

COMMENT

Extract 6.6 marks the beginnings of an important stage in the restructuring of education. Neo-liberal market theorists questioned what they viewed as the high cost and poor productivity of public services in the document, while competition between education providers was envisaged as the route to efficiency and excellence. They argued that a complete overhaul of how education was funded and controlled would be needed, supposedly to put the consumer in charge, and subject providers to the rigours of the market.

The extract also heralds the reconstruction of the subjects of education, in a dramatic shift from children (as pupils) being constructed as the subject of education, to parents (as consumers) being constructed as the subjects of education. This is a critical stage in the transformation of how education is understood, and what its purposes are as part of a larger constellation of welfare provision. Responsibility and control are placed on an entirely different basis. Under the existing arrangements, the key relationship had been between professional (teacher) and client (pupil). In the old organizational settlement teachers exercised professional judgement to decide how and what pupils needed to be taught, and what was in their best interests and those of the wider society. These proposals make parents the arbiters of their children's needs, and the people responsible for ensuring that their needs are met, through their capacity to exercise choice in a competitive market. Schools would be obliged by force of market pressures to provide forms of education which met the preferences of parents.

■ ■ ■

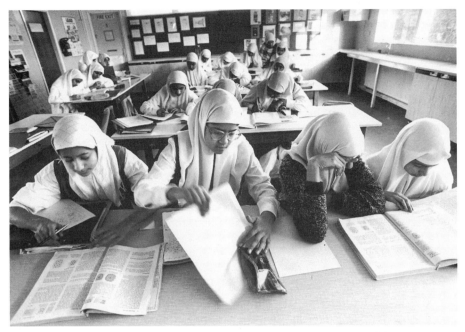

An Islamic school in Yorkshire. Acknowledging difference or fostering separation? Parents are assumed to be the consumers of education, acting in the best interests of their children

Both these intertwined narratives – on restructuring and on the construction of subjects – became part of a powerful set of discourses. Like all discourses they make alternative interpretations seem implausible, because they set a framework within which such alternatives necessarily fare badly. The logic of markets is a powerful discourse. It embodies assumptions which seem unassailable without substituting a different logic. It is taken as read that the primary purpose of education is to provide a service which satisfies its consumers. Parents are assumed to be the consumers, acting in the best interests of their children. It is assumed that they are the best arbiters of what their children need and what a school can provide. It assumes that parents are informed and rational actors who can tell a good school from a bad one. It assumes that parents are best placed to judge which kinds of education will serve the needs of the citizens and employees of the future. It assumes that parents are well placed to govern schools.

So long as these assumptions go uncontested, the chain of reasoning acquires immense power by association with other more familiar market discourses. But once we begin to unpack them, a number of questions arise:

- What does the shift of power from teachers acting in the interests of clients to parents acting as consumers imply?

- If parents are the consumers of education, why is it funded by *all* taxpayers?

- How do parents know what is best for their children?

- What happens to children whose parents are incompetent consumers?

- How does this model of consumption take account of the diversity of educational subjects?

The Omega File proposals signalled the end of the last vestiges of the consensus in education. As Chapter 2 showed, the political, economic and social settlements had already been largely undone by this time. The one settlement on which little had changed was the organizational settlement. In a range of areas of welfare, the power of professionals and the bureaucracy within which their power was embedded, remained largely intact. This bureau-professional axis (see Chapter 2) represented a serious impediment to restructuring. There were two major obstacles. The first was the exclusive, confidential professional–client relationship. In education the key subject in the relationship had to become the parent rather than the child, to challenge the authority of the teacher-professional, and to legitimize the claim to rational action by parents repositioned as consumers. Second, the argument had to shift from the supremacy of specialist knowledge of educational processes (the teacher's) to the supremacy of knowledge of the child as an individual (the parent's). This entailed an appeal to the rights of parents to shape their offspring as they preferred, according to their values and ambitions for them, and not those of professionals. In other words, the shift required refocusing from *the public to the individual good.*

The Omega File attacked the distributions of power embodied by the old organizational settlement. Teachers were denigrated as self-interested and unaccountable. And while self-interest is normalized as part of the discourse of market relations, and elsewhere is celebrated as the engine of progress, it is seen in this instance as invalidating teachers' claims to professionalism. Other routes to breaking bureau-professional power entailed the public questioning of the competency of teachers, allegations of the failure of the comprehensive system, the down-skilling of teacher's professional knowledge through the exclusion of theory in favour of more instrumental forms of initial training and in-service staff development and so on (see, for example, Whitty *et al.,* 1987; Furlong, 1992; Barton *et al.,* 1994; Lawn, 1996). Local education authorities came under attack as part of the wider attack on local democracy described in Chapter 2. They were said to be part of the bureau-professional power bloc, controlling the character of local schools, causing high public spending, and imposing 'politicized' values which challenged some of the key assumptions of social relations and normalities.

Publications such as *The Omega File* had a significant impact not only by reconceiving how educational subjects were constructed, but also on the social organization of schooling. Interestingly, the words 'ability' and 'selection' do not appear. There is no sense of differentiation by ability being significant in the proposed new arrangements. No professional or bureaucrat has the task of deciding what kinds of schools there should be, or who should attend which. Market powers of co-ordination – the matching of supply and demand, energized by self-interest – will decide. The assumption here is that the market is a value-free allocator. Any differentiation is not by assessment of abilities, but by which parents prefer which type of school, and which schools can command the strongest market position. According to this view selection is a two-way process, in which parents choose schools as well as schools choosing students. Ability may turn out to be the most critical axis of market negotiation, but that will fall out of the myriad negotiations which allocate each child to a school place.

This neo-liberal strand of New Right thinking marked a complete break with many of the defining characteristics of state educational provision. It brought into question the terms of all four settlements: social, political, economic and organizational. It proposed a radical restructuring of funding and organization. It proposed a transformation of the subject position of users of state education. And it very significantly altered the parameters of the social organization of schooling.

5 Simulating the market in schools

The proposals of some New Right think-tanks went considerably further than *The Omega File*. Some advocated complete handover to a market system of funding of schools through vouchers (for example, Seldon, 1986), and free market determination of curricula (Sexton, 1988). The state would make residual provision for those without means to participate in the market. None of these proposals was implemented, but the 1980s' reforms tried to simulate the conditions of markets, choice and competition within the funded state system. Equivalents had to be found for independent entrepreneurial providers, competition over customers and resourcing, and maximization of choice based on market information. The 1988 Education Reform Act achieved an approximation of all of these. Local management of schools (LMS) significantly increased schools' autonomy by making them responsible for budgets and free to set their own budgetary priorities. Accountability for performance shifted from the local education authority to the governing body of each school, which is at liberty to act largely independently of local education authority control, or even to become grant maintained, that is, directly funded by central government.

local management of schools

grant maintained
open enrolment

Competition was facilitated by open enrolment, in which parents could choose their child's school, provided this was compatible with the efficient use of resources within the local education authority area, and provided it catered for the age and, significantly, the 'aptitude' of the child. Schools were given some limited freedom to increase rolls, and were rewarded with numbers-driven funding. Customer choice was to be realized through open enrolment and efforts to increase diversity of provision, through grant maintained schools and city technology colleges. Alongside the private sector and voluntary-aided denominational schools, a mixed economy of education was envisaged which paralleled that in other forms of welfare (see Chapter 7). Schools were required to collect and publish information on regular testing and examination performances and other alleged performance indicators. Parents and the local business community took the majority of places on the governing bodies, at the expense of local education authority and teacher representation.

mixed economy

In what ways do you think the Education Reform Act simulated the market effectively?

In what ways does the Education Reform Act seem likely to fall short of creating market conditions?

The creation of different kinds of schools, with some differences in their curricula, published information and the possibility of parental choice of schools were important steps towards creating market conditions. For schools, the pressure of competition through published league tables and the risk of a downward spiral of falling rolls, reduced funding and staffing, a diminished curriculum, poorer results and further declining enrolment became a real prospect – of the kind which drives performance in any competitive market. But parents' rights as consumers are highly circumscribed by locality and by the physical size of schools. Schools' capacities to benefit from market success are similarly limited. Parents lack spending power, schools lack the power to set their own prices in recognition of market conditions and their place within them. Restructured welfare sites such as education are therefore regarded as quasi-markets – that is, attempts to 'mimic' markets in relationships which are nevertheless managed and regulated by the state (see Le Grand and Bartlett, 1994).

quasi-markets

ACTIVITY 6.8

In the light of your reading so far, make some notes on the following questions:

1 What would be the effect of all parents exercising choice in the way suggested by the two guides to choosing a school (Extracts 6.1 and 6.2)?

2 Which parents would you expect to operate most successfully, and which least?

3 What would be the impact on schools of all parents successfully exercising their powers of choice?

COMMENT

To different degrees both guides encourage parents to aim for the schools with high examination results and other positive indicators, which would result in competition for places. Some parents would be better placed than others to assess performance and act on it. High-attaining schools would become oversubscribed and would be tempted to become selective in order to enhance their performance. Schools whose results are poor would find that the best placed parents locally would pursue alternatives, thus beginning the downward spiral of market failure. So different degrees of power affect which schools and which parents fare well and which do not. **Clarke and Cochrane (1998)** point out that discourses, and the ways in which they shape practice, have to be understood as part of the power relations that prevail in societies. Yet the discourse of markets engenders the belief that markets are open to all to benefit equally.

■ ■ ■

Keep the above questions and the issue of power in mind as you read Extract 6.7. It is written by Ball and his colleagues and is an account of their research into market systems and parental choice in education, after the implementation of the 1988 Education Reform Act.

Extract 6.7 Ball *et al.*: 'Market forces and parental choice: self-interest and competitive advantage in education'

- none of the fifteen secondary schools involved in our study can afford to ignore the marketplace. While some are better placed than others, being oversubscribed, there is an awareness that there is a degree of volatility and fashion in parental choice. And the system of year-on-year funding of schools encourages this sense of anxiety. In our interviews with headteachers the need 'not to be complacent' was pointed up by everyone. The discipline of the market bites. Nonetheless, the logic of the market suggests that those schools which are oversubscribed or working more or less at full capacity have less reason to change what they are currently doing, or at least radically to rethink their current practice, than those schools currently significantly undersubscribed. They are, in general terms at least, satisfying their consumers. However, our research clearly indicates that it is a mistake to see patterns of choice as being solely an expression of educational preference in any simple sense. There is no *simple* relationship between enrolment and quality, as some advocates of choice would have us believe ...

- schools are paying a lot more attention to what parents want for their children's education. Or more precisely what schools *think* that parents want. Or even more precisely what schools think that *some* parents want. In a few cases schools are engaging in crude forms of 'market research' or are consulting public relations firms but for the most part the 'responsiveness' of schools is based upon impressions or the emulation of rivals. (All of this still begs the question as to whether parents always know what is best educationally for their children.)

- the publication of examination league tables and other performance indicators has meant that schools are increasingly keen to attract enrolments from 'motivated' parents and 'able' children who are likely to enhance their relative position in local systems of competition. In a sense there is a shift of emphasis from student needs to student performance: from what the school can do for the student to what the student can do for the school.

- in relation to the above there is increasing evidence of a shift of resources away from students with special needs and learning difficulties. Well established and proven systems of SEN [special educational needs] teaching in schools are being dismantled or much reduced in size. Resources are being directed more towards those students who are most likely to perform well in tests and examinations. The reintroduction of setting and streaming proceeds apace. (This is also driven by the introduction of differentiated syllabuses for GCSE and parts of the National Curriculum.) ...

- by contrast we find that working-class parents are more likely to prefer *the* local school for their children. This in part reflects a more limited knowledge of other schools and the economic and familial constraints within which choice of school is set. School has to be 'fitted' into a set of limitations and expectations related to work roles, family roles, the sexual division of labour and the demands of household organization ... *But locality is also a positive value for many working-class parents.* They want their children to go to a school which is easily accessible and does not involve long and dangerous journeys; a school where friends', neighbours' and relatives' children also go; a school which is a part of their social community, their locality ...

- [the capacity of middle class parents to take advantage of the market] is enhanced both by material resources and the right kind of cultural capital. Material resources confer a number of obvious advantages in the educational market place: (1) They maximize opportunities for transport. The range of schools to choose from is more extensive for parents who can afford to pay for long journeys on public transport or who can use private cars or taxis for awkward routes. Although LEAs provide the financially disadvantaged with free passes, these are not generally valid for travel to out-LEA schools. It is also often the case that middle-class areas tend to be better served by public transport; (2) They allow greater flexibility for moving house and thus greatly extended choice of school, that is 'selection by mortgage' continues to operate; (3) They enable coaching for grammar and private school entrance exams as well as payment of school fees and so give greater access to selective schools; (4) Child care opportunities are enhanced so that where parents have more than one child, they can send their children to schools at a distance from one another ...

- whilst material resources greatly enhance choice, having a certain degree of cultural capital 'in the right currency' is indispensable for playing the market successfully. Having the right kind of cultural capital means being knowledgeable about and familiar with the education system and having the confidence to 'work' it. Those who have always 'done well' out of the system themselves – that is, those who have had a 'good education', got 'good jobs' etc., tend to have more confidence in negotiating it. 'Working the system' involves knowing which strategies to use to maximize one's chances of getting a good deal out of it.

(Ball *et al.*, 1994, pp.16–22)

According to Ball *et al.*, markets are highly selective because of extensive differences in people's powers to exercise consumer rights. Partly because this is a quasi-market, not a 'perfect' economic market, a range of social and cultural factors exerts a powerful influence. The discourses of parental choice and consumer rights mask the capacity of the market to allow schools to choose pupils as a corollary of the right of parents to choose schools. In particular market contexts, either consumer or supplier may have an advantage over the other. For some years there have been consistent reports of schools which are not designated as selective making unofficial use of interviews and other procedures to ensure that their out-catchment recruits will add to the mean performance of the school. A significant proportion of grant maintained schools selects students by ability, and many have formally altered their admissions criteria to increase the proportion of entrants selected since opting out (Dean, 1996). But far more prevalent is the self-selection which enables increasing numbers of typically white middle-class parents to place their children outside their local school's catchment area as official and unofficial selection has grown, leaving others to use local provision.

cultural capital   Ball *et al.* refer to the cultural capital conferred on the children of middle-class parents. This means those aspects of dominant middle-class cultures which correspond to the culture of schools. They range from particular kinds of knowledge and ways of speaking, and understandings about how to negotiate with others, to sense of self (see Bourdieu, 1977). Middle-class parents – particularly white ones – are also said to have advantages of social capital (how they interact, who they know) and economic capital (to pay for travel to school, uniforms, books, etc.). If it is only those with the appropriate capitals who can exercise choice, the trend of market transactions will be towards differentiated schools and selection. And these processes of selection are likely to be more subtle and resilient than the old selection for grammar or secondary modern school was. For every parent who absorbs the discourse of markets, there is a predisposition to accept the optimality of their choice and see it as their own action for which they have responsibility. The sense of having been unfairly judged by a crude system which sorts the able from the rest is reduced. Market outcomes appear to be just desserts determined by impenetrably complex and disinterested processes. Hence the subjects of education, the parents, internalize the rationale for any given outcome and are less inclined to challenge its legitimacy. In practice, of course, parents do feel dissatisfied with the outcome of particular market processes as they affect them and their children, but their objections may not be so easily focused as in an explicitly selective system.

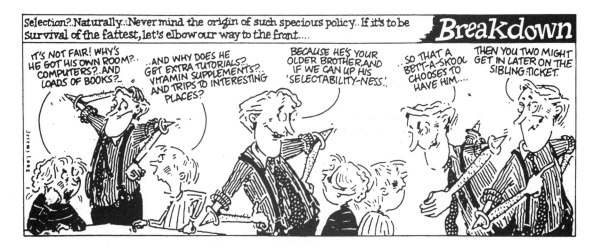

6 Contradictions, contingencies and the power of managers

The effects of the 1988 Education Reform Act are strongly disputed. Research such as that by Ball *et al.* provides important insights but cannot describe the extent of change. There is evidence that the exercise of choice is limited. One survey found that almost 20 per cent of parents did not get their first choice of school (Audit Commission, 1996), and the huge numbers of appeals against non-admission since 1989 (see *Times Educational Supplement*, 1996) almost certainly represent only a small proportion of the parents who were dissatisfied. There is also evidence that many parents do not feel able to interpret data to make an informed choice (Gewirtz *et al.*, 1995), or rely on hearsay about the reputation of schools rather than 'hard' data (Ball and Vincent, 1996). Furthermore, because it prescribes most of what has to be taught in state schools, it can be argued that the national curriculum has seriously curtailed effective choice (see, for example, Sexton, 1988).

Unsuccessful attempts in the mid 1990s to press more schools to opt out, to intensify competition through expansion of grant maintained schools and to establish a grammar school in every town, suggest that the market had not met the aims of its architects. In the eyes of many, despite 18 years in power the Conservative governments of the 1980s and 1990s were unable to transform the structure and social organization of schooling. Their legacy is a hybrid of an enlarged private sector struggling after its 1980s boom; extensive state provision part-centrally controlled; some competition between schools; and a degree of choice for parents which resembles market relations but falls a long way short of them.

This hybrid has resulted in contradictions about how much the state should be involved in educational provision, and whether control should be centralized or localized. The tensions this has produced have resulted in a range of contingent responses which are highly varied locally. The restructuring envisaged by the New Right is incomplete. One explanation is that the structures, discourses and practices of the old settlements are too powerful and too deeply embedded to be overthrown by one ideological shift. An alternative explanation is that the ideologies of the New Right were contradictory. The neo-liberal wing of the

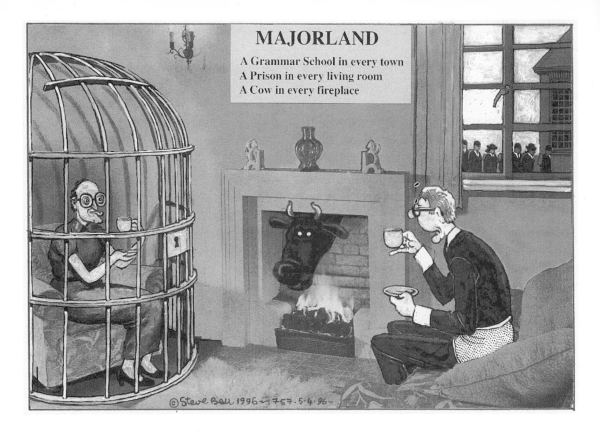

Conservative Party was dedicated to reducing state activity to the minimum compatible with ensuring a safety-net for the seriously disadvantaged. The market was to be given sway in all spheres – not just economic but social, moral and so on. The conservative wing reflected the paternalism and commitment to one nation of traditional conservatism. These two wings were in frequent conflict within the party. Johnson (1991) argues that the 1988 Education Reform Act is the product of a skilful (but less than coherent) political compromise between them, resulting in tensions between the active and the residual state, and between centralization and decentralization. These are important elements of any understanding of restructuring, and they require some exploration of one missing element in the analysis so far: the national curriculum.

The curriculum of any education system has a profound influence on the construction of subject identities, particularly in relation to national belonging and citizenship. Much of the contestation over education as the consensus began to collapse was over the curriculum, and the regimes of discipline and morality which prevailed. In the eyes of many, comprehensivization had, as Extract 6.5 suggested, been accompanied by forms of progressivism which were intended to reduce the advantages of cultural and social capital of white middle-class children, and develop curricula which were either culturally neutral, or which celebrated diverse forms of knowledge, thinking and expression, for example amongst black and Asian children and in working-class culture. These were seen on the Right as compromising the construction of culturally homogeneous educational subjects. In 1978 Conservative MP Norman St John Stevas called for education to enable 'all children … to share and participate in the nation's heritage of cultural and moral values' (quoted in Knight, 1990, p.124). The perceived politicization of the curriculum was also a concern. The curriculum of peace studies, for example, was attacked by another Conservative MP, Olga Maitland, in 1985 as being 'anti-self reliance, anti-initiative, and anti-nation' (quoted in Knight, 1990, p.173). The accumulating response to these concerns was a growing call for a national curriculum. Its introduction was one of the politically less contentious features of the Education Reform Act, with many finding advantage in its potential for standardization and, among other things, improving the employability of the future workforce. But it was also driven by these conservative concerns.

The national curriculum was unprecedented. In its initial form it determined 80 per cent of the school timetable, at a level of detail which radically curtailed teachers' professional autonomy. It excluded a great deal of the curriculum development work of the previous 20 years and had a powerfully conservative influence on the kinds of pedagogy through which it could be taught. The following account highlights the cultural significance of the national curriculum and points to the way in which it constructs subjects.

national curriculum

ACTIVITY 6.9

Read Extract 6.8, which is taken from a chapter in a 1992 Open University course book, *Social and Cultural Forms of Modernity*.

As you read, consider this question: how does the national curriculum construct subjects in relation to national belonging and nationhood?

Extract 6.8 Whitty: 'Education, economy and national culture'

In launching the working group on history, Kenneth Baker, then Secretary of State, stated that 'the programmes of study should have at the core the history of Britain, the record of its past and, in particular, its political, constitutional and cultural heritage' (quoted in *The Times*, 14 January 1989). Attempts to construct a particular sense of national identity, together with a prescribed epistemology to secure adherence to one particular way of reading history, were evident in the debate surrounding the work of the history curriculum working group. Despite recent trends in school history, there were concerted efforts to deny the multiplicity and provisionality of perspectives in favour of an authoritative (or authoritarian) emphasis on 'the facts' ...

Clearly some critics felt that Margaret Thatcher (though not necessarily all ministers or the history working group itself) was trying to embody a version of the nation's past within school history that would construct subjectivities in pupils appropriate to the New Right's political project ...

Neo-conservative concerns are also revealed in other aspects of the debate about the National Curriculum. Particularly interesting are the representations in the debate of the 'others' of Western culture. The Hillgate Group, for example, expressed a concern about the pressure for a multicultural curriculum that 'has been felt throughout the Western world, and most notably in France, Germany, and the United States, as well as in Britain'. They joined with those 'who defend the traditional values of western societies, and in particular who recognize that the very universalism and openness of European culture is our best justification for imparting it, even to those who come to it from other roots' (Hillgate Group, 1987, p.3). While, as we have seen, the Hillgate Group were happy to see the emergence of new and autonomous schools, including Moslem schools, this commitment to market forces was in the context of an insistence that all children 'be provided with the knowledge and understanding that are necessary for the full enjoyment and enhancement of British society'. Nothing, they said, was more important than to 'reconcile our minorities, to integrate them into national culture, and to ensure a common political loyalty, independent of race, creed or colour'. 'Our' culture, being part of the universalistic culture of Europe, 'must not be sacrificed for the sake of a misguided relativism, or out of a misplaced concern for those who might not yet be aware of its strengths and weaknesses' (Hillgate Group, 1987, p.4).

Reference

Hillgate Group (1987) *The Reform of British Education*, London, Claridge Press.

(Whitty, 1992, pp.295, 299)

COMMENT

The brief comments about the national curriculum for history in Extract 6.8 convey a good deal about the ways in which the content of an area of the school curriculum is capable of constructing particular subjectivities. One faction's ambitions in particular (those of the Hillgate Group) recognize the potential of the history curriculum for promoting a sense of Britishness which positions some groups as 'Other', and which requires their adjustment to a dominant version of what it means to belong to this nation. The reference to 'the full enjoyment and enrichment of British society' clearly envisages only one acceptable version of this. Whatever the success of such factions in influencing the history curriculum, Whitty's study led him to the view that developing trends towards plurality, multiplicity and diversity of understandings of nation and national belonging gave way to versions of the past which were presented categorically, and which constructed subjects of a very particular kind.

■ ■ ■

The 1988 Education Reform Act set up a framework of control and management of schools in which local education authorities had a considerably reduced role. At the same time, it created a framework for determining what schools taught and for assessing their performance that gave the central state a considerably enhanced role. While local management of schools was intended to reduce bureaucracy and promote autonomy, diversity and self-reliance, the national curriculum, assessment and inspection entailed bureaucratic complexity, control and imposed standards. State agencies and quangos assumed powers for determining whether schools could opt out, and for funding them directly. But for most schools, control over budgets was devolved, allowing considerable self-determination by the headteacher in particular, as were most powers over the appointment and dismissal of staff, over admissions, and over a wide range of school policies.

Local histories, local political configurations and local social structures have a profound impact on how these contradictions and tensions produce contingent outcomes. It would be hazardous to generalize about the impact of restructuring for the country as a whole. The effects on the social organization of schooling have varied greatly, with some local education authorities completely selective, others completely comprehensive. The impact on the fine-grained multiplicity of experiences which make up the construction of educational subjects is even more difficult to generalize about. The introduction of market reforms undoubtedly had a very wide range of effects, but during the 1980s and 1990s there began to emerge a powerful brake on these diverse effects: managerialism. Managerialism is discussed in Chapter 9 of this book, where it is defined as a set of discourses which draws on a particular knowledge base, legitimates particular goals and underpins a particular ordering of relationships. It has considerably wider meaning than just the power of managers, but it does imply their power to define agendas locally within broad policy frameworks. Headteachers acquire power to determine the interpretation of curricula, the ethos of the school, teaching methods, means of assuring the quality of teaching and so on. They may require the sanction of governors and the co-operation of staff to implement their decisions, but their influence is considerable. However, this increased autonomy in some spheres is circumscribed by centralized regulation in others. This is largely achieved through measures to monitor output, with particular emphasis on adherence to the national curriculum, school performance in assessment published through league tables, inspections, staff appraisal, efficiency targets and so on. In principle, the market, and increased managerial power to interpret broad policies, are intended to result in greater diversity in the character of schools. In practice, managerial use of the same tools and benchmarks tends to reduce diversity (see Gewirtz *et al.*, 1995).

managerialism

Managerialism is the set of relations through which the residue of bureau-professional power is lived out in a world shaped by marketization (Chapter 7 discusses this further). In many respects, managerialism is the reconstitution of the organizational settlement – a new basis on which the forces of professional autonomy are balanced against those of the competitive market. Some commentators see managerialism as the inevitable legacy of incomplete restructuring, the only resolution of tensions and contradictions being to leave each institution to arrive at its own interpretation within given parameters. For others it is a highly provisional set of arrangements, too unstable to survive, because it inherently lacks an underlying vision or set of principles on which to base its drive for efficiency and effectiveness (see Newman and Clarke, 1994). It may be that the vision which takes up where the incomplete processes of restructuring left off is itself coloured by the projects, possibilities and mechanisms which managerialism has come to embody. If a new settlement is possible, which reconciles marketization and some of the abandoned social commitments of the old consensus, it may be one powerfully shaped by managerialism.

7 Inclusion, exclusion, citizens, consumers: the roots of resettlement?

The challenge to forge a welfare resettlement was the major task accepted by the Labour government elected in 1997. Much of the Party's manifesto seemed to capture elements of both the neo-liberal reforms and of the social citizenship commitments of the social democratic consensus, despite the new Labour Party's rejection of the Conservative Right and the Old Left. The Labour Party's manifesto of 1997 contained commitments to the interests of the many not the few, to a

UK of which all feel part, and in which all have a stake, but it also praised the dynamism of the market and advocated enhancing not undermining it. This amounted to 'a commitment to enterprise alongside a commitment to justice' (Labour Party, 1997, pp.1–3). For education this implies commitment to the subject positions of the parent–consumer and the social citizen, two subject positions which are, at least potentially, contradictory. When Tony Blair writes 'what I want for my own children I want for yours' (Labour Party, 1997, p.1) he is apparently fusing his subject position as a parent–consumer, who has choices he is entitled to make, with his subject position as social citizen, concerned for the benefit of all. This fusion nicely captures some of the tensions we have examined in tracing the social organization of school provision from bipartism to the quasi-market. It highlights the question of whether the shift in subject position of parent to that of consumer is compatible with the subject position of children within the professional–client relationship of the old settlements.

ACTIVITY 6.10

Re-read the notes you made in Activities 6.2 and 6.3 and consider the following questions.

1   What subject position did you assume in Activity 6.2: that of a parent or another one?

2   How did the subject position you chose in Activity 6.3 alter your criteria for choosing a school?

3   How did adopting the subject position of 'social citizen' affect your criteria?

COMMENT

It is clear that parenthood is only one of a number of possible subject positions from which to decide what makes a good education. Different positions imply different views and different interests in the outcome. Employers, for example, might have quite specific and narrow preferences for skills. A women's refuge organizer would be likely to stress some social priorities. It could be argued that the only position which encompasses the range of interests is that of social citizen.

■ ■ ■

How do the priorities of the citizen and the consumer–parent differ? One way of answering this question is to look at a specific issue which affects the question of social inclusion and social exclusion, and which also affects the construction of educational subjects. The exclusion of pupils from schools for unacceptable behaviour does both. It has links with wider forms of social exclusion, and it exemplifies well how social institutions define and construct the category of deviant (see **Muncie, 1998**). Recalling **Lewis' (1998)** exploration of how education constructs racialized subjectivities, we should also note that there is extensive evidence that school exclusions fall disproportionately on black males.

As a social citizen you would be likely to want schools to be inclusive institutions which ensure that young people become integrated members of adult society. You might be wary of policies which made 'Others' of any identifiable group, in a way which might extend into adult life. You might well question approaches which defined children as 'problems' and utilized that definition to exclude them, rather than to focus resources to address the difficulties. As consumer–parent, your prime concern might be that your own child was fully integrated and well prepared to be a fulfilled, employable and socially acceptable young adult. You would probably want policies on behaviour which enable your children to learn, both to guide them, and to prevent other children setting a poor example or disrupting teaching.

The subject positions of social citizen and consumer–parent are being used as ideal types here. The premise of this concept of social citizenship is that there is formal equality among all social citizens. The consumer–parent is assumed to be primarily self-interested, in the sense of giving priority to their child's needs to the exclusion of concern about the needs of others. Both positions are assumed to carry equality: equality of status before the law and state in the former, and equality of market choice in the latter. In practice, these positions are considerably more complex. As various authors in **Hughes (1998)** argue, there are a number of contested models of citizenship and of consumerism which would blur these tidy boundaries.

At first sight there is clear compatibility between the priorities of these two ideal types. The status of citizen implies inclusion for all; while the parent wants the best for his or her children. So the agreed task of schools is to include all. The more each parent is able to press for the inclusion of her or his child, the more the totality of children will be included. But this appearance of mutuality is deceptive and breaks down when we look at specific issues such as classroom behaviour.

- First, it assumes a level of agreement about acceptable behaviour which is at odds with the moral and cultural diversity found among a school's population. Moreover, processes of normalization mean that there may be enormous difficulty in differentiating minor transgressions from serious ones. The issue of diverse subjects is critical here.

- Second, some parents will be more successful than others at ensuring that their definition of acceptable standards prevails.

- Third, keeping marginally disruptive students in mainstream classrooms may secure their long-term social inclusion, but may be felt by parents of other children to be impeding academic progress. Conflicts of interest are inherent here.

- Fourth, competition may incline headteachers to exclude pupils whose behaviour threatens the school's reputation or its published examination performance. Informal exclusions which ask the parents of 'difficult' children to find another school are probably even more common (see Gewirtz *et al.*, 1995). Again, processes of normalization are central here.

The appearance of mutuality mistakes a multiplicity of common individual goals for a shared collective goal that reflects agreed social priorities. The market emphasizes differences in the interests of different parents. The normalization of parental interests in discourses about 'what parents want' hides and delegitimizes the concerns of parents whose children are not experiencing schooling as inclusive. The interests of parents in the inclusion of their individual child are always in tension, and often in conflict, with those of citizens inclined towards policies and practices which maximize inclusion for all. The reconstruction of education as a process of consumption had to make *individual* parents – rather than the aggregation of all parents – the subjects of consumption.

In a market system it is impossible to make a collectivity of interests the subject of a process of consumption because the system is premised on individualized judgements, values and actions. But social citizens are members of communities whose positions are constructed through their social relations with others.

On this analysis, it looks doubtful that a resettlement built on fusing the subject positions of citizen and consumer, or principles such as competition and inclusiveness, or enterprise and justice, can work easily. Their priorities constantly pull at each other. It is therefore particularly interesting to look at how Blair and the Labour Party sought to reconcile some of these antitheses. It can be argued that they aimed to find a third way between Right and Left which is not a bland centre ground, but an unprecedented mix of inclusive social citizenship and market dynamism. This quotation from the manifesto indicates this eclectic approach:

> We will put behind us the old arguments that have bedevilled education in this country. We reject the Tories' obsession with school structures: all parents should be offered real choice through good quality schools, each with its own strengths and individual ethos. There should be no return to the 11-plus. It divides children into successes and failures at far too early an age.
>
> We must modernize comprehensive schools. Children are not all of the same ability, nor do they learn at the same speed. This means setting children in classes to maximize progress, for the benefit of high-fliers and slow learners alike. The focus must be on levelling up not levelling down.
>
> (Labour Party, 1997, p.7)

The idea of a third way in education highlights the tensions, struggles and dilemmas which underlie the history this chapter has traced. This short quotation has echoes of the social democratic consensus commitments to universality, good quality provision for all and the comprehensive principle, but it also clearly recalls the essentialism of the discourses of ability of the Norwood Report and the Black Papers (see sections 3.1 and 3.3) and the market commitments to choice and diversity of the New Right. Is a resettlement which balances the citizenship commitments of the social democratic settlements and the consumerist commitments of marketization possible? Or are they irreconcilable, each bound to delimit and eventually undo the project of the other? Is the pursuit of an inclusive citizenship through universal comprehensive education a brake on the pursuit of choice, excellence and diversity? Does the market entail forms of self-interest, exclusivity and residual welfare that are at odds with citizenship?

The contested principles of universalism, mobility, equality of opportunity and meritocracy which made up the social democratic settlements stressed the role of education in combating disadvantages of birth and circumstance, to provide opportunities for the realization of the potentials of all citizens. Yet schooling since the social democratic settlements has continued to reproduce forms of difference which closely reflect the distributions of power, income and status of the wider society and of previous generations. If we take entry into higher education as a significant marker of educational achievement, many deeply entrenched inequalities remain. Most black and some Asian ethnic groups are under-represented. Young African-Caribbean men and Bangladeshis, especially women, are particularly seriously under-represented (Coffield and Vignoles, 1997). Table 6.1 is a stark illustration not only of continuing underachievement by young people from families in the lower and middle socio-economic groups, but also of their markedly reduced capacity to gain a university

Table 6.1 Percentage participation in higher education of 18–19 year olds by qualification and socio-economic group

	Socio-economic group*			
	I–II	*III*	*IV–V*	*Total*
	Percentage of 18–19 year olds with following qualifications			
2 A levels or equivalent	50	27	16	33
2 A levels	41	17	8	24
Other equivalent qualifications	9	10	8	9
	Percentage with following qualifications going to university			
2 A levels or equivalent	77	59	47	67
2 A levels	86	78	71	82
Other equivalent qualifications	40	27	21	30

Total number of people included in sample = 7,423.

Source: Metcalf, reproduced in Robertson and Hillman, 1997, Table 2.3, p.50

* I–II = professional, administrative and managerial; III = non-manual and personal service workers; IV–V = small proprietors and skilled/unskilled manual workers.

place *even* when they have qualifications which are broadly comparable to those of their counterparts from the higher group.

At least until 1998 girls performed markedly better at GCSE than boys, but this advantage was eroded by the time they entered higher education. Even the serious under-representation of young men from lower socio-economic backgrounds in higher education – itself a cause for concern – did not help girls maintain their earlier overall advantage (Coffield and Vignoles, 1997).

These inequalities need to be read alongside signs of real progress since the post-war settlements, particularly in the achievement of girls generally, of the children of Indian and Pakistani parents, and those of upper-middle socio-economic groups. But the stubborn persistence of these deeply socially patterned differences leaves no doubt about continuing constructions of difference.

8   Conclusion

Whether the proposals for a third way can make any impact on these patterned inequalities and exclusions is of course uncertain. But some of the debates about the major turns of education policy which this chapter has traced may provide some indication of possible outcomes. This section looks at some of the early signs of the direction that the Labour government's education policy may take. The section also offers a brief review of the main themes of the chapter. Reviewing past contestations allows us to view the latest policies in their historical context. The central question is whether resettlement can escape from the past or whether a third way is no more than a pragmatic mix of recycled policies.

The history of changing structures of schooling traced in this chapter indicated the movement from the post-war settlements and the high levels of state intervention of the 1960s and 1970s, to the pursuit of marketization in the 1980s and 1990s. Free universal secondary education was a keystone of the social settlement, conceived by some as the leading welfare route to social citizenship, inclusiveness, opportunity and mobility. The balance of forces which allowed this settlement to form around education was delicately poised and far from wholehearted in its commitment, allowing a divisive tripartite system to emerge in the name of inclusion and equal opportunity. But it was based on a sufficiently strong consensus to sustain the shift towards comprehensivization in the 1960s, without the aid of legislation.

The period of unsettlement beginning in the 1970s eroded this consensus. This erosion was partly triggered from outside education, through the attack on high levels of state intervention, high public spending, deteriorating national economic fortunes and the power of organized labour. There were also profound doubts about the structures and character of secondary schooling, particularly the advance of progressive education.

The New Right emerged in the mid 1980s to query fundamental features of the structures of school provision. It partially secured a number of reforms, adopting market principles for the allocation of resources and the determination of control over schooling. These developments were accompanied by reforms intended to raise standards, primarily through market pressures. In practice, many of the reforms have produced new forms of managerialism which outstrip the powers of markets and consumers.

What is to be the third way on the structure of secondary education? The White Paper *Excellence in Schools* (Department of Education and Employment, 1997) was clear that standards, not structures, are the critical issue. The main features of restructuring will remain in place. In effect, the commitment to a quasi-market and choice remain, not simply by default, but with active efforts to smooth the more perversely competitive features of the admissions system to secure more effective parental choice, through enforced local co-ordination. The independent sector, the separate administration of the grant maintained sector, the devolution of control to schools through local management of schools, and the position of local education authorities seem unlikely to change radically. Parent representation on governing schools is marginally enhanced. Diversity is to be fostered, with specialist schools and public–private partnerships encouraged.

Turning to our examination of the social organization of schooling, the post-war settlements reaffirmed the arrangements which pre-dated it and consolidated the old divisions of grammar and secondary schooling. The attack on selection in the mid 1960s was inspired by concerns about wastage of talent, as well as by social concerns. The adoption of comprehensivization, incomplete as it was, ended the separation of children into two or three types of schools, and allowed shared curricula and resources. But it co-existed alongside a selective private sector, it divided children according to their suitability for public examinations, and it left open a range of possibilities for internal selection. Grammar schools survived in a number of areas, and other schemes secured state-funded assisted places in selective private schools for high-achieving children from low-income households. Further erosion of the comprehensive principle came through the introduction of open enrolment and grant maintained schools. Under open enrolment, self-selection, combined with local geography and housing differences and informal selection by schools, exaggerated existing hierarchies of schools. As with the earlier tripartite system, a stratified system began to emerge, justified not through overt discourses of ability, but through complex and ostensibly disinterested market mechanisms.

Here, the third way envisaged by Labour is slightly more distinct from what went before. The relaxation of regulations which allowed the steady drift towards selection in some localities in the mid 1990s is likely to be stemmed. Selection by interview is largely disallowed, but will be difficult to prevent. In addition, the system of support which sends state-funded pupils to selective independent schools ceases. But the existence of such schools is unchallenged, and the future of most grammar schools is likely to be secure. On one front at least, powers of selection will increase, as specialist schools choose students by aptitude for subject rather than 'general academic ability'. Perhaps the most significant development is the intention to abandon mixed-ability teaching within comprehensive schools (Department of Education and Employment, 1997).

Tracing the history of the social organization of schooling demonstrated one important aspect of the construction of educational subjects: as the embodiment of particular abilities. The discourses of Extracts 6.3 and 6.5 portrayed ability as fixed and prescribed by nature. This essentialism characterized the thinking behind tripartism, and the attack on the comprehensive principle. The idea that ability is an essentialist *construct*, that competence is affected by background and context, or may change over time according to circumstance, are left out of consideration. The effect is to legitimize the allocation of educational subjects to differentiated positions in a differentiating education system. These differentiations are likely to imply inequalities in resourcing, staffing and provision which in turn reproduce patterns of advantage and disadvantage between generations and social groupings.

The culture and curricula of schools also construct pupils as unequal subjects, by virtue of the highly differentiated cultural capital they bear. Traditionally, the children of middle-class homes were regarded as greatly advantaged. Many of the projects of progressive education which came under fire in the 1970s were intended to ameliorate the ways in which culture and curriculum acted to disadvantage children of working-class homes, girls and some racialized groups. The assumptions, knowledge and modes of thought and expression which infuse the national curriculum and tests are thought by many to have restored much traditional disadvantage.

Curricula and cultural forms of school life construct senses of national belonging, particularly through literature and history, and the national norms and values they embody. The primacy afforded to Christianity, and in particular Protestantism, as the dominant national religion furthers these constructions. They bind subjects to particular understandings of Welshness, Scottishness or Britishness. But by implication they also exclude those whose ethnicity inclines them to resist, reject, or not understand the norms implied. It is by this means that subject positions of 'Otherness' are constructed.

These constructions have the potential to divide, to exclude, to rank and to devalue subjects and particular subject positions. *Excellence in Schools* makes some gestures towards recognizing the significance of cultural differences, but conceives of pupils as disadvantaged, not the culture of schools as disadvantaging, and offers compensations. Where compensation does not work, the threat of exclusion remains, recalling questions about conflicts between individual and wider social interests in deciding exclusions, and the constructions of excluded subjects they imply. There is no recognition that the nature of the curriculum and assessment might be significant factors in determining how some social groups are constructed, and how this affects their performance. The 'crusade' to improve standards concentrates attention not on the differences in achievement of particular social categories, but on the differences between schools in the performances of socially comparable groups. Differences in performance are viewed as measures of the effectiveness of each school, and the thrust of policy is to secure improvements in each school's effectiveness. The means to this are likely to be more vigorous application of the instruments of managerialism: league tables, targets, active interventionist local education authority monitoring, inspection and, where necessary, school closures.

How do the Labour proposals look in this historical context? On one view this is a vision of a third way which has jettisoned dogma, ideology and old battles, and put in their place commitments which will secure real opportunity, effective inclusion and sound provision for the many not just the few. The vision has taken the best of the past, openly accepted the successes of 1990s' restructuring, and seized the potential of competition and inspection to eradicate poor teaching. The worst excesses of selection will be gradually eroded in favour of greater equity, alongside a realistic recognition of individual differences.

On another view, the fundamental adherence to the restructured system promises not a third way, but a continuation of the persistent patterns of inclusion and exclusion which have changed so slowly and so little over 50 years. Competition, inequalities between schools, choice and devolved powers will remain the dominant features of a system which reproduced disadvantage even when it was comprehensive, and exaggerated its capacities to do so as restructuring took hold. The continued essentialist adherence to discourses of ability and the continuing commitment to the national curriculum and assessment and their managerial enforcement demonstrate poor awareness of why schooling reproduces not just difference but inequality.

Certainly, taken individually, few of the 1997 proposals could be said to escape from the past. The comparisons are striking between the old Labour/ Conservative consensus symbolized by the transition from bipartism to comprehensivization, and the present search for a third way between state and market, and between selection and comprehensivization. Most of the proposals are re-tailored projections of pre-existing policies, or adaptations of abandoned older policies in a new context. The critical question for the next few years will be whether the mix they represent is as contradictory as the forces which brought the end of consensus and the tensions inherent in restructuring; or whether it is a dynamic and refined blend of the best of the past brought to bear upon new times in a spirit of resettlement.

The Professionals

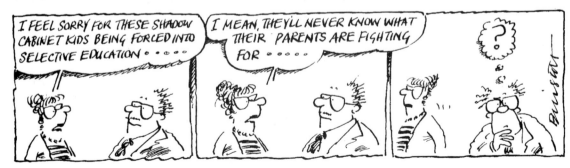

From Education, *February 1996*

The allocation of children to structured places in schools, and their construction through school curricula and cultures, are amongst the most extensive, penetrating and totalizing public acts of social differentiation of any society. They are at the centre of how this society constructs its welfare subjects, how it responds to their diversity, and what kinds of social relations come to prevail as a result. Understanding the construction of welfare subjects means, in part, understanding the educational processes at the heart of their construction.

Further reading

A thorough analysis of the place of education as part of the settlement is provided by the Centre for Contemporary Cultural Studies (1981) *Unpopular Education*. Benn and Simon (1972) *Half Way There* and Benn and Chitty (1996) *Thirty Years On* offer critical assessments of comprehensive and selective secondary provision. The New Right critique is best encapsulated in the Black Papers on Education (see, for example, Cox and Boyson, 1975), and more recently in Green's (1991) *Empowering the Parents*. Probably the most thorough report and discussion of research to date on the effects of marketization on schools and selection is Gewirtz *et al.*'s (1995) *Markets, Choice and Equity in Education*. The Department of Education and Employment's 1997 White Paper *Excellence in Schools* provides the fullest policy statement to date on the Labour government's plans, and is a rich text for analysis in the light of some of the issues raised in this chapter.

References

Adam Smith Institute (1984/5) *The Omega File*, London, Adam Smith Institute.

Atha, A. and Drummond, S. (1994) *The Good Schools Guide* (4th edn), London, Macmillan.

Audit Commission (1996) *Trading Places*, London, Audit Commission.

Ball, S., Bowe, R. and Gewirtz, S. (1994) 'Market forces and parental choice: self-interest and competitive advantage in education', in Tomlinson, S. (ed.) *Educational Reform and its Consequences*, London, Institute for Public Policy Research/Rivers Oram Press.

Ball, S. and Vincent, C. (1996) 'I heard it on the grapevine: "hot" knowledge and school choice', *Times Educational Supplement*, 20 September.

Barton, L., Whitty, G., Miles, S. and Furlong, J. (1994) 'Teacher education and teacher professionalism in England: some emerging issues', *British Journal of Sociology of Education*, vol.15, no.4, pp.529–43.

Benn, C. and Chitty, C. (1996) *Thirty Years On: Is Comprehensive Education Alive and Well or Struggling to Survive?*, London, David Fulton.

Benn, C. and Simon, B. (1972) *Half Way There: Report on the British Comprehensive School Reform* (2nd edn), Harmondsworth, Penguin.

Beveridge, W. (1942) *The Beveridge Report in Brief*, London, HMSO.

Bourdieu, P. (1977) 'Cultural reproduction and social reproduction', in Karabel, J. and Halsey, A.H. (eds) *Power and Ideology in Education*, Oxford, Oxford University Press.

Carr, W. and Hartnett, A. (1996) *Education and the Struggle for Democracy: The Politics of Educational Ideas*, Buckingham, Open University Press.

Centre for Contemporary Cultural Studies (1981) *Unpopular Education: Schooling and Social Democracy in England since 1944*, London, Hutchinson.

Chitty, C. (1992) *The Education System Transformed*, Manchester, Baseline.

Clarke, J. and Cochrane, A. (1988) 'The social construction of social problems', in Saraga (ed.) (1998a).

Clarke, J., Cochrane, A. and McLaughlin, E. (eds) (1994) *Managing Social Policy*, London, Sage.

Coffield, F. and Vignoles, S. (1997) 'Widening participation in HE by ethnic minorities, women and alternative students', Report 5 of National Commission of Inquiry into Higher Education, *Higher Education in the Learning Society* (Dearing Report), London, HMSO.

Cox, C., Balchin, R. and Marks, J. (1989) *Choosing a State School*, London, Hutchinson.

Cox, C. and Boyson, R. (eds) (1975) *Black Paper 1975*, London, Dent.

Dean, C. (1996) 'More pupils opt for the GM sector', *Times Educational Supplement*, 12 July.

Department of Education and Employment (1997) *Excellence in Schools*, White Paper, Cmnd 3681, London, HMSO.

Furlong, J. (1992) 'Reconstructing professionalism: ideological struggle in initial teacher education', in Arnot, M. and Barton, C. (eds) *Voicing Concerns*, Wallingford, Triangle.

Gewirtz, S., Ball, S.J. and Bowe, R. (1995) *Markets, Choice and Equity in Education*, Buckingham, Open University Press.

Green, D.G. (ed.) (1991) *Empowering the Parents: How to Break the Schools Monopoly*, London, Institute of Economic Affairs.

Green, G.K. (1975) 'Why comprehensives fail', in Cox and Boyson (eds) (1975).

Hughes, G. (ed.) (1998) *Imagining Welfare Futures*, London, Routledge in association with The Open University.

Johnson, R. (1991) 'A new road to serfdom? A critical history of the 1988 Act', in Education Group II, Department of Cultural Studies, *Education Limited*, London, Unwin Hyman.

Jones, K. (1989) *Right Turn: The Conservative Revolution in Education*, London, Hutchinson Radius.

Knight, C. (1990) *The Making of Tory Education Policy in Post-war Britain, 1950–86*, Brighton, Falmer.

Labour Party (1997) *New Labour: Because Britain Deserves Better* (election manifesto), London, Labour Party.

Lawn, M. (1996) *Modern Times: Work, Professionalism and Citizenship in Teaching*, Lewes, Falmer Press.

Lawson, J. and Silver, H. (1985) 'Education and social policy', in McNay, I. and Ozga, J. (eds) *Policy Making in Education: The Breakdown of Consensus*, Oxford, Pergamon in association with The Open University.

Le Grand, J. and Bartlett, W. (1994) *Quasi-markets and Social Policy*, Basingstoke, Macmillan.

Lewis, G. (1998) 'Welfare and the social construction of "race"', in Saraga (ed.) (1998a).

McClure, J.S. (1968) *Educational Documents: England and Wales 1816 to the Present Day* (5th edn), London, Methuen.

McCoy, L. (1998) 'Education for labour: social problems of nationhood', in Lewis, G. (ed.) *Forming Nation*, *Framing Welfare*, London, Routledge in association with The Open University.

Muncie, J. (1998) '"Give 'em what they deserve": the young offender and youth justice policy', in Langan, M. (ed.) *Welfare: Needs, Rights and Risks*, London, Routledge in association with The Open University.

Newman, C. and Clarke, J. (1994) 'Going about our business? The managerialization of public services', in Clarke *et al.* (eds) (1994).

Robertson, D. and Hillman, J. (1997) 'Widening participation in higher education by students from lower socio-economic groups and students with disabilities', Report 6 in National Committee of Inquiry into Higher Education, *Higher Education in the Learning Society* (Dearing Report), London, HMSO.

Saraga, E. (1998a) *Embodying the Social: Constructions of Difference*, London, Routledge in association with The Open University.

Saraga, E. (1998b) 'Abnormal, unnatural and immoral? The social construction of sexualities', in Saraga (ed.) (1998a).

Seldon, A. (1986) *The Riddle of the Voucher*, London, Institute of Economic Affairs.

Sexton, S. (1988) 'No nationalized curriculum', *The Times*, 9 May.

Times Educational Supplement (1996) 'Parents "deceived" over choice', 9 August.

Whitty, G. (1992) 'Education, economy and national culture', in Bocock, R. and Thompson, K. (1992) *Social and Cultural Forms of Modernity*, Cambridge, Polity in association with The Open University.

Whitty, G., Barton, L. and Pollard, A. (1987) 'Ideology and control in teacher education: a review of recent experiences in England', in Popkewitz, T. (ed.) *Critical Studies in Teacher Education*, Lewes, Falmer Press.

CHAPTER 7

The Reshaping of Social Work and Social Care

by Sharon Pinkney

Contents

1   Introduction

You will realize by now that defining key terms is often difficult, that their meanings can be slippery. Within social work and social care various definitional issues arise. One is about the terms used to identify different people or groups of people who use social care services. These include terms such as 'the elderly', 'the mentally ill', 'the mentally handicapped' or 'the disabled'. These terms and others have been highly contested and the language of welfare has changed accordingly. Also worth noting here is that when we write 'the' in front of a term, the group becomes homogenized.

Can you think of examples of other terms that reflect the contestation around language within the area of social work and social care?

The terms people use tell us something about their perspective. It is clear when we study changes in language that terms such as 'the elderly' and 'the mentally ill' are culturally and historically specific **(Clarke and Cochrane, 1998)**. It is important to remind yourself of these points, particularly when you read reports and extracts. Within this chapter I will settle, albeit uneasily, for using 'elders', 'people with a disability' and 'people experiencing mental ill-health'. Similarly the word 'client' will be avoided and I will use 'service-user' instead. It is important to remember, however, that these terms are still contested and their usage remains unsettled.

ACTIVITY 7.1

What do you understand by the terms 'social work' and 'social care'?

Within most of the social policy literature they are used interchangeably and this leads to confusion about the meaning of the terms. Spend a few minutes thinking about these two terms and make a note of what they mean to you.

COMMENT

You may have defined *social work* to include services provided by social services departments (SSDs) or social work departments (SWDs) (Scotland), involving support and protection for children, families, people with a disability, people experiencing mental ill-health or elders. These services may be either wanted or unwanted by the service-user. According to this definition, then, social work includes services provided by the state, usually through the local authority SSD or SWD. Some of you may have mentioned that social work can also be provided by voluntary or charitable organizations.

informal care

formal care

Social care is perhaps a more slippery concept than social work. You may have included the provision of care for people with a range of difficulties, provided by family, friends or neighbours. In the literature this is often referred to as informal care. Where agencies such as health or social services departments are involved it is likely to be called formal care. Even these distinctions raise difficulties, however, as some informal carers are paid. **Barnes (1998)** argues that provision and access to social care are both disputed. Social care is a problematic and contested concept, but will be used in this chapter in a broad sense to cover care provided by a range of sources, including statutory, private, voluntary and informal sources, within the context of the mixed economy of welfare. *Social work* is one of the sources of *social care*, mostly falling within the statutory sector; together these are often referred to as 'the personal social services'.

■ ■ ■

This chapter aims to:

- ■ Examine social work and social care as an area of contestation within the general reconstruction of welfare. This will involve you in looking at some of the continuities, challenges and changes within social work.

- ■ Trace the threads from earlier chapters on the way the settlements, old and new, can be used as an organizing framework, to see the contestations and unevenness within social work and social care.

- ■ Use the ideas of the mixed economy of welfare and marketization of welfare to help you understand the changes taking place within social work and social care.

- ■ Introduce you to two key pieces of legislation to illustrate the complexities, dilemmas and challenges in social work and social care.

- ■ Use the 'new welfare subjects' framework introduced in Chapter 2 to look at the way social work/care has marginalized and excluded some groups.

2 Histories of social work and social care

The main focus of this chapter is the changes in social care during the 1980s and 1990s. As you will see, these changes came about for a number of reasons and the pressure for change came from various directions. Before looking at some of this in more detail, you need to grasp some of the key aspects and themes of the organizational structure of social work prior to the changes.

Even within this limited discussion we will be talking about 'histories' rather than 'the history'. The use of the plural rather than singular is an important signifier of the way history is being viewed within a contested framework, one which acknowledges that there are many different versions of history, which are often contradictory. What emerges is a multi-layered account of the development of social work. The outcomes of these contestations are complex, but that is not to say that there are never any winners and losers. The outcomes are usually less clear-cut than we might imagine at first glance.

histories

2.1 The early histories of social work

Since the nineteenth century a range of specific personal services has been developed to offer support to individuals who are seen to have special needs, resulting either from illness, disability or from their individual or social circumstances. The main groups which have traditionally been offered such services are elders, people with either learning or physical disabilities, people suffering from mental ill-health and children. It is clear that the construction of 'need' for each of these groups has been the subject of debate and contestation

(Langan, 1998a). In some instances support may be requested, whereas in other situations the services may be viewed as stigmatizing and undesirable.

In the nineteenth and early part of the twentieth centuries much of the formal support for the groups above was provided by the voluntary sector, and especially by charities. The existence of the private and voluntary sectors in the nineteenth and early twentieth centuries illustrates that there has always been a mixed economy of welfare. In the nineteenth century the Charity Organization Society (COS) and other similar organizations became responsible for the co-ordination of services within the voluntary sector **(Mooney, 1998)**.

One of the important legacies for social work which remains from the days of the COS is the casework method. This was developed as a way of maintaining records on families where charitable support was offered and where the COS worker was visiting at home. One of the main features of this method is the individualized nature of the relationship between the COS worker (or social worker) and the family, most often the mother, who was seen to have prime responsibility for care and for bringing about improvements in the family's situation. This focus on the individual obscured the environmental, social, political and economic factors which may have contributed to the difficulties. The COS also established the idea of home visiting as a routine way of intervening in and regulating the lives of the poor. Both health visitors and social workers continue to use this as a central method today, particularly in work with children and families.

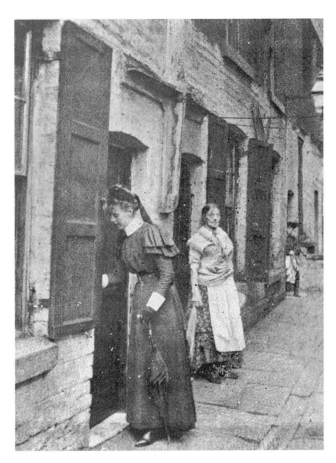

Home visiting by a charity worker in nineteenth century Manchester

The classical conception of the welfare state as it developed in the UK after the Second World War was centred on a set of state-provided social services in four areas: health, education, housing and income maintenance. Despite the existence of numerous children's, welfare and health services, the personal social services were added as the fifth social service only in the early 1970s. The length of time it took to develop a coherent framework for the personal social services could be an indication of the complex and fragmented nature of the services which were in place prior to 1970.

Before the 1940s, when the development of state welfare services began in earnest, most 'social workers', as they were then being called, were situated within the voluntary sector. After the 1940s they gradually moved into the state social services' agencies which were located within local authorities. In the period between the 1940s and the early 1970s responsibility for local authority services was fragmented between children's, welfare and health departments.

The development of state social services from the 1940s onwards did not curtail the activity of either the voluntary or private sectors, which flourished alongside the state sector. An example of this would be the National Society for the Prevention of Cruelty to Children (NSPCC) which was established in the nineteenth century. Another example would be the successor to the COS which was the Family Welfare Association. Similarly, voluntary organizations such as MENCAP, Age Concern and Mind have been active in the provision of support to people with learning disabilities, elders and people experiencing mental ill-health.

2.2 The Seebohm Report

One of the most significant features of the recent history of social work was the Seebohm Report of 1968, which reviewed social services in England and Wales (Department of Health and Social Security, 1968). In Scotland the Kilbrandon Committee (1961–64) had already proposed a set of reforms, which led to the establishment of Social Work Departments (SWDs) (Scottish Home and Health Department, Scottish Education Department, 1964). The Kilbrandon Report was addressing particular concerns regarding juvenile delinquency, but the outcome of both reports was fairly similar. Some of the pressures and challenges which led to the creation of the Seebohm Committee were:

- The existence of two separate and mostly unrelated services – child health and health and welfare – each with its own distinct organization, policies, procedures and problems.

- 'Clients', as they were then known, often needed services from both the child health and the health and welfare spheres, and the existence of separate services created difficulties and confusion. The creation of 'a single door on which to knock' therefore became one of the key objectives.

- The problem of co-ordination across disparate and fragmented services. Many of the topical issues and problems were seen to transcend the organizational boundaries. An example of this was 'juvenile delinquency', which was becoming a growing preoccupation with politicians, the media and policy-makers.

- Social workers themselves were part of the pressure for change because in the quest for greater professional standing they were keen to develop a more coherent and unified structure.

The Seebohm Report led to the reorganization in 1970 of the fragmented provision of the personal social services, bringing these services under one umbrella, which was the local authority Social Services Department (SSD) in England and Wales.

It seemed unsurprising, therefore, given the pressures for change, that Seebohm recommended a unified structure for the delivery of the personal social services as well as endorsing the fusion of the diverse tasks carried out by social workers into the role of the generic social worker. Implementation of Seebohm took place in the 1970 Local Authority Social Services Act.

One of the important features of the changes introduced to social work during the years following Seebohm and Kilbrandon was the gradual move away from specialist services to generic services. This is linked to the idea of 'a single door on which to knock.' Social workers were expected to be able to hold expertise and skills in a wide range of different areas. The pendulum has since swung back towards specialist services, but for the period between 1970 and the 1980s social work was generic rather than specialist in nature.

2.3   Radical critiques of social work

Radical critiques of social work came from within social work itself, from service-user groups and also from the government and the New Right. Here I will look briefly at some of these critiques.

The influence of community social work methods, and the development of what became known as 'patch' social work, gained popularity in the period between the late 1960s and the early 1980s. This involved the idea that social workers should ideally live in the area in which they worked; develop local knowledge and expertise; become involved in local community organizations; and work towards structural change rather than locating social problems at the individual level. Alongside this there was a widely held belief that social problems could be alleviated by state provision of welfare services. This optimism can be viewed within the context of a post-Second World War consensus on welfare which included a commitment to the eradication of poverty. Most of these critiques were premised upon a Marxist analysis and viewed class inequality as the main problem to be overcome (see Corrigan and Leonard, 1978; Brake and Bailey, 1980). These approaches were themselves later criticized for not acknowledging the inequalities that derived from other social divisions, particularly those of gender, 'race' and disability.

Parallel to these developments within social work, the women's movement was gathering strength and feminist perspectives exerted considerable influence over the emerging shape of social work. In a later period, between the 1970s and 1990s, black perspectives in the form of anti-racist social work criticized social work for being Eurocentric and reinforcing racist stereotypes of black and other communities defined as 'ethnic minority' (see **Saraga, 1998b**; **Lewis, 1998a**). The outcome of these challenges from 'the margins' remains controversial, although it is possible to see in places that critiques of social work regarding class, gender, 'race', sexuality and disability did challenge the organization and content of social work training as well as the way social work itself was organized and delivered. But in general we can see that social work tends to reproduce rather than challenge inequalities. One example of this could be the fact that social work assessments are mainly carried out on women who are living in poverty, yet the material conditions have seldom been a factor within these assessments.

Chapter 2 provided a general discussion of the way in which these challenges to social work were appropriated by what became known as the New Right. A different set of radical critiques that emerged from the New Right changed the way welfare was conceived and delivered in the period between the 1970s and 1990s. The Thatcher governments attempted to restructure welfare in various ways, in particular by introducing market mechanisms into all aspects of the welfare state. The New Right agenda radically altered the ethos and practices within the welfare state. What was at stake was the way the state sector itself was organized. It is important to bear in mind the wider context of the mixed economy of welfare here, the idea that welfare is delivered by a range of agencies and institutions, including private, voluntary and the family, not just the state. The rearticulation of the mixed economy of welfare by the New Right was also about a reconfiguration of social relations of welfare – that is, between the state and citizens. The role of the family and voluntary and private provision in welfare was vigorously promoted. Family care was viewed as the right and proper form of care in most cases. Wilding states:

mixed economy of welfare

> If one takes the view that a – perhaps the – key theme in Thatcherism is dislike of the state then the idea of the mixed economy of welfare offers a window of opportunity for change acceptable to public opinion. The state is redefining its responsibilities rather than abandoning them, but statism, and indirectly the idea of public responsibility – is being weakened.

(Wilding, 1992, p.21)

For the personal social services, this shift in ethos and practice meant the introduction of market mechanisms into the state sector itself. Several themes emerged during the late 1970s and 1980s which were to be critical in shaping the future of social care.

First, the introduction of the purchaser–provider split became a key organizing principle for various forms of welfare. In social care this meant the state taking on the role of purchaser, with the private and voluntary sectors, or more perversely other sectors of the state, taking on the role of provider. The objectives of this split were to encourage competition between the state and the private and voluntary sectors and the reduction of expenditure by the state. Spending on personal social services was the second (to education) largest category of local authority expenditure in 1976, and this meant it was an obvious target for reductions. 'Cutbacks' became part of the language of welfare during this period.

purchaser–provider split

Wilding (1992) argued that the real issue was not about cuts, which focused the debate on complex and always disputable calculations about expenditure, but instead was about the appropriate levels for welfare provision. The focus on expenditure meant an obscuring of the legacy of Thatcherism, which for Wilding includes falling standards, services which are desperately stretched for resources and the establishment of a lower and shabbier base-line. At the time of writing it is too early to see how the Labour government elected in 1997 will deal with the issue of resourcing welfare services, though early indications suggest that the lower, shabbier base-line referred to by Wilding will persist into the next decade.

The second set of concerns grew out of the desire to encourage a move away from state provision towards the private, informal or voluntary sectors.

This in turn was linked with the idea of the local authority as an 'enabling' authority, assisting individuals to move away from dependency on state welfare.

A third theme which emerged during this period was of a different nature, related more to the role of social workers themselves, who were often viewed as misguided 'do-gooders' who sometimes did more harm than good. Another view of social workers saw them as self-interested professionals whose main interest lay in protecting themselves and improving their status and rewards.

The fourth aspect was that social workers' professional status and knowledge was challenged by the suggestion that all they did was what any sensible adult could do. Here, the New Right understanding of common sense was set up against the idea of professionalism, and social workers were constructed as lacking common sense.

Fifth, there were changes in the aims, purposes and values of welfare that were more subtle and less easy to evaluate. Between the 1940s and 1970s the aims and values of the public sector were varied and complex, but it is possible to argue that there was a general concern to reduce inequalities, to promote an ethic of fairness, to combat poverty and to assert and promote the rights of citizenship. During the 1980s there was a gradual move away from the notion of universal provision, from free services as a right of citizenship, and towards a greater stress on charges for services, as well as the targeting of services to the very poorest.

Although these perspectives and arguments for change within welfare came out of New Right and Conservative Party policy from the mid 1970s, viewing them as arising from that direction only would be too simplistic. The Labour Party had at that time also made their view clear that welfare state expenditure was too high. The shifts which were about to take place within welfare had a wide resonance across various political parties and policy-making bodies. The challenges to social care need to be viewed within the context of the shifts and restructuring processes which were taking place within welfare generally.

The restructuring of social work and social care came later than the reorganizations of housing, health, income maintenance and education. The survival of personal social services as a monopoly provider of services throughout the 1980s may be attributed to the complexity of legal, organizational and professional structures (see Langan and Clarke, 1994). The restructuring which took place in the 1990s came about partly as a result of legislative change in the form of The Children Act 1989 and the NHS and Community Care Act of 1990, both of which covered England and Wales and which together provided the framework and the rationale for change. We will be looking at the impact of these Acts, because both of them changed the internalities as well as the externalities of social work. Social work itself was changed and, perhaps more important in this context, social work relationships with other agencies and organizations were radically altered too. It is interesting that despite the fierce criticisms of social work, both of these Acts assumed that SSDs and SWDs in Scotland would continue as what was called the 'lead agency', albeit in a radically different form.

3   The community care revolution

The 1989 White Paper *Caring for People* (HMSO, 1989), and the subsequent NHS and Community Care Act 1990, initiated a process of fundamental change in the way community care services were provided. It is important to remember, though, that the promotion of community care and the reduction in institutional care is not a new phenomenon, and in the case of some aspects of service provision, such as mental health services, the present movement began as early as the 1930s **(Barnes, 1998)**.

Personal social services had been subjected to hostile media attention and to fierce public criticism throughout the period of the late 1970s and 1980s. Much of this hostility was based on perceived failings of social workers in provision for people with disabilities, people suffering from mental illness and elders. As we saw earlier, these criticisms of social work came from 'the margins'. The other, often more powerful critiques came from 'the centre' and included New Right criticisms of social work. These latter criticisms were more influential in shaping social work's future. From this perspective much hostility was directed at the apparent failure of social workers in the child protection arena, and SSDs were seen as inefficient and expensive and in some areas wasteful of resources. A second criticism here was that managers of social services were inadequate at making plans, setting targets and deciding priorities.

3.1   Management magic

In the reconstruction of welfare generally, and community care in particular, management was given a key transformational role. The structure, culture, languages and practice of social care all changed dramatically. It was noted that 'this "cultural revolution" of community care captured precisely the magic of management – the ability to recast old assumptions and patterns into a new configuration which promises happy endings' (Langan and Clarke, 1994, p.90).

Management was viewed as essential to the reforms which were required to take place within SSDs. It seems unsurprising, therefore, that management should be the focus of many of the reports and recommendations from semi-autonomous agencies such as the Audit Commission and the Social Services Inspectorate. The Audit Commission, established in 1983, was responsible for a series of investigations into local authorities. Their reports criticized inefficiency and managerial weakness. The Commission offers detailed advice to SSDs which, although not legally binding, carries enough weight to be difficult to ignore.

In a similar vein the Social Services Inspectorate (SSI), which is a branch of the Department of Health, carries out inspections of local authority services, inspecting both quality and management. The SSI adopted a standards-based approach to inspections. The standards do not have formal legal status but are drawn variously from legislation, government policy, 'achievable best practice supported by research' and 'beliefs and values current in Social Services' (Social Services Inspectorate, 1993, p.14). Another role for the SSI is in ensuring that local policy and practice is consistent with central policy directives, thus ensuring that standards and control from the centre are maintained. Again, as with the Audit Commission, the SSI standards have no legal force themselves, but various consequences would follow an unfavourable SSI inspection; the Secretary of State could, for example, order an inquiry if concerns were raised.

ACTIVITY 7.2

Because of the importance of both the Audit Commission and the Social Services Inspectorate, this chapter uses them as sources of extract material so that you can gain an insight into the way in which social work was reshaped as well as develop skills in the critical analysis of official reports. Extract 7.1, taken from a 1986 Audit Commission report, is particularly concerned with community care. As you read it make notes on the central arguments by considering the following:

1   Reflecting back on earlier material on language and definitional issues, underline any words which are problematic.

2   What are viewed as the main grounds for concern in making community care a reality?

3   What are viewed as the underlying problems which need to be tackled to make the shift towards community care possible?

4   What is being said about resources for community care?

Extract 7.1 Audit Commission: 'Making a reality of community care'

Summary
Every year, some £6 billion is spent from public funds providing long-term care support for elderly, mentally ill or mentally or physically handicapped people excluding the cost of acute hospital care and GP services …

These clients are cared for in a wide range of settings, from their own homes to National Health Service (NHS) hospital. Broadly, services can be considered as part of a 'spectrum' of care; for example Exhibit 1 illustrates some of the alternative forms of accommodation available to mentally handicapped people away from the family home and typical total public sector costs (£ per week) in each case:

The policy of successive governments has been to promote community-based services allowing the reduction of long-stay hospital provision. This is generally considered better in most situations. It is also more economical in many cases … At the same time, there will always remain a very important role for hospitals (although on a reduced scale) in caring for a small number of very severely handicapped people; and residential care will continue to play an important role in the spectrum of care. 'Community Care' is about changing the balance of services and finding the most suitable placement for people from a wide range of options. It is not about imposing a community solution as the only option, in the way that institutional care has been the only option for many people in the past.

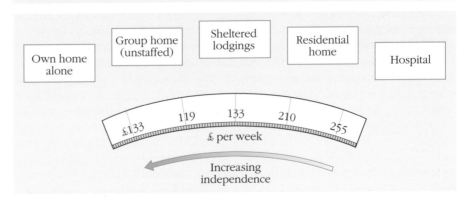

Exhibit 1: Spectrum of care settings

Although there has been worthwhile progress in some areas, and most authorities have at least made a start, care in the community is far from being a reality in many places:

(a) Progress with the build-up of community-based services has generally been slow, and in some places is not keeping pace with the run-down of long-stay institutions in the NHS ...

(b) A very uneven pattern of local authority services has developed, with the care that people receive as much dependent on where they live as on what they need ...

(c) Over 300,000 people still live in residential settings. The reduction in NHS facilities has been offset by the growth in private residential homes where some residents are entitled to receive help with their fees from Supplementary Benefits ...

At best, there seems to be a shift from one pattern of residential care based on hospitals to an alternative supported in many cases by Supplementary Benefit payments – missing out more flexible and cost-effective forms of community care altogether. At worst, the shortfall in services will grow, with many vulnerable and disabled people left without care and at serious personal risk.

Although more money could always be spent to advantage, the current levels of expenditure from public funds could provide a community-based service for elderly, mentally ill and handicapped people. But some underlying problems must be tackled first:

– While the Government's policies require a shift from hospital-based (health) services to locally-based (local authority and health) services, the mechanisms for achieving a parallel shift in funds are inadequate ...

– Meanwhile, local authorities are often penalised through the grant system for building the very community services which government policy favours and which are necessary if the NHS is to be in a position to close its large long-stay psychiatric hospitals and release the capital assets – conservatively valued at over £500 million.

– The funds being made available to bridge the transition phase are limited ...

– Supplementary Benefit policies fund private residential care more readily than community-based care of which there is still relatively little in the private sector. Partly as a result, private and voluntary homes are expanding very rapidly ...

– Responsibility for introducing and operating community-based services is fragmented between a number of different agencies with different priorities, styles, structures and budgets who must 'request' co-operation from each other. For community care to operate these agencies must work together. But there are many reasons why they do not, including the lack of positive incentives, bureaucratic barriers, perceived threats to jobs and professional standing ...

– Staffing arrangements are inadequate. A new impetus in training and a different approach to manpower planning are required ...

It is therefore not surprising that joint planning and community care policies are in some disarray. The result is poor value for money ...

However, in spite of the many obstacles, effective community care is being promoted in a number of authorities ...

Specifically, the Commission believes that the following actions are required:

(i) A rationalisation of funding policies must be undertaken from the centre so that the present policy conflicts are resolved ...

(ii) Adequate short-term funding must be provided to avoid the long-term waste of two inadequate services struggling along in parallel indefinitely.

(iii) Social security policies must be co-ordinated with community care policies, and present conflicts and 'perverse incentives' encouraging residential rather than community care removed.

(iv) A more rational organisational structure must be established; local responsibility, authority and accountability for delivering a balanced community-based care service for different client groups need to be more clearly defined.

(v) The organisational structures of the different agencies need to be aligned and greater managerial authority delegated to the local level.

(vi) Staffing arrangements must ensure provision of an appropriate supply of properly trained community-based staff.

(vii) Provision for cost-effective voluntary organisations must be sufficient to prevent them being starved of funds for reasons unrelated to their potential contributions to the support of clients and those caring for them in the community.

The objective of any changes should be to create an environment in which locally integrated community care can flourish – because it is at this level that community care works …

The one option that is not tenable is to do nothing about present financial, organisational and staffing arrangements. Redeployment of the assets released by the rundown of long-stay hospitals, combined with the projected increase of 37% in the number of very elderly people over the next ten years presents a 'window' of opportunity to establish an effective community-based service to provide the care needed for frail elderly, mentally ill, mentally handicapped and physically handicapped people. If this opportunity is not taken, a new pattern of care will emerge, based on private residential homes rather than a more flexible mix of services which includes residential care where appropriate. The result will be a continued waste of scarce resources and, worse still, care and support that is either lacking entirely, or inappropriate to the needs of some of the most disadvantaged members of society and the relatives who seek to care for them.

(Audit Commission, 1986, pp.1–5)

COMMENT

The first thing you may have noticed in Extract 7.1 is the use of terms such as 'mentally handicapped', 'physically handicapped' 'and 'mentally ill' which, as you saw earlier, have been contested and problematized. The Audit Commission expressed the view in this report that there were several grounds for concern regarding the shift towards community care. They felt that progress was slow and that there was an uneven response from different parts of England and Wales. The underlying problems were seen as the mismatch of resources, the perverse effects of social security policies, organizational fragmentation and confusion and inadequate staffing arrangements. The result of all of this was 'poor value for money'. The issue of resources was dealt with here by sweeping aside concerns about proper funding for community care. Instead it was seen that 'the current level of public funds' were adequate and could support the changes.

The following quotation, taken from later in the same report, is interesting in the way it refers to financial considerations. Under the heading 'potential benefits of community care' it states: 'Quite apart from value for money considerations, the scale of the benefits that could follow from successful introduction of community-based care of frail elderly, mentally ill, physically handicapped, and mentally handicapped people is immense' (Audit Commission, 1986, p.65).

The assumption implicit in the report is, therefore, that community care will save money, but alongside that there will be other benefits. What is clear is that the cost-saving implications are the first consideration.

■ ■ ■

3.2   The marketization of welfare

Although local authority SSDs and SWDs were given the role of lead agencies in community care, there was a built-in requirement that their provision would decline as care was increasingly provided from a variety of sectors, including informal, voluntary and private. Johnson (1990) argued that the NHS and Community Care Act was being directed at privatizing community care services via the promotion of contracts as well as imposing the purchaser–provider split on local authorities. The Act also propagated the virtue of internal markets, with different parts of the service buying and selling to and from each other. This drive to introduce the market mechanism into the personal social services via internal markets, competitive contracts, contracting out of services and promoting competition between various sectors was not unique to this area of welfare; similar processes had taken place within hospitals, schools and universities, for example.

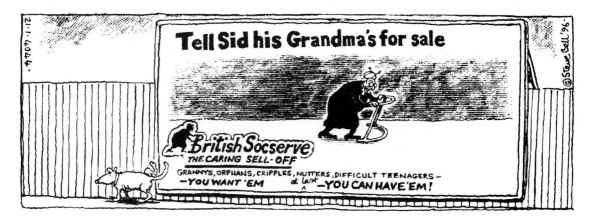

The creation of care managers within SSDs was part of a strategy to implement the mixed economy of welfare in social care. They were to commission the purchase of services from a variety of sources, including private and voluntary organizations as well as local authority services. This shift from social worker to care manager required a radical rethink of the role of social workers.

care managers

What do you think is the significance of this shift from social worker to care manager?

The care manager was made responsible for assessing individual needs and organizing a suitable 'package of care services'. As Smale *et al.* point out, 'A package of care is not like a basket of goods and services: it is actually a fluid set of human relationships and arrangements ...' (quoted in Hoyes *et al.*, 1994, p.26). The care manager was viewed as much more than just a renamed social worker, and, importantly, the role of the care manager could be carried out by other professionals such as home care organizers.

customers

This change towards care management, with its combination of needs-led assessment and targeted resources, was claimed to offer greater flexibility as well as transferring power to 'customers'. As argued in earlier chapters, the New Right was successful in constructing a range of new welfare subjects within this discourse of the customer or consumer (see also **Clarke, 1998**). Within community care it carries within it the supposed transfer of power from the state to the 'customer'. Again, as with care management, this signifies more than a change of language. The idea of the social service-user as 'customer' is problematic for a number of reasons. One is the argument that, unlike the marketplace, the customers here cannot go elsewhere for their goods, neither do they have real purchasing power because it is the care manager who purchases on their behalf. Other users are reluctant customers, who would not choose the services for themselves. Some commentators have stated that 'the position of users is that of a quasi-customer, exercising consumer sovereignty at second hand through the care manager' (Langan and Clarke, 1994, p.86). Wistow *et al.* (1994, pp.99–112) noted the important point that 'social care is different – the culture of the market has limited relevance' and argued that it is difficult to predict the form which social care markets will take, or the extent to which they would promote governments' objectives of cost savings, quality, choice and equity. Although the language of community care often appears to be user led and customer oriented, the real ambiguities become apparent with a closer examination of some of the issues around the relationship between community care and resources.

3.3   Resources and social care

In practice, care managers are often left to juggle within their constrained but supposedly flexible budgets, aiming to provide care packages based on their assessment of needs. It is at this point that disputes arise between service provider and service-user, particularly when the latter's idea of need does not correspond with the former's assessment of their needs. Mandelstam and Schwehr (1995) have argued that, amongst the talk about rationing, setting priorities, eligibility criteria and targeting of resources to those deemed most in need, there could be a tendency to forget how rationing actually affects people. Bathing, for example, is traditionally viewed as low priority, with people waiting months or even years to be assessed and offered assistance. How many of us would manage without a bath or shower for months or years and still regard it as a low priority?

Social services have a duty to consult with health authorities about community care plans and to ask health authority staff to participate in community care assessments, but basically the duties of health authorities are not specifically covered by the community care legislation. Health services are therefore not officially defined as community care services, even though in practice they are essential to community care. Discharge from hospital provides a good example of the complicated decisions which involve both health and social services. There are many examples of cases where hospitals decide to discharge patients to nursing accommodation, where the patient becomes liable for fees on the grounds that they do not need active medical treatment (Mandelstam and Schwehr, 1995). The pressure to clear hospital beds often leads to conflicts between the various professionals involved.

Local authorities have always operated within limited resources and service provision has often been affected as a result. Given that authorities have wide discretionary powers as to how they meet needs, the argument arises that services will be budget rather than needs led. The authority is required to record information about areas of 'unmet need', which led to concerns that authorities would be legally challenged. As a result, the subsequent guidance made the distinction between 'unmet need' and 'unmet preference'. The basis of this approach is the assumption that the word 'need' triggers off a duty to provide services. This guidance was met with great cynicism and evidence can be found of euphemistic terminology being used to avoid reference to unmet need, such as 'issues and tasks causing problems'; 'issues identified'; 'service shortfalls'; or 'service preferences deficit' (Mandelstam and Schwehr, 1995, p.160).

One of the biggest problems was the context of shrinking resources at a time of escalating demand for services. Demographic changes, particularly an ageing population, together with economic recession resulting in increased unemployment, homelessness, poverty and distress, led to an increase in demand for social care services, at a time when public expenditure on these services was being reduced. Brian Cavanagh, chair of social work on Edinburgh City Council, said, 'The vulnerable are competing with the vulnerable for diminished resources at a time of rightfully heightened expectations' (*The Herald*, 11 October 1996, p.16). Market economics have transformed every public service, but the question remains whether this is an appropriate model for meeting social care needs.

The focus on managerialism in social care became a way of devolving responsibility for these difficult decisions to a very local level, with care managers often responsible for managing their own budgets. This was hailed as a great breakthrough, 'the freedom to manage', blurring the fact that it was central government that made decisions on resourcing for local authorities, who in turn decided the level of resources social services received. Strategic managers within social services divided up the budget and passed responsibility to the level of front-line management, who then had to ensure that they provided services within the budget allocated to them. It is at this point that the conflict over resources became most apparent, with front-line workers placed in the stressful position of rationalizing decisions to disgruntled service-users, who understandably felt they had an entitlement to a service as a right of citizenship. It was in this way that the new-found 'freedom to manage' became a double-edged sword.

3.4 Working in partnership

There are inherent difficulties for the various agencies working together in the interests of the service-user. Community care talks of a 'seamless service' between the various agencies and different parts of the state, such as housing, health, social security and social services. In 1995 the Department of Health (1995a) reported that organizational boundaries often posed difficulties in addressing needs in an effective, efficient and co-ordinated way. This report emphasized the need for joint commissioning, which is the process whereby different agencies co-ordinate their activities. This was said to be beneficial because it delivered a 'seamless' service from a user and carer perspective.

joint commissioning

Can you see any difficulties in the process of joint commissioning?

The language of partnership tends to underestimate the real difficulties in working together. Various sectors within the state each have their own organizational culture, ethos, priorities and working practices. The interface between social services, other welfare sectors and private and voluntary organizations is where these tensions are often played out. Service-users are often at a loss to understand what this tension is about, since they are interested in being provided with a service rather than concerned about which organization is going to provide it.

4   New subjects in social care

At this point it is helpful to think back to some of the issues raised in earlier chapters and revisit the idea of the post-war settlements in the UK. Chapter 2 argued that the 'old' social settlement marginalized and excluded some groups, but that this was challenged by various 'new social movements'. Chapter 2 also argued that in the process of the restructuring of welfare, some of the terms of the challenges were appropriated by sections of the New Right. This tension between, on the one hand, contestations and, on the other, appropriations led, in part, to the creation of new welfare subjects.

4.1   The familialization of welfare

The Thatcher governments wanted to promote vigorously the role of the family as well as voluntary and private sectors in welfare services, thereby playing down the role and significance of state provision. The emphasis was on the family as one of the key providers of welfare. Wilding (1992, p.20) noted: 'there have been eulogies – though nothing much more tangible – for the individuals, largely women – who devote themselves to caring for elderly and dependent people … family care is promoted as the right and proper form of care.'

Although the UK did not have an explicit family policy in the 1990s, it is clear that many of the policies in place carried within them certain normative assumptions about the nature and role of the family. This normative family is a nuclear family, where a man and woman are married and live together with their biological children. This obscured the real diversity of families, which include lone parents, gay or lesbian couples with or without children, extended families, step-families following divorce or death and remarriage, and so on (see **Lentell, 1998**). Community care implicitly reinforced the role of families in providing care and carried within it these normative assumptions about the family, upon which the welfare state has always been premised **(Hall, 1998)**.

The assessment of carers in the putting together of community care packages has become one of the key areas of contestation in social care. It is at this precise point that the boundaries between the public and the private became blurred **(Lewis, 1998b)** as the state transfered responsibilities to the family. In principle, community care recognized the important role played by informal carers such as parents, children, partners or friends, and the resourcing implications of enabling the carer to care. It also recognized that the caring role was usually carried out by women. In practice, however, shortfalls in resourcing often meant that the carer was in effect left to get on with it.

Finch and Mason (1992) made an extensive study of the nature of family responsibilities and the way in which the state redrew the boundaries between state and family responsibility during the 1980s. Importantly, their research showed that the responsibilities and obligations which people feel will be variable and, as such, cannot be assumed within social policy. Another finding was that generally people do not want to have to rely on their relatives for extensive help, that they would prefer 'intimacy at a distance' – close relationships which do not involve dependency. Finch and Mason argued, therefore, that family responsibilities are much more complex than we would imagine at first sight.

4.2 'Race' and social care

The NHS and Community Care Act states that 'Because of their cultural background, some users may need services of a special type or kind, services geared to the requirements of the majority may not always be appropriate' (para. 3.22). The White Paper that preceded the Act acknowledged that the policy would have to take account of 'minority interests' and be planned in consultation with a diversity of service-users and communities (HMSO, 1989). This suggests that some users will have special needs, with the implication that these are different needs from the rest. This construction of black and other communities' needs as 'special needs' is problematic **(Lewis, 1998a)**.

It is important to note the way the term 'ethnic minority' is being used within the discourse of community care as a fixed and rigid category and not as a social construction. It is in this way that the needs of 'black' communities are essentialized **(Lewis, 1998a)**. Walker and Ahmad (1994, p.50) noted the way in which 'minorities are homogenized for the purposes of magnifying the "welfare burden" or blanketing their needs under "special provision" or the rubric that "they look after their own". In these ways the ideology of the mythological family and the imaginary community serves both inclusive and exclusive purposes.' What becomes apparent is the way that community care involves slippery idealizations of the family and the community.

In reviewing the literature relating to Asian and African-Caribbean carers, Atkin and Rollings (1992) argue that the needs of black carers have generally been ignored; that is, within the context of carers' needs being marginalized. They challenge the stereotype of the caring black family which 'looks after its own', and the related assumption that resources from the public purse should not be used to offer additional support, on similar grounds to those argued by Finch and Mason (1992). Both argue that the idea that everyone has a family that is willing and able to look after them is fundamentally flawed. Atkin and

Rollings go on to point out that, although the extended family is still common amongst people of South Asian origin and descent in the UK, there is also a significant proportion of South Asian people who live alone, or have no family in the UK outside of their immediate household. Walker and Ahmad (1994, pp.65–6) similarly argue that 'changes in family structures and geographical dispersal of kin, housing problems and economic imperatives combine to make it no wiser to assume traditional care networks in black communities than can be assumed in the population generally.' The impact of immigration and the way this disproportionately affects and divides black families would also need to be taken into account if we were to consider the availability of families to provide care.

Community care has been viewed as a mixture of threat and opportunity, the threat being the gulf between self-defined need and resources. Black communities are already starting from a disadvantaged position in relation to access to welfare services in the form of health, education, housing and other benefits; the effect of community care is to further marginalize their varied and diverse needs. The opportunities, on the other hand, can be seen as the creative possibilities for opening up planning and consultation processes to a diversity of groups and communities. As part of an agenda for action, Atkin and Rollings stated that:

> Successful community care, in a multi-racial society, cannot therefore rely merely on an understanding of black users' views … perceptions of black people do not occur in a void but are interpreted, framed and acted upon by service providers, using judgments which may be inherently racist. This, in effect, provides the context in which black user views will be incorporated …
>
> We need to avoid the danger that race issues become insulated and isolated from general discussion of social care issues, thereby marginalizing the needs of black people. The issues of the range, quality and accessibility of service provision, although having to reflect different needs, are relevant to all. Rather than being regarded as a 'special needs' group, race must become an integrated part of the future debate on social care.
>
> (Atkin and Rollings, 1992, pp.70–1)

The policy tension in this context was how to find a path which acknowledged and challenged racism, and simultaneously avoided the pitfalls of constructing racial or ethnic difference as indicative of essential difference.

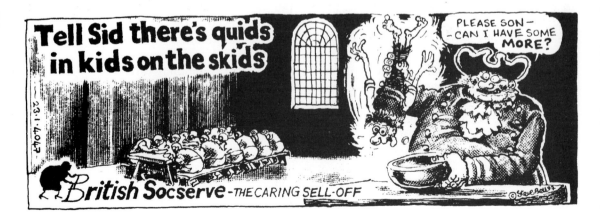

5 The refocusing of children's services

As with the community care legislation, The Children Act 1989 (England and Wales) was introduced during a period of intense change and fierce criticism of social work. In order to understand the changes that have been introduced it is necessary to understand where the pressures for change came from. This chapter argues that the discourse of managerialism, so evident in community care, has had similar consequences in services for children.

5.1 The pressure for change

During the 1970s social workers came under increasing public scrutiny. For example, the death of Maria Colwell in 1973, while living with her family but known to social services, and the subsequent inquiry provoked a hostile media reaction. Inquiries focused on social work practice and procedures, and the terms of reference for each inquiry report excluded a discussion of *why* children are abused: 'It becomes almost as if child abuse is caused by lack of communication, missing memos or whatever other problems an inquiry has uncovered. Perhaps this helps also to explain the phenomenon of social workers being blamed for child deaths as if they were personally responsible for them' (Frost and Stein, 1989, p.49).

Part of the crisis for social work at this time was that each inquiry report made recommendations, without reference to earlier reports. The outcomes were many and varied but the contradictions inherent within the reports meant that there was some confusion about what actually needed to be done. During this period social workers were continually being asked to assess their practice within a hostile climate. Demoralization, confusion and defensive practice, with the aim of avoiding professional risk taking, became widespread.

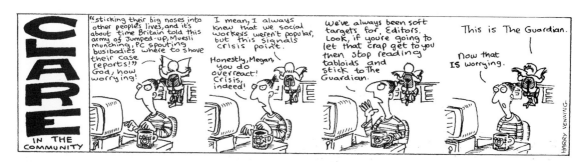

It is important to understand the way in which the inquiry reports impacted upon social work practice, because they were so significant in shaping legislation, policy and practice. The earlier reports tended to focus on individual children who were killed by either a parent or step-parent, while the later reports were more often about sexual or 'ritual' abuse. We will look at two examples, the Beckford and Cleveland Reports, mainly because both had major significance in shaping social work with children and their families, but also because of the contradictions inherent within each about the role of social work.

5.2   The inquiry reports

Jasmine Beckford was born in 1979. As a result of concerns, Jasmine and her younger sister were placed with foster carers in 1981 and both were made subject to care orders. After a period with foster carers the decision was made to return both children to the care of their mother and step-father. Jasmine died in 1984, aged four. Her step-father was later convicted of manslaughter. The inquiry into Jasmine's death, led by Louis Blom-Cooper, reported in 1985 (London Borough of Brent, 1985). The major criticisms of social workers to emerge from this report (known as the Beckford Report) were as follows:

- too slow to intervene to prevent the child's death;
- regarded the parents rather than the child as their 'client';
- too willing to accept the parents' explanations for injuries or bruises;
- too optimistic in their interpretation of events within the family;
- the child's needs were sometimes lost as social workers became drawn into support for the parents;
- failed to use their authority.

The Beckford Report raised the issues of the role of social work itself, in particular the tension between the dual mandate of care and control. The potential for conflict and confusion between the social policing role and the befriending and supportive role of social work was acknowledged, but generally social workers were viewed as reluctant to use their statutory powers.

Various commentators have noted that social workers are not simply law enforcement officers and that the area of child care law is ambiguous and open to interpretation. Social workers are not provided with a clear-cut 'mandate' for intervention, as characterized by Beckford and other inquiry reports. The view of social work presented within the report leads the reader into misunderstanding and oversimplifying the nature of the relationship between social workers and service-users. Frost and Stein (1989) argue that this narrowing of the social work role, to law enforcement, detracts from other roles such as, for example, prevention, support and counselling. They go on to argue that the report was written with the benefit of hindsight, as well as being written as if the social worker was working with only this one case at the time. This decontextualization of practice was unhelpful.

One of the wider implications of the inquiry reports was the idea that complete protection of children in their families was not possible without further intrusion by the state into the family. This issue of the boundaries between the state and families was significant since 'Child abuse … helps to define the "good" family and the boundary of state intervention into households' (Frost and Stein, 1989, p.48).

ACTIVITY 7.3

Read Extract 7.2, which is taken from *The Family: Is it Just Another Lifestyle Choice?* published by the Institute of Economic Affairs, a New Right think-tank. As you read, consider the view of the causes of child abuse being proposed.

Extract 7.2   Carlson: 'Liberty, order and the family'

Analysis of still other current social pathologies drives home the critical importance of the intact family and the enormous social price exacted by a growing number of divorced or mother-headed families. Turning to child abuse, for example, David G. Gil observes that:

> The data … suggests an association between physical abuse of children and deviance from normative structure, which seems especially strong for non-white children.

An investigation of 214 parents of battered babies in Britain found that they 'are likely to be reared in broken homes', with pre-marital pregnancy, illegitimacy, and absence of the child's father among the most common 'precursors of baby battering'. Even remarriage seems unable to help. A research team at McMaster University established in 1985 that:

> preschoolers living with one natural and one step-parent were *40 times* more likely to become child abuse cases than were like-aged children living with two natural parents.

Making the point a different way, in 1985 a NIMH study found that violence against children is actually *decreasing* in America's intact families.

To strengthen families

Nonetheless, the number of such families is falling in the United States, both relatively and in absolute terms. The economic incentives and political pressures have made it ever more difficult for such families to function, and fewer adults are able to sustain the effort. The consequence is the swelling level of the predictable social pathologies reported in the media: criminal behaviour; adult and juvenile suicide; drug abuse; poor educational achievement; the physical abuse of children; and the breakdown of urban civility.

(Carlson, 1993, pp.51–2)

COMMENT

In Extract 7.2 the Institute of Economic Affairs (IEA) argue that 'deviant' families, such as lone parents, divorced or step-families, are more likely to abuse their children. In addition, 'non-white children' are seen to be especially vulnerable. Child abuse is being constructed here as one of the consequences of the breakdown of the normative family and of 'urban civility'. These arguments may be familiar to you as part of 'the underclass theory' **(Lentell, 1998; Morris, 1998)**.

The IEA goes on to argue that 'families must be allowed to become more powerful … families can be strengthened in this way only as they are allowed to reclaim some of the functions they have lost.' For the IEA the agenda must include 'A prudent reduction and reform of the state's child protection system, restoring the preference given to the natural rights of parents' (Carlson, 1993, p.53). Note here how it is the rights of parents, not children, which are to be strengthened, which is in direct contradiction to the Beckford Report's emphasis on children's rights over those of parents. This tension between the rights of parents and those of children has continually been played out in the inquiry reports, policy and legislation.

■ ■ ■

The Cleveland Report, in contrast to Beckford, focused on the alleged sexual abuse of a large number of children. In a period of five months during 1987, 121 children were diagnosed by two paediatricians, Dr Marietta Higgs and Dr Geoff Wyatt, as being sexually abused. The main criticisms to emerge from the report into the Cleveland crisis were:

■ Social workers were too quick to intervene to 'protect' children.

■ Children were being removed from home in circumstances which were dubious, in particular in 'dawn raids' where children were removed in the early hours.

■ Social workers were not working with parents or carers in a way which would enhance co-operation.

■ The medical tests used by paediatricians to diagnose sexual abuse became highly contested.

Interestingly, the report that emerged from Cleveland (Secretary of State for Social Services, 1988) referred back to the earlier reports, in particular to Beckford. It acknowledged that social workers had been criticized in the Beckford Report for not intervening to protect children and the effect of this could clearly be seen in Cleveland. The lessons learnt from Beckford were seen to backfire. One of the key questions we need to ask here is: to what extent can social workers legitimately intervene in families? The Cleveland Report acknowledged the difficulties faced by social workers in that they would be criticized if they intervened to remove the child unnecessarily, but that they are also criticized if they do not intervene and the child is either injured or killed. 'The contradiction of Cleveland is that society has demanded that the professionals do something about child sexual abuse, and yet it won't forgive them when they do or when they don't' (Campbell, 1988, p.13).

The media and the local Labour MP, Stuart Bell, took on a particularly hostile attitude towards social work during the crisis. It became, as Nava (1988) has noted, a moral panic in which the two paediatricians became the scapegoats, or 'folk devils' (see, for example, Cohen, 1972).

ACTIVITY 7.4

What do the news headlines from 1987 given in Figure 7.1 show about the media perception of social workers and the paediatricians involved?

One of the most powerful criticisms from the media during the Cleveland crisis was the argument that huge numbers of children were removed from their homes unnecessarily. It is worth pausing for a moment here to examine this a little further. In 70 per cent of cases the cause for concern about sexual abuse was accepted by the courts or by the families themselves. Out of the 118 children removed on 'place of safety' orders, the courts eventually decided that social workers 'got it wrong' in only 26 cases, involving 12 families (Kelly, 1988). Campbell argues that 'dreadful discoveries' about sexual abuse arose from the Cleveland crisis. These were that:

> it takes place inside rather than outside families and neighbourhoods ... that the perpetrators aren't dangerous strangers ... they're the men we all know, not so much the outcasts as the men in our lives, respectable dads, neighbours, stockbrokers and shop stewards, judges and jurors. They are men of all ages, races, religions and classes.
>
> (Campbell, 1988, p.5)

Overboard on child abuse

The danger of labelling parents guilty until proved innocent

Freed children taken back from family

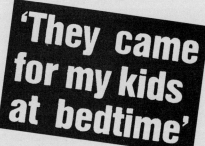
'They came for my kids at bedtime'

The making of Doctor Marietta Higgs, crusader

Figure 7.1 Headlines from the Daily Mail, News on Sunday *and* The Independent *during the 1987 Cleveland crisis (Source: Nava, 1988)*

The other area that Cleveland forced an acknowledgement on was that sexual abuse was much more widespread than the normative idea of the family would suggest and, crucially, that it crossed class boundaries. These arguments make it problematic to view child abuse as a homogeneous category and make it necessary to separate out physical and sexual abuse, where the explanatory frameworks need to be very different. Acknowledging the different part played by social class, gender, and social and environmental factors would be a positive step towards understanding why abuse occurs.

In 1997, 10 years on, a re-examination of events in Cleveland took place. *The Observer* reported that:

> Many of the papers came out emphatically for the Stuart Bell happy-families package. They treated Marietta Higgs as a fiend, and characterised the sexual abuse diagnoses as part of a radical feminist conspiracy. Salem was invoked, so was Orwell. Accused parents were interviewed on the unexamined assumption that they were innocent and injured, especially the many who appeared middle class, articulate, liberal, 'nice'.

> (Nicci Gerrard, *Observer Review*, 25 May 1997, p.4)

A 1997 television documentary (*The Death of Childhood*, May 1997, Channel 4) argued that the effect of the crisis was that children were returned home despite a strong belief by social workers, health visitors, doctors and a child psychologist that they had been abused. In effect some of the children may have been returned to abusers. All records relating to the children who were part of the original investigation were destroyed, and in this way the past was erased. This silence, 10 years on from the Cleveland crisis, was startling.

It is worth noting the different criticisms of social work within these inquiry reports because they reflect the ambivalence held by the media and the public about the nature and role of social work. The earlier reports were about individual children and their families and tended to 'pathologize' and locate responsibility at the level of the individual. It became possible therefore to construct these individuals as 'sick', 'mad' or 'bad'. Whichever way they were seen, it was possible to distance oneself from the individual or family concerned and never examine wider issues, such as the inequalities between children and adults, the difficulties for children in being heard, or the environmental or structural inequalities, such as poverty, which may sometimes be significant in explaining why physical abuse occurs. This obscuring of wider social inequalities, such as those linked to class or gender, becomes unhelpful in understanding the *why* questions. In contrast, the later reports focused attention on whole communities rather than individuals and it was no longer possible to pathologize in the same way. This led to an examination of the widespread nature of sexual abuse and the way in which it was not possible to identify who would be 'at risk' in the same way as with physical abuse.

A further and important outcome from the later reports was the backlash against feminist critiques in social work, critiques which had become influential during the 1970s and 1980s. Feminist academics and social workers had been active in many areas of social work and had in particular challenged the way that systems theories and family therapy, the dominant theories in social work in the 1980s, had meant that societal problems were located only at the level of the individual or the family. Many SSDs had incorporated feminist critiques into their policies and procedures. The SSD in the London Borough of Islington was one of a number of authorities that led the field in acknowledging feminist criticisms in their work with children and families (Boushel and Noakes, 1988). After Cleveland, however, there was a retreat from feminist-influenced policy, procedures and practice in most authorities. The point made in section 2.3 about challenges to social work from 'the margins' having limited success is relevant here, and it is possible to see a distancing from feminist critiques after Cleveland.

One of the outcomes of the inquiry reports was the introduction of detailed guidance, and many felt that social work became more bureaucratic and procedural. It was as though the use of checklists would prevent abuse and provide safety, in the sense that social workers would feel reassured that they had acted reasonably. Another outcome was the shift to a socio-legal model for child protection, where legal experts came to dominate **(Saraga, 1998b)**.

It can be argued, then, that the pressure for change in the organization of services to children and their families came from a number of directions, but not least from the outcome of the cluster of inquiry reports.

5.3   The Children Act 1989 (England and Wales)

The Children Act 1989 was introduced after almost two decades of fierce criticism of social work, as well as growing unease within social work itself about its role and responsibilities in relation to work with children, and in particular about child protection.

ACTIVITY 7.5

Some of the key principles of the Children Act 1989 are listed below. As you read them think about and note how they reflect the various criticisms of social work discussed earlier.

- Social workers should aim to work in partnership with parents/carers as well as with other agencies. (Parental participation in child protection case conferences is one example of an initiative which has been developed from this.)

- There was an assumption of minimal intervention, which became known as the no-order principle. What this meant in practice was that a court order, such as supervision or care orders, should not be sought unless thought to be absolutely necessary and where voluntary agreements for work with the family have been tried and failed.

- The interests and welfare of the child should be paramount.

- The child's 'race', religion, language and culture should be taken into account when assessing or making a placement for a child.

- There should be a reduction in delays in proceedings that could prejudice the welfare of the child. This arose from criticisms that long delays in providing assessments for care proceedings had caused additional stress on the child and family concerned.

COMMENT

Even from this brief examination of some of the principles which underpin the Children Act, it is possible to trace the threads of earlier criticisms of social work and to see the way these criticisms have manifested themselves within the legislation. With the no-order principle, for example, it can be seen that some of the earlier criticisms of social work were picked up, particularly those raised within the Cleveland inquiry, that social workers had misused their powers and been too quick to seek legal orders. Similarly, the principle of the children's interests being paramount reminds us of earlier criticisms of the child being 'lost' in the work with the parents.

Criticisms of social work, as in other areas of welfare, are contested. It is interesting to examine the way some criticisms emerged as more dominant and influential in shaping social work, while others were either lost or silenced within the same legislation. One way of viewing this is to examine the way that some features of the legislation are permissive, which means SSDs *should* take this into account (such as the 'race', religion, language and culture principle), whereas others are obligatory, which means SSDs *have* to take this into account (such as the child's interests being paramount). In general terms it can be seen that those criticisms which came from 'the margins' have been only partially successful in shaping the outcomes, or they have shaped them in a different way than intended. Challenges from 'the margins' created a powerful critique of social work practice which, although uneven in impact, challenged some practices. What is clear, however, is that the criticisms from 'the centre', such as the inquiry reports or the New Right critique of welfare, have generally been more powerful in shaping the legislation, procedures and practice of social work.

■ ■ ■

The Children Act received a mixed response within social work and from other professionals involved in work with children. It was welcomed by some social workers and viewed as a comprehensive and coherent piece of legislation which provided a legal framework for the protection and promotion of the interests and welfare of children. Others argued that it simply reasserted what was already considered to be 'good practice'. Ahmad argued that the Act provided an opportunity to reform child care work and that the potential for enhancing anti-racist social work should not be underestimated (MacDonald, 1991).

The contradictions within the legislation are noteworthy. Although the Act acknowledges diversity within and across families, including cohabiting parents and step-parents, it gives little formal recognition to gay or lesbian parenting, although it has been used by lesbian parents to gain joint residence orders. Similarly, it is possible to use the Act to remove the perpetrator of abuse rather than removing the child from the home, which could be viewed as a small victory for feminist perspectives, which argued that removing the child amounted to blaming the victim. The Children Act (Scotland) 1995 is more explicit in that it has 'an exclusion order' which will be used, where appropriate, to exclude alleged abusers from the child's family home (*Children in Scotland: Children (Scotland) Act 1995 – Information Pack* (1995).

5.4   Working together?

One of the key documents to shape work with children and their families was published in 1991. *Working Together Under the Children Act 1989* focused on the area of inter-agency co-operation in child protection and became central in providing guidance and advice on multi-agency working and decision-making within social work.

ACTIVITY 7.6

Read Extract 7.3, which is taken from *Working Together Under the Children Act 1989*, a document produced by the Department of Health with the Home Office, the then Department of Education and Science and the Welsh Office. Keep the following questions in your mind as you read:

1   Who are viewed as the main agencies involved in protecting children?

2   How are social workers' powers constrained by the guidance in this document?

3   Is it possible to see the way the criticisms of social work mentioned earlier are incorporated into the guidance?

Extract 7.3 Department of Health: 'Working together under the Children Act 1989'

Legal framework

1.10 Fveryone who is concerned in a professional capacity with the protection of children needs to have a clear understanding of the main points of child care law as it applies to the care and protection of children, and its implications for the discharge of their respective responsibilities. They should be aware, in particular, that legislation places the primary responsibility for the care and protection of abused children and children at risk of abuse on local authorities …

1.11 Other agencies besides local authorities have statutory duties or powers and all agencies have specific functions and professional objectives. In working together for the protection of children, however, they need to understand that they are not only carrying out their own agency's functions but are also making, individually and collectively, a vital contribution to advising and assisting the local authority in the discharge of its child protection and child care duties …

1.13 The difficulties of assessing the risk of harm to a child should not be underestimated. It is imperative that everyone who deals with allegations and suspicions of abuse maintains an open and inquiring mind …

Part 4: Role of agencies involved in child protection

Introduction

4.1 This section deals with the roles of agencies and other associated groups in relation to child protection and how their duties and functions should be organised in order to contribute to inter-agency co-operation for the protection of children … The responsibility for protecting children should not fall entirely to one agency: awareness and appreciation of another agency's role will contribute greatly to collaborative practices.

Social services

4.2 Social services departments have a wide range of duties and responsibilities to provide services for individuals and for families. The services which they are required to provide encompass people of all ages, abilities and social groupings. Social services departments provide services for people living in the community in their own homes and they also provide residential and day care services. In addition they have regulatory functions in relation to services provided by the voluntary and private sector and they may also work collaboratively with these bodies.

4.3 The child protection work of social services departments should be considered in the wider context of all the department's work and more precisely in the context of its child care services. Field workers engaged in child protection work are also involved in a wide range of other child care work and they often work with other client groups. They are aware of the wider child care facilities provided and known to the department and can draw on these in order to provide support and treatment services for children who have been abused. These include day care facilities, residential accommodation and foster homes.

4.4 Local authorities are under a statutory duty to investigate where they have reasonable cause to suspect that a child is or is likely to suffer significant harm or is subject to an emergency protection order or police protection. The social services department carries these responsibilities on behalf of the local authority. They do not do this alone and of necessity call on the expertise and knowledge of other agencies and professionals ...

The police

4.11 Police involvement in cases of child abuse stems from their primary responsibilities to protect the community and to bring offenders to justice ...

Police/social services consultation

4.16 Although in cases of child abuse both the police and social services have as their foremost objective the welfare of the child, their primary functions, powers and methods of working are different. Whilst the police will focus on the investigation of alleged offences, the social services are concerned with the welfare of the child and other members of the family.

4.17 Difficulties will be encountered in joint inter-agency investigations but these can be minimised by the selection of specialist staff who undergo appropriate inter-agency training ...

Health services

4.18 All those working in the field of health have a commitment to protect children, and their participation in inter-agency support to social services departments is essential if the interests of children are to be safeguarded. Health professionals are major contributors to the inter-agency care of children which extends beyond the initial referral and assessment, into child protection conference attendance, participation in planning and the ongoing support of the child and family. There will always be a need for close co-operation with other agencies, including any other health professionals involved ...

The role of the midwife and health visitor

4.23 Medical, nursing and midwifery staff have a part to play, but the major roles are played by the midwife and health visitor working together. Parents are responsible for the well-being and protection of their children. The encouragement to take a responsible attitude to the care of their children and to seek appropriate help and support will do much to prevent child abuse. Child abuse is less likely if there is an affectionate and positive relationship between the parents and baby ...

All hospital staff

4.24 Staff in hospital departments see children in the course of their normal duties and need to be alert to indications of child abuse. Abused children may attend hospital accident and emergency departments as a consequence of injuries inflicted on them ...

Primary and community health services

4.25 Health surveillance programmes are a well-recognised part of the primary services for children. Parents are encouraged to bring their children to child health clinics where health visitors and doctors will be involved in monitoring the child's health and development ... These and other community health staff are well placed to identify children who are being harmed or who may be at risk of harm and should be aware of the signs and symptoms of abuse, and the procedures to follow ...

General practitioners

4.31 General practitioners have a vital role in the protection of children. As family doctors, working closely with health visitors, and other members of the primary health care team, they are well placed to identify at an early stage family stress which may point to a risk of child abuse, or to notice in the child indications of significant harm … General practitioners' extensive knowledge of the family background enables them to make a particular contribution to child protection conferences and to the long term support of the child and family …

Probation service

4.34 Probation officers may become involved in cases of child abuse as a result either of their responsibility for the supervision of offenders including those convicted of offences against children, or of their responsibility to the court for the supervision of children following marital breakdown. They may be able to identify potential cases and bring in other agencies when, through their work, they become concerned about the safety of a child …

The education service

4.35 The education service does not constitute an investigation or intervention agency, but has an important role to play at the recognition and referral stage. Because of their day-to-day contact with individual children during school terms, teachers and other school staff are particularly well placed to observe outward signs of abuse, changes in behaviour or failure to develop …

Day care services

4.41 Day nurseries, playgroups, out of school clubs and holiday schemes, and childminders, are likely to have an important part to play in helping parents under stress cope with their children's behaviour, to support them and give them a respite and thus prevent abuse …

National Society for the Prevention of Cruelty to Children (NSPCC)

4.44 Uniquely amongst voluntary bodies the NSPCC has a power to apply for care, supervision and child assessment orders in its own right. The NSPCC is a charitable organisation whose Royal Charter places upon it 'the duty to ensure an appropriate and speedy response in all cases where children are alleged to be at risk of abuse or neglect in any form'. Social workers employed by the NSPCC have a central concern to identify and prevent cruelty to children …

Other voluntary organisations

4.45 A wide range of voluntary organisations provide services, including telephone helplines, to help parents under stress and children at risk. Some of these are national, such as Childline, which provides counselling for children with problems; others are for the support of parents, such as Parentline, or are locally based …

The community

4.47 The community as a whole has a responsibility for the well-being of children. This means that all citizens should remain alert to circumstances in which children may be harmed. Individuals can assist the statutory authorities by bringing cases to their attention. Relatives, friends and neighbours of children are particularly well placed to do so, but they must know what to do if they are concerned.

(Department of Health, 1991, pp.2–3, 15–24)

Working Together Under the Children Act 1989 provided a framework for social work to be one of a number of key organizations involved in decision-making in the child protection arena. In the light of the events in Cleveland it can be seen as an attempt to balance the rights of parents with the need to protect children. On the one hand this multi-agency framework could be viewed as introducing further bureaucratic and professional constraints on social workers. Another view would see it more positively, as an extension of previously existing 'good practice'. Both the Children Act 1989 and *Working Together* assumed that social work would be the key agency involved in protecting children, although they formalize the roles and responsibilities of each of the other agencies involved. The parallels with community care are notable here, with the assumption that no one agency has monopoly of power or decision-making. This suggests that the mixed economy of care exists in children's services as it does in services to adults.

The role of the courts in questioning the rationale and decision-making of recommendations in reports also meant that the powers of social workers were constrained in a new way. The framework provided by the legislation increased central government control over the shape of the services provided. In addition, the focus on inter-agency work reduced social workers' authority, autonomy and discretion. This links in with the idea of social workers themselves as 'new subjects' in social care, in that their autonomy and powers were curtailed in relation to other agencies such as the police, legal experts and medical practitioners (see Chapters 1 and 2).

The difficulties and tensions created by inter-agency working should not be underestimated. These tensions are often played out in child protection case conferences, which are the formal arena for decision-making in child protection. Each professional enters this arena with a different background, training, organizational structure, supervision, experience and interest in the child or family. These differences often lead to tensions and conflict, which in themselves may often deflect from the interests of the child. These difficulties are not unique to children's services, but are also observed in community care, particularly in the tension between health and social services.

■ ■ ■

5.5 Children in need versus child protection

The discussion of children's services so far has mainly centred around child protection, but it is important to remember that the Children Act 1989 provided a framework for preventive and supportive work with children and families as well as child protection. As with community care, it was envisaged that this support could be provided either by the state itself or by a range of other providers, either private, voluntary or the family, with social workers being in a co-ordinating or commissioning role. This distinction between children in need and child protection is a critical one if we are to understand the way social work was reconstructed in the period between the 1970s and 1990s. The distinction crucially impacts upon resources, and the criticism has often been made that children in need are neglected as resources are channelled into child protection instead. **Saraga (1998b)** argues that how the needs of children are defined and which children are seen to require welfare provision is socially constructed and varies historically and according to socio-economic circumstances.

The Children Act can be viewed as seeking to strike a delicate balance between, on the one hand, promoting support services for families with children in need and, on the other, protecting children deemed to be at risk of abuse. Some have suggested that the Act reflects rather than resolves many of the inherent contradictions of social policy, particularly as it relates to children and families. While the Act provides a clear legislative framework, which was welcomed by many professionals who work with children and families, and was acknowledged as providing the basis for a progressive welfare approach, it could not resolve many of the underlying conflicts which exist between the state, the family and the individual parent or child (Jack and Stepney, 1995).

Contrary to the spirit of the Children Act 1989, children in need sometimes have to be identified as being at risk of abuse before they qualify for services at all. Department of Health commissioned research which focused on SSDs' response to children in need showed that generally SSDs are experiencing problems in giving any priority to cases which are outside of the child protection area. In the authorities examined, child protection cases were talked of as the 'core business'. The demand-led context, general defensiveness and safeguarding against criticism and hostility meant that staff found it difficult to support children in need if they were not deemed to be at risk of 'significant harm'. Social workers felt they had sometimes to accentuate parts of the 'children in need' case to ensure that they qualified for support services. Financial managers confirmed that up to 80 per cent of their children's service's budget was directed towards child protection, whereas the remaining 20 per cent went towards promotional or support services (Department of Health, 1993).

In the light of the pressures and criticisms following implementation of the Children Act 1989, in particular that services must be preventive and supportive as well as being targeted at children deemed to be at risk of harm, most authorities had to rethink their approach. The development of children's services plans was an attempt to balance the different parts of the legislation, including both support and protection for children. The publication of these plans was made mandatory in England and Wales in March 1996. In Scotland they were already mandatory under the Children (Scotland) Act 1995. Again, the parallels between children's services plans and community care plans is striking, in that both assume a separation of purchaser and provider roles, and both assume that services will be provided within a framework of a mixed economy, that is, by a variety of agencies.

The development of children's services plans is a reflection in part of a developing understanding that 'no one department or agency has a monopoly on meeting the needs of individual service-users' (Sutton, 1995). Sutton goes on to argue that children's services plans represented an ideal opportunity to plan targeted services for children in need. The idea was that local authorities, child health services and the private and voluntary sectors would collaborate in the planning of integrated services for children. It was possible that other areas of activity such as play, road design, traffic management and environmental planning would be acknowledged as contributing in important ways to children's well-being. Some of the potential conflicts and complexities involved in multi-agency work mentioned earlier made the development of children's services plans a challenge for the agencies involved. It is also worth noting that managerial and bureaucratic solutions were being proposed here, though the problem was one of scarce resources, stretched to their limit.

children's services plans

Public spending constraints meant that there was a tendency towards narrowing definitions of risk and need. Social workers have often argued that the threshold of risk, particularly in relation to child protection, had constantly been raised. Competition for scarce resources resulted in preventive and supportive work being devalued, in a culture where performance targets, measurement of outcomes, and the demand for greater efficiency mitigates against preventive work, which by its very nature is difficult to quantify in this way. The dilemmas facing social workers in providing services to both children in need as well as child protection has not gone unnoticed. As one social worker stated:

> The Children Act specifies two categories: children in need and children at risk, and they want the department to deliver services to both groups. But there has always been and will continue to be, even more overtly, a hierarchy: you can't ignore the children at risk to offer services to children in need, because there's no resources for children in need.

(quoted in Novak and Sennet, 1995)

During the late 1990s a major debate emerged in the UK about how policies and practice for child protection and children in need could be integrated. Increasingly the tension between these two areas was being played out through policy-makers, managers and practitioners in social care. The Children Act 1989 was clear in providing a framework for child welfare in the widest sense; that is, in a way which included protection, prevention and support services. In the early years of implementation, however, a consensus of opinion developed which was that services to children in need were neither adequate nor desirable.

In 1994 the Audit Commission published *Seen But Not Heard: Co-ordinating Community Child Health and Social Services for Children in Need*. This report, together with the Department of Health report *Child Protection, Messages from Research* (Department of Health, 1995b), informed an agenda for change, particularly in the balance between child protection and child support. Both of these reports were highly significant in shaping child welfare services. One of the most critical aspects of the Department of Health report was the suggestion that valuable time and resources were being focused on child protection investigations, a large proportion of which did not result in child protection registration and therefore provided little benefit to the child or the family. One of the studies cited in both reports noted the series of filters which operated in relation to child protection investigations, where only 15 per cent of referred children were placed on the child protection register. In 44 per cent of cases the investigation led to no further action at all, neither registration, monitoring, nor support services of any kind (Gibbons *et al.*, 1995). This research has been interpreted as support for the idea that most social work intervention is wasteful of resources and that these resources could be more usefully employed in offering practical support to families and children.

One of the consequences of the attempt to rebalance child protection and support for families is the way it highlights perfectly the relationship between resources and service provision. Changing definitions of risk and need directly impact upon who will and will not receive a service (see **Langan, 1998b**). It is important to remember that the context here is one where the construction of child abuse is highly contested and these contestations have been, and will continue to be, played out in relation to policy, procedures, guidance and practice.

Read Extract 7.4, which is taken from the 1995/96 annual report of the Social Services Inspectorate (SSI). Make notes on the following questions as you read:

1   What changes did the SSI argue needed to take place?

2   Can you see the continuities and contradictions with criticisms raised earlier in this chapter?

3   Do you think bureaucratic and managerial solutions are being sought here?

Extract 7.4 Social Services Inspectorate: 'Progress through change'

Services for children and families

Introduction

4.1 Following implementation of the Children Act and Criminal Justice Acts, the main priority for children and families work is to secure effective, efficient and economical delivery of services within the framework of the legislation. Inspection, policy implementation and development work on children's services again absorbed a substantial share of SSI's resources …

Developing children's services planning

4.2 Planning for children's services needs to be developed jointly by local agencies. In June the Government announced it would make an Order requiring the production and publication of children's services plans. The order was made in March 1996 and guidance on good practice was also issued in March …

4.3 Children's services plans will form a central part of SSI's work in the coming year, and will underpin many other initiatives such as work on information, and costing needs and services. The focus will be on a multi-agency approach to planning, emphasising the importance of education and health service involvement.

Study of children's services plans

4.4 In December SSI published the second part of a development project to examine the contents of published plans and explore issues involved in their production. The study carried four key messages:

- it is as important to get the **planning process** right as to produce the published plan. The written plans are important, but can only be as good as the process of planning of which they are a product.

- inter-agency co-operation requires a shared understanding of **values, principles and definitions of need**, as well as compatible planning cycles. Agencies need to appreciate one another's different roles in relation to children, and recognise that co-operative planning is more than just agreeing about definitions and language.

- the task of **measuring need** is difficult, but measurement is essential for making comparisons with existing provision of services and determining policies, priorities and costs. Further work is required on the technical difficulties related to measuring of needs and costs.

- the three key disciplines, health, education and social work, must develop a **common language** in order to have a shared understanding of child care need …

Organisation of children's services

4.7 Over the last two years, an SSI project has looked at the organisational structure of services for children in social services departments. Early work suggested that about half of the departments had re-organised services for children along similar lines to services for adult users – with some degree of separation between purchasing and providing functions. The main findings of the pilot study in 4 local authorities in 1995 were:

- generally financial control was left with the providers, calling into question the rationale for the structural split;
- problems of co-ordination between purchasers and providers were experienced with a potential risk to users and waste of staff resources;

The main messages for the future are:

- departments should carefully consider the purpose of internal market arrangements for children's services;
- the development process for children's services plans could provide a vehicle to consider any changes;
- top management must give attention to arrangements for staff accountability and delegation of budgets ...

Refocusing child protection in the context of children in need

4.9 SSI together with Department colleagues and the Association of Directors (ADSS) has contributed to the debate on the need to redefine child protection within the overall provision for children in need. The coming year will see further opportunities for debate on how policy should in future be focused ...

Children in need: inspections 1993/95

4.16 The main findings from a report of eight inspections of service responses to children in need were:

- cases of children in need tended to receive **insufficient priority** unless they came within the definition of child protection;
- departments failed to define clear **priorities for action**;
- inexperienced staff were operating the **duty system**;
- some duty systems were **inefficient**;
- referring agencies believed it was necessary to make a **child protection referral** in order to access services.

The report recommends to authorities:

- a clear **corporate approach** to the development of children's services plans;
- better **measurement of demand** for services, referrals, service outputs and unmet need;
- clearly defined **performance criteria** for children's services;
- improved **inter-agency understanding** of responsibilities.

4.17 ... In all authorities these services were overshadowed by the competing demands of child protection. This reinforces the current debate on the need for a new approach to children's services.

(Social Services Inspectorate, 1996, pp.25–7, 29–30)

The SSI's *Progress Through Change* echoed the message from the previous year's Department of Health (1995b) research which called for a shift away from child protection to a more preventive and supportive approach. One of the concerns voiced here was the idea that organizational change has often meant that the voices of the 'client' are sometimes lost. It is unclear here whether the 'client' is the child or the family. The report also places local authority social services within the wider context of the mixed economy of social care and acknowledges that SSDs are often the purchasers rather than the providers, who are more likely to be the private or voluntary sectors. In an interview with *The Guardian*, Laming, Chief Inspector of the SSI, said that he was not dodging the resources issue, that there had been problems, but that he believed authorities could help themselves by striking a better balance between services and spending (*The Guardian*, 10 July 1996).

Many practitioners of social care would state that it is precisely this difficulty with resourcing which prevents the services being developed in a fashion that is consistent with good practice. Laming stated that he was looking for concrete evidence of change in the delivery of children's services. Referring to the eight inspections of services relating to children in need, the report says that such children were accorded insufficient priority unless they fell within a definition of child protection: 'In all authorities, these services were overshadowed by the competing demands of child protection' (Social Services Inspectorate, 1996, p.30). While this is consistent with earlier reports, and with criticisms from within and external to social work, it does not resolve the basic dilemma which faces practitioners and managers, which is how to integrate services in a way that will provide both protection and support to children and their families. Many see this as further evidence of a double bind, similar to the 'damned if they do and damned if they don't' idea.

Language such as 'priorities for action', 'corporate approach', 'measuring need' and 'performance criteria' helps us to understand that the SSI saw bureaucratic and managerial solutions to the difficulties authorities faced. The issues of provision of services within severely constrained budgets is less noticeable.

■ ■ ■

6   Conclusion

The changes which were introduced into social work and social care did not go unchallenged, although some challenges had a greater impact than others. These contestations, particularly as they emerged around diversity and difference, were important because they provided us with a vision of welfare as shifting, changing, dynamic, uneven and multi-layered. Studying social welfare within this conceptual framework provided greater understanding of the complexity and contradictions within welfare, as well as an opportunity to generate resistance and a vision of alternative approaches.

It is important here to remind ourselves that the backdrop and context to these debates was the way social care had been influenced and shaped by the changing economic, political, social and organizational climate. The framework of the 'settlements' and 'new subjects' provided you with a way of understanding the changes, continuities, contradictions and challenges in social care within the period between the 1970s and 1990s. By examining social care through community care and services to children and families you were able to see the way the settlements were uneven *within* social care. By looking at other areas of welfare such as education and health it is possible to see this unevenness across the various areas and agencies.

The marketization of welfare, with the increasing use of private and voluntary sectors as well as the state sector, the contracting out of parts of the service and the privatization of other areas, has meant that the pace of change has been rapid. Given the drive towards 'efficiency' and cost-cutting measures across all sectors of welfare, together with the constant reorganization of services to cope with the increasing complexity of the legislation as well as budgetary constraints, it seems unsurprising that social care workers often felt demoralized and stressed. Novak and Sennet (1995) reported that this sense of change, which often felt like loss, was characteristic of the 'contract culture', and that as conditions of poverty and stress for service-users become more acute, the services provided become more legalistic and bound by statutory frameworks. One social care worker is quoted by them as saying:

> I don't think it was what Seebohm had in mind in the early 1970s, and I certainly don't think it was what was had in mind at the end of the war with the Beveridge Report. It's a welfare state that has changed beyond recognition, and a local authority that has changed beyond recognition.

(quoted in Novak and Sennet, 1995)

6.1   Imaginary futures?

One possible way forward would be for SSDs to relinquish some of their role by concentrating on being the purchasers of services and acting in a commissioning role, which is the way some authorities interpreted the legislation and guidance. Within community care this seems almost inevitable. In children's services it has long been acknowledged that providing support and child protection services from the same team is difficult in practice (Parton, 1997). Some feel that voluntary organizations, such as the NSPCC, may be better placed to investigate child abuse, thereby freeing up social services to co-ordinate support. In relation to child protection it could be argued that the police are in a better position to investigate as they are most skilled in gathering evidence. An alternative proposal could be that other agencies, from the private or voluntary sector, provide the support services, leaving SSDs with a role which is consistent with the purchaser–provider separation, and involves care managers as co-ordinators of child welfare services, parallel to developments within community care services. Each of these suggestions would only partially resolve the difficulties. In part they reflect the narrowing focus within social care, which obscures the wider issues of inequalities which are prevalent across all areas of welfare.

Further reading

Feminist Review (spring 1988) contains a discussion of child sexual abuse from feminist perspectives. In particular, the Mica Nava article on Cleveland and the press is illuminating. Frost and Stein (1989) provide a useful and thorough account of the politics around child welfare. Marion Barnes' (1997) book on social and community care provides an in-depth account of this sector. Finch and Mason (1992) provide an excellent piece of research on gender and community care, while Atkin and Rollings (1994) review the literature on community care and 'race'.

References

Atkin, K. and Rollings, J. (1992) 'Informal care in Asian and Afro/Caribbean communities: a literature review', *British Journal of Social Work*, vol.22, no.4, pp.405–18.

Atkin, K. and Rollings, J. (1994) *Community Care in a Multi-Racial Britain: A Critical Review of the Literature*, London, HMSO.

Audit Commission (1986) *Making a Reality of Community Care*, London, HMSO.

Audit Commission (1994) *Seen But Not Heard: Co-ordinating Community Child Health and Social Services for Children in Need*, London, HMSO.

Barnes, M. (1997) *Care, Communities and Citizens*, Harlow, Addison Wesley Longman.

Barnes, M. (1998) 'Whose needs, whose resources? Accessing social care', in Langan (ed.) (1998a).

Boushel, M. and Lebacq, M. (1992) 'Towards empowerment in child protection work', *Children and Society*, vol.6, no.1, pp.38–50.

Boushel, M. and Noakes, S. (1988) 'Islington social services: developing a policy on child sex abuse', *Feminist Review*, no.28, pp.150–7

Brake, M. and Bailey, R. (1980) *Radical Social Work and Practice*, London, Edward Arnold.

Campbell, B. (1988) *Unofficial Secrets. Child Sexual Abuse: The Cleveland Case*, London, Virago Press.

Carlson, A. (1993) 'Liberty, order and the family', in Davies, J. (ed.) *The Family: Is It Just Another Lifestyle Choice?*, London, Institute of Economic Affairs Health and Welfare Unit.

Children in Scotland: Children (Scotland) Act 1995 – Information Pack (1995) produced with the assistance of Kay Tisdall, Centre for the Study of the Child and Society, University of Glasgow.

Clarke, J. (1998) 'Consumerism', in Hughes, G. (ed.) *Imagining Welfare Futures*, London, Routledge in association with The Open University.

Clarke, J. and Cochrane, A. (1998) 'The social construction of social problems', in Saraga (ed.) (1998a).

Cohen, S. (1972) *Folk Devils and Moral Panics: The Creation of the Mods and Rockers*, London, MacGibbon and Kee.

Corrigan, P. and Leonard, P. (1978) *Social Work Practice under Capitalism: A Marxist Approach*, London, Macmillan.

Department of Health (1991) *Working Together Under The Children Act 1989: A Guide to Arrangements for Inter-Agency Co-operation for the Protection of Children from Abuse*, London, HMSO.

Department of Health (1993) *Definition, Management and Monitoring of Children in Need*, London, HMSO.

Department of Health (1995a) *An Introduction to Joint Commissioning*, London, HMSO.

Department of Health (1995b) *Child Protection, Messages from Research*, Dartington Social Research Unit, HMSO.

Department of Health and Social Security (1968) *Report of the Committee on Local Authority and Allied Personal Social Services* (The Seebohm Report), Cmnd 3073, London, HMSO.

Feminist Review (1988) 'Family secrets: child sexual abuse', special edition, no.28.

Finch, J. and Mason, J. (1992) *Negotiating Family Responsibilities*, London, Routledge.

Frost, N. and Stein, M. (1989) *The Politics of Child Welfare: Inequality, Power and Change*, Hemel Hempstead, Harvester Wheatsheaf.

Gibbons, J., Conroy, S. and Bell, C. (1995) *Operating the Child Protection System*, London, HMSO.

Hall, C. (1998) 'A family for nation and empire', in Lewis (ed.) (1998c).

HMSO (1989) *Caring for People: Community Care in the Next Decade and Beyond*, Cmnd 849, London, HMSO.

Hoyes, L., Lart, R., Means, R. and Taylor, M. (eds) (1994) *Community Care in Transition*, York, Joseph Rowntree Foundation.

Jack, G. and Stepney, P. (1995) 'The Children Act 1989 – protection or persecution? Family support and child protection in the 1990s', *Critical Social Policy*, issue 43, vol.15, no.1, pp.26–39.

Johnson, N. (1990) *Reconstructing the Welfare State: A Decade of Change, 1980–1990*, Hemel Hempstead, Harvester Wheatsheaf.

Kelly, L. (1988) 'Talking about a revolution', *Spare Rib*, August, no.193, pp.8–11.

Langan, M. (ed.) (1998a) *Welfare: Needs, Rights and Risks*, London, Routledge in association with The Open University.

Langan, M. (1998b) 'The contested concept of need', in Langan (ed.) (1998a).

Langan, M. and Clarke, J. (1994) 'Managing in the mixed economy of care', in Clarke, J., Cochrane, A. and McLaughlin, E. (eds) *Managing Social Policy*, London, Sage.

Lentell, H. (1998) 'Families of meaning: contemporary discourses of the family', in Lewis (ed.) (1998c).

Lewis, G. (1998a) 'Welfare and the social construction of "race"', in Saraga (ed.) (1998a).

Lewis, G. (1998b) 'Review', in Lewis (ed.) (1998c).

Lewis, G. (ed.) (1998c) *Forming Nation, Framing Welfare*, London, Routledge in association with The Open University.

London Borough of Brent (1985) *A Child In Trust: Report of the Panel of Inquiry Investigating the Circumstances Surrounding the Death of Jasmine Beckford* (The Beckford Report), London Borough of Brent.

MacDonald, S. (1991) *All Equal Under the Act? A Practical Guide to the Children Act 1989 for Social Workers*, Leeds, Race Equality Unit.

Mandelstam, M. and Schwehr, B. (1995) *Community Care Practice and the Law*, London, Jessica Kingsley.

Mooney, G. (1998) '"Remoralizing" the poor?: gender, class and philanthropy in Victorian Britain', in Lewis (ed.) (1998).

Morris, L. (1998) 'Legitimate membership of the welfare community', in Langan (ed.) (1998a).

Nava, M. (1988) 'Family secrets; child sexual abuse', *Feminist Review*, no.28.

Novak, T. and Sennet, H. (1995) *Changing Social Work*, unpublished paper, University of Bradford.

Parton, N. (ed.) (1997) *Child Protection and Family Support: Tensions, Contradictions and Possibilities*, London, Routledge.

Saraga, E. (1998a) (ed.) *Embodying the Social: Constructions of Difference*, London, Routledge in association with The Open University.

Saraga, E. (1998b) 'Children's needs: who decides?', in Langan (ed.) (1998a).

Scottish Home and Health Department, Scottish Education Department (1964) *Report of Committee on Children and Young Persons* (The Kilbrandon Report), Cmnd 2306, Edinburgh, HMSO.

Secretary of State for Social Services (1988) *Report of the Inquiry into Child Abuse in Cleveland* (The Cleveland Report), Cmnd 412, London, HMSO.

Social Services Inspectorate (1993) *Raising the Standard: The Second Annual Report of the Chief Inspector, 1992/3*, London, HMSO.

Social Services Inspectorate (1996) *Progress Through Change: The Fifth Annual Report of the Chief Inspector, 1995/6*, London, HMSO.

Sutton, P. (1995) 'Policy: children's services plans', *Community Care,* 7–13 December, pp.16–19.

Walker, R. and Ahmad, W. (1994) 'Windows of opportunity in rotting frames? Care providers' perspectives on community care and black communities', *Critical Social Policy*, issue 40, vol.14, no.1, pp.46–69.

Wilding, P. (1992) 'The public sector in the 1980s', in Manning, N. and Page, R. (eds) *Social Policy Review 4*, London, Social Policy Association.

Wistow, G., Knapp, M., Hardy, B. and Allen, C. (1994) *Social Care in a Mixed Economy*, Buckingham, Open University Press.

CHAPTER 8

What Sort of Safety-Net? Social Security, Income Maintenance and the Benefits System

by Allan Cochrane

Contents

1 Why income maintenance matters

This chapter is about systems of income maintenance. In other words it is about social security, national insurance, pensions and welfare benefits. Just saying that can be enough to put off even the most dedicated of readers. The very notion of income maintenance seems to translate important issues of personal economic survival into the dry language of book-keeping. The term 'income maintenance' itself somehow seems designed to obscure its social meaning.

income maintenance

Yet even the most modest aims of state-run income maintenance policies highlight their importance. These can be divided into three main elements: the relief of poverty, the protection of accustomed living standards and the smoothing out of income over the life cycle (Barr and Coulter, 1990, p.275).

relief of poverty

1   Policies directed towards the relief of poverty are those which aim to ensure that individuals or households do not fall below certain commonly agreed minimum living standards; that is, below the poverty line. These standards vary from time to time. And, for one reason or another, the accepted minima sometimes also vary between different categories of people. This is expressed, for example, in the Victorian distinction between the 'deserving' and 'undeserving' poor. Barr and Coulter (1990) give income support as an example of a policy directed towards the relief of poverty, and the level of income support (previously called supplementary benefit, and before that national assistance) is often used to define the poverty line.

protection of living standards

2   Policies directed towards the protection of living standards are those whose purpose is to ensure that 'no one has to face an unexpected and unacceptably large drop in their standard of living' (Barr and Coulter, 1990, p.275). Such policies include sickness benefit for those in work, or the jobseeker's allowance for those who are unemployed and looking for work.

smoothing income out over the life cycle

3   Policies directed towards smoothing income out over the life cycle would include those which are concerned to provide adequate pensions for older people (including occupational and private pensions), but might also include forms of financial assistance to parents with young children (for example, child benefit).

At different historical moments each of these three elements has been of greater or lesser centrality to policy debates and welfare outcomes, but some or all of them affect all of us at some time in our lives.

Income maintenance policies may also, as Barr and Coulter note, involve broader strategic ambitions to reduce inequality through the redistribution of wealth, or to encourage social integration. They may be intended to transform or influence the ways in which people behave; for example, by reinforcing certain forms of 'moral' behaviour, or by encouraging people into the labour force. Even if these wider ambitions are not taken into account, however, the nature of income maintenance policies is fundamental to a rounded understanding of the UK welfare system. The approaches taken by governments and popular attitudes towards issues of income maintenance have been of fundamental importance in shaping the welfare settlements discussed in the first two chapters of this book and in determining the ways in which welfare is actually experienced.

Approaches to income maintenance both reflect dominant understandings of welfare *and* help to shape them. Income maintenance policies are actively socially constructed in the sense that they are the product of complex processes of interaction between groups and of political conflict. But because they attribute meaning to certain income levels, they also themselves help to construct particular issues as 'problems' that require social policy intervention. They help to define who is 'poor' and who is not, who is 'deserving' of sympathy (and welfare support) and who is not. They help to frame the ways in which we interpret and understand the social world and what is possible within it. So, for example, a shift in emphasis away from viewing income maintenance policies as a means of reducing social inequality, towards one which stresses their role in encouraging individuals back into the labour market, reinforces as well as reflects sharply different approaches to social policy.

This chapter considers both the debates which have helped construct income maintenance policies *and* the ways in which those policies have helped to define and redefine the 'problem' of income maintenance. Here, the intention is to put the humanity back into the debates and to explore the underlying issues which make them so important. The aim of the chapter is to rescue income maintenance from the statisticians, while recognizing the significant contributions they have made.

The chapter is divided into two main sections, each of which explores one particular aspect of the debates about income maintenance. The first focuses on the broader historical context, relating contemporary debates back to those which underpinned the emergence of income maintenance policies in the nineteenth and twentieth centuries; the second looks at the changes which were introduced in the 1980s and 1990s, changes that emphasized the costs of welfare and sought to reduce them dramatically, as well as challenging what was described as a 'dependency culture'. The emphasis of the chapter is on the UK experience, and it is important to note that countries with other systems may have followed quite different trajectories (see, for example, Cochrane and Clarke, 1993; Ginsburg, 1992). A brief concluding section asks whether we are seeing the emergence of a new set of welfare settlements which incorporate different notions of income maintenance.

2 Situating contemporary debates: the past in the present

There are two main defining 'moments' which provide a vital context for the contemporary history of income maintenance in the UK. The first relates to the 'new' (Victorian) Poor Law ('new' because it replaced the 'old' Elizabethan Poor Law), which was sustained in some form until the Second World War; the second relates to the Beveridgean settlements of the immediate post-war period (see Chapter 1). The debates surrounding these rather extended 'moments' cast long shadows across contemporary debates. The arguments developed in this chapter look back rather further than the post-war settlements discussed in the first two chapters of the book because the echoes of the nineteenth-century Poor Law in contemporary debates are so loud and powerful that they cannot be ignored. Two fundamental but related questions are raised by this glance back into the past. Are we seeing the rebirth of the Poor Law (and experiencing the death-throes of the Beveridgean settlements), or is a new settlement emerging?

2.1 'Less eligibility' and the means test

At the beginning of the twentieth century, the assumptions that underlay the UK's income maintenance system were relatively clear. The stress was on the first of the three elements of income maintenance policies identified in section 1, the relief of poverty. The approach combined self-help, charity and state support. Poverty was widely understood to be a problem of the poor – it was their duty not to be poor. The poor were frequently divided into the two categories of the 'deserving' and 'undeserving'. Only the 'deserving' poor were, in principle, entitled to some form of support or relief (see **Mooney, 1998; Morris, 1998; Gazeley and Thane, 1998**).

less eligibility

Poor Law

The able-bodied poor were a particular focus of concern because it was believed that they ought to be in paid employment, and if they were not it was almost certainly because they chose not to be. In the last resort, support would be provided, but it was vital to ensure that no-one was ever in a better position through the receipt of poor relief than she or he would have been through employment, even of the most casual form. This was called the 'less eligibility' principle, because those in employment should never be 'less eligible' (that is, in a less prosperous position) than those on relief. In practice this sometimes meant that families were broken up, with men and women being segregated in separate workhouses, or it meant the payment of low levels of what was called outdoor relief (that is, outside the workhouse) for those undertaking heavy manual labour. The purpose of the 1834 Poor Law in England and Wales and similar legislation introduced in Scotland in 1845 was to discourage welfare dependency, or what was then called 'demoralization', and to encourage a sense of moral responsibility among the poor. The Poor Law system was intended to ensure that low-paid and casualized labour remained more attractive than life on poor relief.

The main emphasis of policy was on individual responsibility, with a particular assumption that every man should seek to provide for himself and 'his' family. The notion of the male breadwinner, and the assumption that his wage was a family wage, meant that there was no additional benefit for households 'headed' by men on low wages. Indeed it was a fundamental principle of the Poor Law that relief should not be used to augment the income of those receiving low pay, whether to subsidize employers or support families.

At the same time it was accepted that motherhood might help to move a poor woman into the 'deserving' category, although only if she behaved appropriately (see **Hall, 1998**). The idealized image of poverty (reflected in late Victorian painting) was that of a widow struggling to bring up her children by undertaking piecework at home (preferably sewing or laundry). Such people would, of course, be prime targets for charitable attention through the Charity Organization Society and other agencies (see **Mooney, 1998**). If not in paid employment of some sort, women were assumed either to be dependent on their husbands or entitled to some form of financial support for the maintenance of their children if the father was dead or otherwise absent.

The stress on individual responsibility also meant that it was assumed that individuals would find ways of protecting the living standards of their families against the threat of sickness or unemployment, and of providing for themselves in old age. The need to save in the good times and to insure against the bad was taken for granted, and there was a patchwork of private insurance companies and mutual ('friendly') societies to provide these services for people in regular employment. It was only in the first decades of the twentieth century that the state became directly involved in the second and third elements of income maintenance identified in section 1. The National Insurance Act of 1911 meant that in return for national insurance payments male manual workers had a right to relief when out of work through sickness, and this was later extended to periods of unemployment (see **Gazeley and Thane, 1998**). Old age pensions were introduced in 1908, although in practice the principles involved remained those of the Poor Law. Only those without other 'means', assessed through a strict means test, were eligible, and the payments themselves were at the same rate as outdoor relief.

The two key principles, therefore, remained, first, that poor relief below what might be earned from wages should be available only to those with no other source of support and, second, that other forms of income maintenance should be covered by means of insurance. However, the principle of individual responsibility was eroded by the introduction of compulsory national insurance.

Income maintenance was a live political issue throughout the inter-war period, not least because of the impact of mass unemployment. The strain on the existing system was enormous. The insurance-based forms of unemployment benefit were unable to cope with the scale of demand. The extra costs which had to be met led the government to reduce benefit levels very sharply in the 1930s. Those who had never been in the scheme (around half of the workforce), of course, benefited not at all, and after their initial period of entitlement even those who had contributed became ineligible for benefit. As a result, over two million people became dependent on the Poor Law in the early 1930s.

The operation of the Poor Law was initially managed through locally based boards of guardians created for this sole purpose in England and Wales and through parish councils in Scotland. These were elected bodies and there were soon major tensions between what the guardians and parish councillors wanted to do in order to represent their constituency and the assumptions that underlay the Poor Law. The payment of relief to the able-bodied poor without the requirement that they be placed in workhouses became more and more common, and in some cases levels of payment rose significantly. To some extent the dominant social construction which 'blamed' unemployment on those unable to find work was being challenged by the people entrusted with managing the Poor Law. There was substantial conflict between central and local government, and between elected officials and local businesses (who paid rates) over levels of relief. Probably the most famous rebellion was based in Poplar in London's East End in the 1920s (where the guardians were imprisoned for setting rates at levels deemed too high by the district auditor – see Branson, 1979), but there were similar conflicts in places such as Bedwellty in South Wales and others, popularly labelled 'little Moscows', such as the Vale of Leven near Glasgow (see Macintyre, 1980). The board of guardians' system was abolished in 1929 and responsibility was transferred to the public assistance committees (PACs) of local authorities. In Scotland responsibility was transferred from the parish councils to county council PACs.

Throughout the inter-war period the means test remained a powerful mechanism for regulating and policing individual households. The principle that any potential source of income would be counted against benefit was fundamental, and women and children were automatically assumed to be

means test

dependent on male members of the household, eligible for benefit in their own right only if there was no adult male present. Many household goods – such as pianos – which could be sold were counted against benefits. Although spending on relief still rose during this period, means testing meant that the PACs and their employees were highly unpopular with those reliant on relief. By the mid 1930s a new national board, the Unemployment Assistance Board, had been created. The Board sought to force benefit rates down. Its existence also implied the recognition that financial assistance was a more permanent feature of the income maintenance scene than could be coped with through local agencies. (The changing pattern of unemployment and policy responses to it is discussed in more depth in **Gazeley and Thane, 1998**.)

ACTIVITY 8.1

Extract 8.1, taken from George Orwell's *The Road to Wigan Pier*, describes the operation of the system of means testing at the end of the 1930s. It is particularly effective in highlighting some of the ways in which the means test operated and the ways in which people learned to survive. As you read, make notes on the main effects of the means test, as Orwell sees them.

Extract 8.1 George Orwell: 'The road to Wigan Pier'

The Means Test is very strictly enforced, and you are liable to be refused relief at the slightest hint that you are getting money from another source. Dock-labourers, for instance, who are generally hired by the half day, have to sign on at a Labour Exchange twice daily; if they fail to do so it is assumed that they have been working and their dole is reduced correspondingly. I have seen cases of evasion of the Means Test, but I should say that in the industrial towns, where there is still a certain amount of communal life and everyone has neighbours who know him, it is much harder than it would be in London. The usual method is for a young man who is actually living with his parents to get an accommodation address, so that supposedly he has a separate establishment and draws a separate allowance. But there is much spying and tale-bearing. One man I knew, for instance, was seen feeding his neighbour's chickens while the neighbour was away. It was reported to the authorities that he 'had a job feeding chickens' and he had great difficulty in refuting this. The favourite joke in Wigan was about a man who was refused relief on the grounds that he 'had a job carting firewood.' He had been seen, it was said, carting firewood at night. He had to explain that he was not carting firewood but doing a moonlight flit. The 'firewood' was his furniture.

The most cruel and evil effect of the Means Test is the way in which it breaks up families. Old people, sometimes bedridden, are driven out of their homes by it. An old aged pensioner, for instance, if a widower, would normally live with one or another of his children; his weekly ten shillings goes towards the household expenses, and probably he is not badly cared for. Under the Means Test, however, he counts as 'lodger' and if he stays at home his children's dole will be docked. So, perhaps at seventy or seventy-five years of age, he has to turn out into lodgings, handing his pension over to the lodging-house keeper and existing on the verge of starvation. I have seen several cases of this myself. It is happening all over England at this moment, thanks to the Means Test …

But in the industrial towns the old communal way of life has not yet broken up, tradition is still strong and almost everyone has a family – potentially, therefore, a home. In a town of 50,000 or 100,000 inhabitants there is no casual and as it were unaccounted-for population; nobody sleeping in the streets, for instance. Moreover, there is just this to be said for the unemployment regulations, that they do not discourage people from marrying. A man and wife on twenty-three shillings a week are not far from the starvation line, but they can make a home of sorts; they are vastly better off than a single man on fifteen shillings. The life of a single unemployed man is dreadful. He lives sometimes in a common lodging-house, more often in a 'furnished' room for which he usually pays six shillings a week, finding himself as best he can on the other nine (say six shillings a week for food and three for clothes, tobacco and amusements). Of course he cannot feed or look after himself properly, and a man who pays six shillings a week for his room is not encouraged to be indoors more than is necessary. So he spends his days loafing in the public library or any other place where he can keep warm. That – keeping warm – is almost the sole preoccupation of a single unemployed man in winter …

A working-class bachelor is a rarity, and so long as a man is married unemployment makes comparatively little alteration in his way of life. His home is impoverished but it is still a home, and it is noticeable everywhere that the anomalous position created by unemployment – the man being out of work while the woman's work continues as before – has not altered the relative status of the sexes. In a working-class home it is the man who is the master and not, as in a middle-class home, the woman or the baby. Practically never, for instance, in a working-class home, will you see the man doing a stroke of the housework. Unemployment has not changed this convention, which on the face of it seems a little unfair. The man is idle from morning to night but the woman is as busy as ever – more so, indeed, because she has to manage with less money. Yet so far as my experience goes the women do not protest. I believe that they, as well as the men, feel that a man would lose his manhood if, merely because he was out of work, he developed into a 'Mary Ann'.

(Orwell, 1937, pp.70–3)

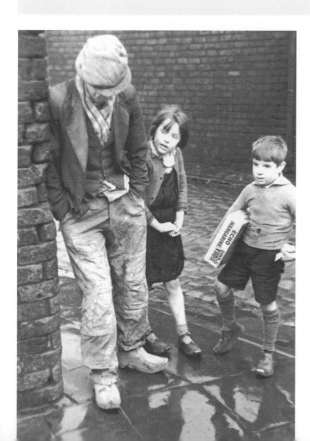

Unemployed in Wigan, 1939

Orwell's main points relating to the means test and its operation are:

- Relief is withdrawn if there is any evidence that a claimant is getting income from any other source. Strict rules are applied. Some of the consequences can be absurd (for instance, Orwell's examples of chicken feeding and the 'joke' about carting firewood).

- Evasion is difficult, although some attempts are made to evade the rules (for example, the use of accommodation addresses).

- Families are broken up so that individuals will be eligible for benefit, rather than being defined as dependants (for example, the example of a pensioner who may otherwise be defined as a 'lodger' with his children).

- The life of a single man on benefit is likely to be worse than that of a married couple. (As a result, says Orwell, 'a working class bachelor is a rarity.')

Orwell describes all this from the point of view of an outsider. He comes from a middle-class background, in which, he suggests, 'the woman or the baby' is in charge of the household, while in a working class home 'it is the man who is the master', even when unemployed. Although tempting, this is probably not the place to explore the nature of Orwell's home life, but his positive attitude to the arrangement he identifies in working class homes is fairly clear. If Orwell is right, then it is clear that it was only because of the supportive role of women in the home that the Poor Law system worked at all.

■ ■ ■

By contrast with Orwell, Max Cohen describes his own experience as an unemployed single man in *I Was One of the Unemployed*. Extract 8.2 describes the moment at which Cohen moves from unemployment benefit to poor relief. As you read the extract, try to identify the main justifications used by the public assistance committee official for questioning Cohen's eligibility for assistance.

Extract 8.2 Max Cohen: 'I was one of the unemployed'

The Relieving Officer drew before him a nice, new, clean file, and a number of lengthy forms. With a sort of sensuous enjoyment he prepared himself to fill in the forms.

One by one, with slow solemnity, he made his inquiries. There were the usual questions as to my name, age, and address and circumstances, how long I had lived at my present address, where I had been previously, and where I had been before that, why I left Forgeton. Finally came the crucial question:

'Are you single or married?'

I braced myself for trouble.

'I'm single.'

'Oh. You're single? We don't give relief to single men.'

'What do you mean – you don't give relief to single men?' I snapped. 'The question of whether I'm single or married doesn't affect the question of whether you grant me relief or not. It only affects the amount of relief.'

Outwardly I might have appeared angry, domineering, but inwardly I was filled with anxiety as to the effect my words would have on him. My heart sank, for he appeared unmoved.

'Have you no relatives who can help you in any way?'

'No.'

I was damned if I was going to be parked on to relatives of mine who had not enough to maintain themselves.

'Well' – he shrugged his shoulders unconcernedly – 'you won't get any relief from us. We're not allowed to give relief to single men.'

'Don't tell me that!' I said derisively. 'You know yourself you're compelled by law to give relief to those who are without means of support. It's a criminal offence,' I went on wildly, determined to shake him somehow. 'And if *I* can't get you to give me relief, I'll take the matter up with those who can.'

Again he seemed unmoved. I felt as though I were expending my energies punching a large, well-stuffed cushion.

'Anyway,' he said casually, 'you're destitute. You'll have to go to the workhouse.'

A pang of fear smote me. The workhouse? A yawning gap seemed to open beneath my feet.

'You don't know what you're talking about,' I said desperately. 'Destitute? A destitute person is someone who has nowhere to live. I have a definite place of abode. Therefore how can I be destitute?'

I had no idea whether this definition and other statements I had made that afternoon were correct. I had a vague idea that what I was saying might be correct, but I was not sure.

'Maybe you have a fixed place of abode,' he said sardonically. 'But how are you going to pay the rent if you have no means of support?'

'That's my business!' I snapped.

'No,' he said shaking his head slowly, 'I'm afraid you'll have to go to the workhouse.'

He seemed quite definitely to enjoy this prospect of my future. Once again I felt appalled. Nevertheless I could not give up. I must get relief out of him somehow. How? Somehow.

'I'll tell you,' I exclaimed, very nearly shouting, 'that you're acting contrary to the law by refusing me relief. You're satisfied yourself that I'm in need of relief, and yet you refuse it. You won't get away with it. I'll get the matter taken up.'

'Well anyway', he said in a manner half casual, half weary, 'I'm not going to give you any relief. That's final. If you want to, you can fill up this form. I don't know that it'll do you any good. Here.' He tossed a form towards me. 'Fill it up outside.'

I grabbed the form, and, as in a fever, hurried outside with it. I had had numerous forms to fill up before now, but they were all pygmies compared with this one. It was a giant, a Colossus of forms. It probed into every conceivable detail of a man's history. It ranged from his name, age, address and relatives, to illnesses and disabilities, pensions, and each separate section of the armed forces to which he might or might not have been attached. I was, however, accustomed to filling up forms, and even this form did not daunt me. I filled it up in record time. Then I re-entered the room …

My Relieving Officer … took the form, but did not even glance at it. Then from under the papers on his desk he took a small piece of paper, about the size of a postcard. He tossed it negligently towards me.

'Here,' he said carelessly, 'that's all the relief you'll get.'

I was astounded and overwhelmed with sensations of victory. I almost staggered from the room in my excess of joy. So I had won! After his obdurate, careless and negligent insistence that he was not going to give me any relief, the fact that he had given me at least something almost overpowered me after the tension and feverish anxiety of the interview. Then I glanced at the form and discovered it was for six shillings. Even this as an amount to live on for a whole week in no way damped my ardour. I went out drunk with victory.

(Cohen, 1945, pp.147–9)

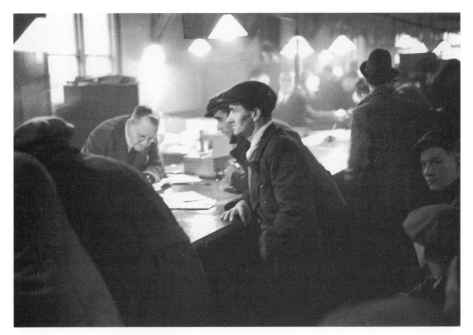

Attending a Labour Exchange, 1939

COMMENT

The move to poor relief implies a substantial change in Cohen's position. The notion that he is entitled to any benefits disappears almost as soon as he leaves behind his vestigial relationship to unemployment benefit. As a single, able-bodied man Cohen is now subject to the full rigours of the Poor Law. If he wants support he is in danger of being forced into the workhouse or having to find a relative who will support him. Despite his readiness to argue and defend himself, his dependence on the arbitrary decision-making of officials is highlighted by the way in which he is given a form (worth six shillings) which can be used to purchase groceries. In other words he receives no allowance for rent.

■ ■ ■

2.2 Beveridge and social security

As Chapter 1 argues, Beveridge, along with Keynes, has become the symbol of the post-war settlements. Indeed, the post-war welfare state is frequently seen as the child of Beveridge. Although the Beveridge Report itself, published in 1942, was narrowly focused on 'social insurance and allied services', it was a major bestseller (Beveridge, 1942). It provided the basis for post-war legislation on national insurance, and set out a series of wider assumptions which underpinned the emergent system.

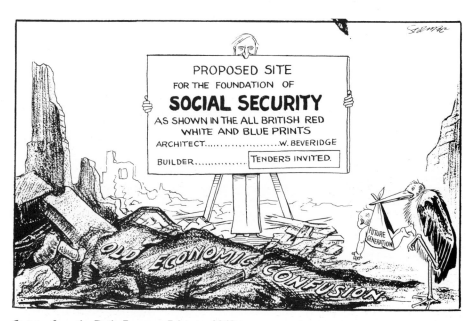

Cartoon from the Daily Express, *February 1943*

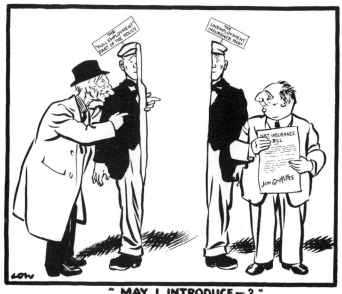

Cartoon from the Evening Standard, February 1946

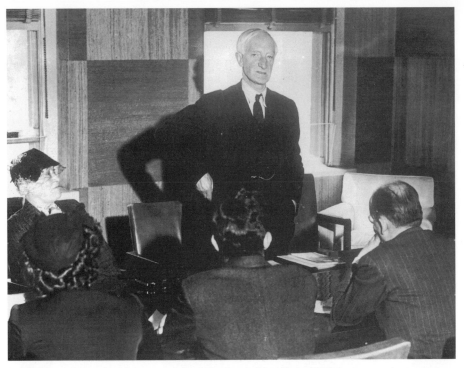

Beveridge explaining his plan at a press conference in New York, 1943

ACTIVITY 8.3

Extract 8.3 is taken from the Beveridge Report. It spells out some of the main features and assumptions underlying Beveridge's approach to income maintenance and social security, based on the attempt to achieve 'freedom from want' as a defining characteristic of post-war UK society. It is an integrated approach, in contrast to the system which had developed piecemeal in the years up to 1939. As you read, consider the following questions.

1   What are the key elements of Beveridge's 'plan for social security'?

2   To what extent and in what form does the 'less eligibility' principle survive?

3   What are the underlying assumptions about the positions of men and women?

Extract 8.3 Beveridge: 'Social insurance and allied services'

409   ... The Plan for Social Security ... is a plan to win freedom from want by maintaining incomes ...

Any Plan for Social Security in the narrow sense assumes a concerted social policy in many fields, most of which it would be inappropriate to discuss in this Report. The plan proposed here involves three particular assumptions so closely related to it that brief discussion is essential for understanding of the plan itself. These are the assumptions of children's allowances, of comprehensive health and rehabilitation services, and of maintenance of employment ...

Assumption A: children's allowances

410   The first of three assumptions underlying the Plan for Social Security is a general scheme of children's allowances. This means that direct provision for the

maintenance of dependent children will be made by payment of allowances to those responsible for the care of those children. The assumption rests on two connected arguments.

411   First, it is unreasonable to seek to guarantee an income sufficient for subsistence, while earnings are interrupted by unemployment or disability, without ensuring sufficient income during earning. Social insurance should be part of a policy of a national minimum. But a national minimum for families of every size cannot in practice be secured by a wage system, which must be based on the product of a man's labour and not on the size of his family. The social surveys of Britain between the two wars show that in the first thirty years of this century real wages rose by about one-third without reducing want to insignificance, and that the want which remained was almost wholly due to two causes – interruption or loss of earning power and large families.

412   Second, it is dangerous to allow benefit during unemployment or disability to equal or exceed earnings during work. But, without allowances for children, during earning and not-earning alike, this danger cannot be avoided. It has been experienced in an appreciable number of cases under unemployment benefit and unemployment assistance in the past. The maintenance of employment – last and most important of the three assumptions of social security – will be impossible without greater fluidity of labour and other resources in the aftermath of war than has been achieved in the past. To secure this, the gap between income during earning and during interruption of earning should be as large as possible for every man. It cannot be kept large for men with large families, except either by making their benefit in unemployment and disability inadequate, or by giving allowances for children in time of earning and not-earning alike …

Assumption B: comprehensive health and rehabilitation services
426   The second of the three assumptions has two sides to it. It covers a national health service for prevention and for cure of disease and disability by medical treatment; it covers rehabilitation and fitting for employment by treatment which will be both medical and post-medical … The case for regarding Assumption B as necessary for a satisfactory system of social security needs little emphasis. It is a logical corollary to the payment of high benefit in disability that determined efforts should be made by the State to reduce the number of cases for which benefit is needed. It is a logical corollary to the receipt of high benefit in disability that the individual should recognize the duty to be well and to co-operate in all steps which may lead to diagnosis of disease in early stages when it can be prevented …

427   The first part of Assumption B is that a comprehensive national health service will ensure that for every citizen there is available whatever medical treatment he requires, in whatever form he requires it, domiciliary or institutional, general, specialist or consultant, and will ensure also the provision of dental, ophthalmic and surgical appliances, nursing and midwifery and rehabilitation after accidents …

Assumption C: maintenance of employment
440   There are five reasons for saying that a satisfactory scheme of social insurance assumes the maintenance of employment and the prevention of mass unemployment. Three reasons are concerned with the details of social insurance; the fourth and most important is concerned with its principle; the fifth is concerned with the possibility of meeting its cost.

First, payment of unconditional cash benefits as of right during unemployment is satisfactory provision only for short periods of unemployment; after that, complete idleness even on an income demoralizes. The proposal of the Report accordingly is to make unemployment benefit after a certain period conditional upon attendance at a work or training centre. But this proposal is impracticable, if it has to be applied to men by the million or the hundred thousand.

Second, the only satisfactory test of unemployment is an offer of work. This test breaks down in mass unemployment and makes necessary recourse to elaborate contribution conditions, and such devices as the Anomalies Regulations, all of which should be avoided in a satisfactory scheme of unemployment insurance.

Third, the state of the labour market has a direct bearing on rehabilitation and recovery of injured and sick persons and upon the possibility of giving to those suffering from partial infirmities, such as deafness, the chance of a happy and useful career. In time of mass unemployment those who are in receipt of compensation feel no urge to get well for idleness. On the other hand, in time of active demand for labour, as in war, the sick and the maimed are encouraged to recover, so that they may be useful.

Fourth, and most important, income security which is all that can be given by social insurance is so inadequate a provision for human happiness that to put it forward by itself as a sole or principal measure of reconstruction hardly seems worth doing. It should be accompanied by an announced determination to use the powers of the State to whatever extent may prove necessary to ensure for all, not indeed absolute continuity of work, but a reasonable chance of productive employment.

Fifth, though it should be within the power of the community to bear the cost of the whole Plan for Social Security, the cost is heavy and, if to the necessary cost waste is added, it may become insupportable. Unemployment, both through increasing expenditure on benefit and through reducing the income to bear those costs, is the worst form of waste.

441   … Assumption C requires not the abolition of all unemployment, but the abolition of mass unemployment and of unemployment prolonged year after year for the same individual.

(Beveridge, 1942, paras 409–12; 426–7; 440–1)

COMMENT

Beveridge spells out three crucial assumptions as the foundation on which his scheme builds. The first of these is the existence of children's allowances; the second the existence of an effective national health and rehabilitation service; and the third is the maintenance of employment. Beveridge argues that only once these assumptions have been met can an effective system of social insurance and income maintenance be achieved, both because demands on the system will be limited (for example, because health services will be improved to reduce the need for sickness and disability benefits) and because there will be sufficient tax income from employment to sustain the real costs of benefits.

One of the arguments Beveridge uses for the pursuit of high employment policies is that he wishes to ensure that there can be a genuine test of unemployment; in the absence of mass unemployment it becomes much easier to judge whether people are actively seeking employment and to penalize them if they are not. As in the case of the Poor Law, therefore, Beveridge makes crucial assumptions about the labour market and its operation. But in this case the emphasis is on stability and security, rather than the maintenance of low-waged employment.

The argument is still based around a male breadwinner model: it is assumed that it will be the man in each household who is in the labour force and preferably in employment. But there is no assumption that his pay will be a 'family wage', because his wages will be 'based on the product of a man's labour and not the size of his family.' So children's allowances (which were initially introduced as family allowances and then became child benefit) are needed to ensure that sufficient income is available, smoothing out income over the life cycle through a universal benefit rather than through insurance.

male breadwinner model

According to Beveridge, one justification for a system of children's allowances is that, at least if the allowances are high enough, it helps to ensure that people out of work do not receive more than they do when in work. The alternative would have been to pay significantly higher levels of national assistance to unemployed people with children than to those without, but this might mean that people in low-paid sectors of the labour market would be better off if they did *not* have jobs than if they did.

■ ■ ■

The 1946 National Insurance Act which enacted some of the Beveridge principles assumed that a wide range of benefits would be paid as a 'right' to those who had contributed to the scheme (that is, those in employment). These included sickness and invalidity benefits, unemployment benefit, pensions and maternity grants. A flat rate contribution would be paid, in return for flat rate benefits. There was no direct link between the amount of individual contributions and benefit payment. As suggested in the Beveridge Report, it was implied that women and children would gain through the income from employment or the national insurance entitlements of the men in their households. Although they were never set at levels high enough to make this possible, family allowances were intended to ensure that household incomes would cover the additional costs associated with maintaining children, so that each household would need only one (male) earner. A further safety-net of national assistance was made available for those without access to employment for whatever reason, but it was assumed there would be very few of these.

National assistance replaced the old Poor Law-related activities, with a national assistance board being set up to oversee provision. National assistance was intended to ensure that those receiving it had sufficient income to support their basic needs. In practice, because the rates of national insurance-related benefits were set at very low levels, many of those in receipt of them also required national assistance. Unlike social insurance, national assistance was calculated to take account of dependants. It was also calculated according to a strict means test so that no more was paid out than was 'required'.

The new system, therefore, built on the old, but the key principle underlying social insurance was that all of those who contributed were entitled to benefit. In that sense it was universal, although the extent of the universality was severely restricted. Those who were in part-time employment, in casual employment or not in paid work were excluded (although it was assumed that they would benefit as dependants of those who were included). In practice that meant that very few women benefited directly.

social insurance

National assistance rates were set at low levels (below those hoped for by Beveridge), but the old assumption that they should be forced down to rates below subsistence to encourage people to go to work was largely overcome. Although the new arrangements had multiple ambitions, for the first time they more or less explicitly included an emphasis on the reduction of social and economic inequality and a commitment to a generalized improvement of living standards for those with low incomes.

2.3   From Poor Law to Beveridge

Historical debates about income maintenance continue to have a very powerful resonance in contemporary debates. Here we have focused particularly on the UK case, first considering the operation of the Poor Law introduced in the middle of the nineteenth century, and second the implications of the Beveridge reforms. Each approach represents a different social construction of the problems being addressed, as well as a different policy approach to dealing with them.

As its name suggests, the Poor Law approach to income maintenance was concerned with managing the poor. Some responsibility for maintaining the incomes of the 'deserving' poor was recognized, but it was felt that the 'undeserving' poor should receive no help. The importance of individual responsibility was stressed and it was a fundamental principle that no-one should be better off in receipt of poor relief than she or he would be if in employment. The system was organized mainly at local level.

Other aspects of income maintenance (for example, to cover periods of sickness, unemployment or old age) were managed through insurance-based systems. The state became involved in providing forms of employment-based social insurance in the early years of the twentieth century, but that was only relevant to those with access to regular employment.

The Poor Law basis of income maintenance systems was formally changed only by the reforms introduced by the Labour government in the late 1940s, although many aspects of the system had already changed in practice in response to the mass unemployment of the 1930s. Responsibility for income maintenance was increasingly removed to national level. Nevertheless, some key features of the Poor Law approach did survive, particularly in the form of the means test and the notion of 'less eligibility'.

The Beveridge reforms had a different starting-point. Their core principles were insurance based, involving most of the working population and their 'dependants'. Social insurance, rather than the management of the poor, was to be the way forward. This was, of course, possible only on the basis of a number of fundamental assumptions – in particular, the payment of children's (or family) allowances, the creation of a national health service and the maintenance of something close to full employment. On that basis it would be possible to even out the variations of income faced by most people across the life cycle, and to guarantee that all those genuinely seeking work would be able to find it.

Beveridge also supported a scheme of means-tested national assistance for those who might fall through the insurance-based safety-net (that is, those whose access to employment was likely to be limited for one reason or another), but the assumption was that very few people would be in this position. Unlike the Poor Law system, there was also an assumption that the new arrangements would lead to a higher degree of social equalization.

Both approaches effectively assumed a male breadwinner model. But in some ways the Beveridge approach was still more family oriented. Under the Poor Law, families might be broken up to ensure that the 'less eligibility' criterion was met. Beveridge, by contrast, was concerned with the maintenance of household or family incomes. So, for example, the introduction of family allowances (which were not means tested) was intended to ensure that men with low wages could maintain their families even when they had several children. In other words, the state would help to generate a 'family wage' without women having to take paid employment. Their domestic role was, therefore, reinforced in the Beveridge model.

Although the discussion so far has not directly focused on the relationship between income maintenance and the settlements outlined in Chapter 1, the process of change which has been charted can usefully be revisited in these terms. The transition from Poor Law to Beveridge can also be seen as a move towards a new configuration of welfare settlements.

The political settlement associated with the Poor Law at the end of the nineteenth century was based around a reluctance to interfere with the operation of labour markets (and more generally in the working of economic markets). Alongside this was an economic settlement based around the operation of a competitive 'free' market in a global economy in which the British Empire was still one of the dominant players. The social settlement reflected in the Poor Law was based around individual responsibility, with the assumption of a male breadwinner on whom dependants were expected to rely; only in extreme cases was any income support to be expected. The organizational settlement was one which combined charitable assistance with highly localized arrangements for providing support through parishes and Poor Law boards of guardians; welfare subjects were defined in terms which divided them between the deserving and undeserving poor.

These arrangements were already under strain in the early twentieth century, but the different elements increasingly came under challenge in the 1920s and 1930s. Although the political rhetoric continued to stress individual responsibility and (in principle at least) the market was treated as sacrosanct, mass unemployment made it difficult to sustain the existing social settlement or the organizational regime associated with it. However, a new approach to income maintenance only emerged alongside the settlements arising from the Beveridge Report. The political consensus suggested that the state had some responsibility for maintaining the incomes of its citizens at an acceptable level, although the responsibility of individuals for their own welfare (and those of their dependants) continued to be fundamental. This was underpinned by a Keynesian commitment to the maintenance of 'full employment' as part of an economic settlement. The social settlement assumed the existence of 'normal' families in which women and children were dependent for their income on the employment of their husbands and fathers in secure jobs. The organizational arrangements were based on a highly centralized bureaucratic and rule-based system, with government officials determining who was eligible for benefits and at what rates.

3 From threadbare safety-net to personal responsibility

3.1 Income maintenance and welfare

By the mid 1970s, the UK's income maintenance system had changed still further, in the sense that policies were no longer principally concerned with a marginalized or excluded population. It was no longer restricted to the relief of poverty – that is to providing support (or a safety-net) for those on very low incomes. On the contrary, its operation affected the middle classes as much as members of the working class or those defined as poor. The smoothing out of income over the life cycle had become as important as the relief of poverty. All families with children were in receipt of some sort of benefit through the family allowance, while after retirement age everybody was eligible for a basic state pension. All of those in employment were eligible for sickness benefits, and many people had drawn on unemployment benefit at some time in their working lives.

The shift towards an income maintenance system which covered all sections of the population also encouraged a move beyond Beveridge. This was apparent in a number of key ways. There was a move away from the flat rate contributions which had been assumed by Beveridge; an earnings-related pensions scheme was introduced (SERPS) to provide a supplement to the basic pension; child benefit, paid as a flat rate to mothers, was introduced to take the place of family allowance and the child tax allowance; family income supplement was introduced to help low-paid people who were in employment; state pensions were index-linked to earnings or price rises, whichever was the higher; and national assistance was renamed supplementary benefit, which may not have made much difference in practice to those in receipt of benefit, but did seem to represent an acknowledgement that supplementary benefit was a benefit like others, not just a means of managing the residual poor.

In principle the insurance principle continued to underpin the state's system of income maintenance, and brought the involvement of most of the working population, although it remained far less likely for women to be members of the contributory schemes. However, because the contributions were earnings related, while in many cases the benefits (except SERPS) were not, it also became more and more difficult to distinguish between income tax and national insurance. In practice, the benefits system was funded from taxation rather than directly from contributions. The national insurance fund existed in a highly notional sense only and never covered the full cost of benefits. In practice, national insurance contributions were treated as if they were taxes, and while it was possible for governments to increase contribution levels without being accused of raising income tax, an increase in employee contributions had the same effect on an individual's disposable income as a rise in income tax.

The importance of private arrangements also increased dramatically in the post-war period. With the help of tax relief, occupational pensions rose to cover over 50 per cent of the working population by the end of the 1960s. So, the insurance principle was of growing importance for those in employment, through private schemes effectively licensed by the state.

Another very important factor in the period from the late 1940s up to the mid 1970s was that economic prosperity, reflected in full employment and a growing rate of participation of women in paid employment, helped to make income maintenance seem less of a problem.

Almost as soon as the new arrangements were consolidated in legislation, however, the economic crises of the mid 1970s heralded their demise. First there was a renewed emphasis on the high cost of state provision of all sorts, and welfare provision in particular. In 1976 the government was forced to seek a major loan from the International Monetary Fund and the first stirrings of economic monetarism found their expression through the mouth of Denis Healey, who was then Labour Chancellor of the Exchequer. Even before the rise of the New Right it was becoming common to describe state spending as a bad thing, because it was perceived to be unproductive, and, worse than that, a drain on productive activity (Bacon and Eltis, 1976). It was (very) soon an accepted part of the dominant political discourse that the public sector share of the economy was too high and the private sector share too low. Nowhere was this more apparent, perhaps, than in debates on benefits, social security and even pensions. The key point being made was that the country could not afford to meet the costs of its income maintenance system.

This understanding has helped to provide the context for policy-making since the late 1970s. As a result, a number of changes were made to benefit levels. The earnings-related supplements to unemployment benefit and sick pay were abolished in the early 1980s, and a range of other minor changes accumulated during the 1980s and 1990s to reduce levels of support and periods of entitlement still further. The Supplementary Benefits Commission (set up in 1966) was abolished, regulations on supplementary benefit were tightened and it was relabelled income support. In the late 1980s family income supplement was abolished and replaced by family credit, and child benefit was effectively frozen. Because the earnings of those in employment rose consistently faster than prices, governments were reluctant to raise state pensions at the same rate, so pension increases have been tied to prices rather than earnings. Although by the late 1990s SERPS had not been abolished as initially proposed in a government Green Paper of the mid 1980s, levels of benefit were restricted, and a further shift towards private occupational pensions was encouraged.

The details of the benefits system are, of course, vitally important to those whose incomes rely on it, but few people can remember the particular features of the various benefits, the changing names or the rules on entitlement. For our purposes, the following general trends which can be identified since the late 1970s are more significant.

- Hills notes that the social security system 'includes at least 37 separate benefits; the two comprehensive guides to its rules published by the Child Poverty Action Group together have over 950 pages; over 100,000 people are employed to run it; its administration cost £3.5 billion in 1996/7' (Hills, 1997, p.39).

- The period between the mid 1970s and early 1990s was a time of a thousand cuts in benefit levels, although overall spending on social security actually rose over the same period because of the increased numbers of people in receipt of benefit of one sort or another.

- At the same time, there were continued attempts to redefine who was eligible for which benefit, and a growing obsession with identifying people attempting to 'defraud' the system. There were successive attempts to launch anti-fraud initiatives and to define entitlement more narrowly. So, for example, because of the increased rate at which people were claiming invalidity benefit in the early 1990s, it was replaced in 1996 with incapacity benefit, which involved much tighter medical checks and rules on entitlement. Similarly, the introduction of the jobseeker's allowance in 1996 (alongside a number of earlier schemes) had as one of its purposes the aim of more accurately identifying those who were unemployed and looking for work. It was an attempt to require people claiming benefit to show that they were actively seeking employment, and it restricted the period for which unemployed people could claim the benefit (see Novak, 1997, for a critical analysis of the introduction of the jobseeker's allowance). Because those in receipt of benefit have been defined as untrustworthy, some benefits never actually pass through their hands. Since the early 1980s, housing benefit (which replaced the housing element of supplementary benefit) has been paid directly to the public and private sector landlords of those nominally receiving it.

■ The reorganization of government departments (for example, through the formation of the Benefits Agency, the Northern Ireland Social Security Agency, the Employment Service and the Child Support Agency) has also been justified in part by the claim that the new agencies will be more effective at rooting out fraud, as well as being more efficient and responsive. (Chapter 9 contains a relevant, extended discussion on the role of managerialization.)

The public waiting room of a DSS office, South London

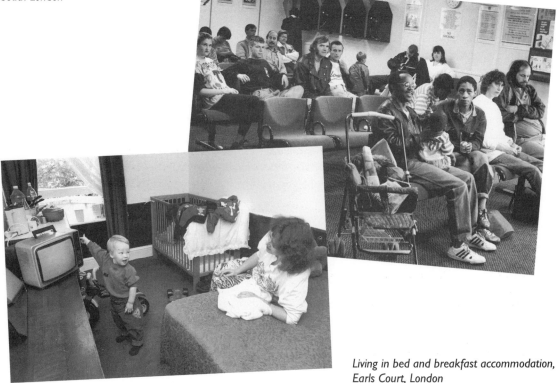

Living in bed and breakfast accommodation, Earls Court, London

ACTIVITY 8.4

Extract 8.4 is taken from a leaflet produced by the Benefits Agency. It summarizes two of the main benefits available to people on low incomes in 1997: income support and family credit. The Benefits Agency is responsible for the management of social security benefits in Great Britain; the Northern Ireland Social Security Agency has that responsibility in Northern Ireland. (Although legally separate, social security legislation in Northern Ireland 'seems to meet the same policy objectives as in the rest of the UK' – Ditch, 1993, p.76.)

The precise benefits available in any one year will vary as legislation changes them, so it is important not to assume that these particular benefits will exist in perpetuity. At the time of writing, for example, family credit is about to be replaced by forms of tax credit for working families. However, focusing on the ways in which potential recipients are informed about what is available can help us to identify the principles that underlie the benefits system at any one time. It may also make it easier to see the extent to which the different benefits fit together. In reading the extract, try to identify the main conditions on which the benefits are made available.

Extract 8.4 Benefits Agency: 'Which benefit'

Income Support
Income Support is a social security benefit for people aged 16 or over whose income is below a certain level **and** who are not working 16 hours or more a week (and do not have a partner who works 24 hours or more on average a week) **and** who are not required to be available for work because, for example, they are:

sick or disabled

or a lone parent or foster parent

or 60 or over

or getting Invalid Care Allowance for looking after someone.

You must be:

habitually resident in the United Kingdom, the Channel Islands, the Isle of Man or the Republic of Ireland

or treated as habitually resident in the United Kingdom.

Income Support can be paid to top up other benefits, or earnings from part-time work (including self-employed work), or if you have no money coming in at all.

Your right to Income Support does not depend on National Insurance contributions.

You cannot normally get Income Support if you are working for 16 hours or more on average a week, or your partner (if you have one) works for 24 hours or more on average a week. (Partner means someone you are married to or whom you live with as if you are married to them.)

You, or you and your partner together, must not have over £8,000 in savings. Savings between £3,000 and £8,000 will affect the amount you can get. Special rules apply if you live in a residential care home or nursing home …

If you are still at school
You can't normally claim Income Support for yourself if you are still at school. But you can if you are aged 16 or over but under 19 and any of the following applies to you:

you are looking after your own child

or you are an orphan and no one is looking after you

or you are so disabled that even if you were available for work you would be unlikely to get a job

or you are not living with your parents or anyone acting in their place and are not being kept by them, and either you are not in touch with them, or they are separated from you for reasons that can't be avoided.

How much you get

The amount you get depends on, among other things, how old you are, whether you have a partner, whether you have any dependent children and how old they are, whether you or anyone in your family has any disabilities, how much money you and your partner have coming in each week, and how much you, or you and your partner together, have in savings.

Your Income Support payment may be made up of three parts:

- a **personal allowance** for yourself and your partner (if you have one) and one for each child or young person that you or your partner look after

- **premiums** for groups of people with special needs, such as families with children, people with disabilities, people over 60 and people who are getting, or are entitled to get, Invalid Care Allowance …

- **housing costs** to help with mortgage interest and certain other housing costs not met by Housing Benefit. Mortgage interest payments may be paid direct to your lender …

If your child's other parent lives elsewhere

The DSS Child Support Agency (CSA) is responsible for the assessment, collection, review and enforcement of maintenance for children in many cases.

If you or your present partner are awarded Income Support, income-based Jobseeker's Allowance, family credit or Disability Working Allowance, and you are a parent with care of a child/children whose other parent lives elsewhere in the UK, you will be required to apply for child maintenance if asked to do so by the CSA. An exception may be made where the CSA accepts that there is a risk of harm or undue distress occurring to you or any of the children who live with you if you are required to apply …

Family Credit

Family Credit is a tax-free benefit for working families with children. It is **not** a loan and does not have to be paid back.

Your right to Family Credit does **not** depend on National Insurance contributions.

Who can get it?

To get Family Credit, you must be responsible for at least one child under 16 (or under 19 if in full-time education up to, and including, A level or equivalent standard).

You **or** your partner (husband, wife, or someone you live with as if you are married to them) must be working at least 16 hours a week. You can get it whether you're employed or self-employed, a couple, or a lone parent.

You don't have to be on a very low income or have a very large family to be able to get Family Credit.

You, or you and your partner together, must not have over £8,000 in savings. Savings between £3,000 and £8,000 will affect the amount you can get.

How much you get

The amount of Family Credit you get depends on:

- how many children you have and their ages

- your family's net earnings and other income

- any savings you or your partner may have

- in certain circumstances, the amount of childcare charges you pay

- the number of hours you or your partner work.

You get the same amount whether you are a one-parent or two-parent family.

(Benefits Agency, 1996, pp.12–17)

COMMENT

Income support provides a basic level of income for those who need it, but entitlement is restricted to those 'who are not required to be available for work.' (Those who are unemployed and required to be available for work need to apply for a different benefit – the jobseeker's allowance.) The examples given in Extract 8.4 show that very specific categories of people only are likely to be entitled to receive income support. In a sense, the rules on income support help to define what it is to be one of the 'deserving' poor. The section headed 'If your child's other parent lives elsewhere' discusses the role of the Child Support Agency, indicating that, where parents are separated or divorced, the absent parent is required to contribute to the maintenance costs of the children. This both reduces the costs of benefit payments (since maintenance above a certain level is counted against income support) and, since most absent parents are men, reflects the continued understanding that children and their mothers are, to some extent at least, dependent on their fathers and male partners.

Family credit was a benefit paid to people in low-paid jobs, who have children under 16 or under 19 in full-time education. There seem to be two principles underlying it: first, it encourages people to enter the labour market, even where pay is low; second, it is intended to provide extra support to those with children. In that sense it is consistent with Beveridge's approach, since it does not disadvantage those in work. It could also be argued, however, that it is a form of subsidy to employers who pay low wages, and that is an issue to which we return below.

Income maintenance for people on low incomes is, as Extract 8.4 suggests, a complex system which requires a high degree of regulation and assessment. The extract provides only brief summaries of the rules and entitlements to access. The next stage for any claimant is to fill in forms which are than assessed in detail by the agency responsible. Moreover, income support and family credit are just two of a range of different benefits. It is also possible, for example, to draw on the social fund, which operates to provide 'one-off' grants or loans to people facing particular, narrowly specified, short-term difficulties (such as cold weather payments or crisis loans).

3.2   The rediscovery of personal responsibility

Although a concern about costs and levels of spending has provided a continuing backdrop to the development of policies for income maintenance, it has not been the only one, or even the most significant one in policy terms. Alongside that concern, since the early 1980s there has been a renewed stress on personal responsibility and a criticism of welfare for encouraging dependence on the 'nanny state'. This has found a clear reflection in a growing emphasis on the need for households and families to provide for their own futures through insurance of one sort or another. There has, for example, been a gradual and continuing growth in occupational pensions, subsidized by the state through forms of tax relief, and this has been accompanied by the promotion of private pensions by government. The notion of dependence on state welfare was being socially constructed as a social problem at the same time as labour market insecurity and low incomes were gradually redefined as private problems.

The argument for substantial reform of the pensions system – and a continued move away from state provision – has been reinforced by the view that the numbers of pensioners relative to younger people who are in employment will shift dramatically over the next 40 to 50 years (Hills, 1997, pp.11–13). According to this argument, the amount of tax that will have to be raised to cover pensions will be unsustainable, and it will not longer be possible to maintain the implicit contract between the generations which underpins the payment of state pensions out of tax income. This threat, described as a 'demographic timebomb', is used both to justify a continued downward pressure on state pensions in real terms and to encourage individuals to take out private schemes. In other words, the argument combines a strong moral element – individuals must take responsibility for themselves and their future – with a powerful financial one – tax income will not cover the expected real costs of maintaining the existing system.

Hills (1997, pp.12–13) shows that some of the fears about a demographic timebomb are actually unfounded, at least in their extreme form. Although a higher proportion of the UK's population will be over 65 in 2040 than in 1990, Hills notes that the rate at which this shift will take place will be much slower in the UK than in most other welfare states (such as Germany, Japan and the USA), because a relatively high proportion of the UK's population in the 1990s was over 65 (see Figure 8.1). Even if associated costs such as health workers' salaries, as well as benefit and pension levels, are included, Hills (1997, p.12) calculates that the ageing of UK society would only 'imply spending growth at a rate of 0.32 per cent per year.' Similarly, although the Government Actuary has forecasted a significant increase in payments under the State Earnings Related Pensions scheme (SERPS) (from £1 billion in 1990/91 to £15–16 billion in 2040/41), Hills notes that, when the associated reduction in the need for income support for some along with increased taxes for others is taken into account, the overall effect over 50 years will amount to only 0.8 per cent of one year's national income (Hills, 1997, p.13). In other words, in this case at least, the shift towards new arrangements probably has less to do with the need to make major financial savings than it has to do with attempts to change dominant understandings of the ways in which welfare should operate.

A similar set of arguments was applied to the field of child support. The Child Support Act 1991 specified the responsibility of both parents to provide financial support for the upbringing of their children, even where one parent

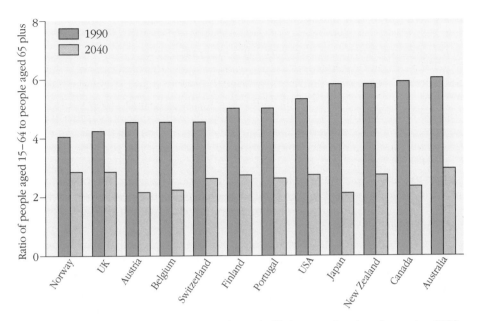

Figure 8.1 Number of people of working age for each elderly person in selected countries, 1990 and 2040 (Source: Hills, 1997, p.12, Figure 6)

(called the 'absent' parent in official documents) is no longer living with them. The Child Support Agency and the Child Support Agency (Northern Ireland) have the specific responsibility for ensuring that the 'absent' parent makes the necessary contributions when the 'parent with care' is in receipt of income support, and can also act on behalf of the 'parent with care' in other circumstances if requested to do so. Child support legislation has the intended effect both of reducing social security (income support) payments to 'parents with care' and of highlighting the responsibility of the 'absent parent' for his or her children. In practice, of course, it also reinforces the notion that women (the overwhelming proportion of 'parents with care') are dependent on their relationship with men (the overwhelming proportion of 'absent parents') for the income they receive. Again, the approach powerfully combines 'moral' arguments about responsibility, with 'financial' arguments about saving taxpayers' money.

3.3   From welfare to workfare

During the 1980s and 1990s the availability of benefits at rates which meet anything more than the subsistence needs of those in receipt of it was increasingly defined in policy debates as a disincentive to working (and, therefore, escaping poverty through paid employment). A two-pronged approach to resolving this was adopted: first, benefit levels were squeezed dramatically and rules on entitlement were more tightly drawn; second, schemes such as the jobseeker's allowance were launched to target advice and to require at least some of those receiving benefit to move into employment within a certain period. The notion of workfare (borrowed from the USA) has become increasingly attractive across the main political parties (Labour, Conservative and Liberal Democrat). Workfare implies that in return for benefit individuals will be required to undertake work

workfare

or training generally provided through training and enterprise councils (England and Wales) or local enterprise companies (Scotland) at local level, or the Training and Education Agency in Northern Ireland (Peck, 1997).

The notion of workfare is based around a reassessment of the ways in which the labour market operates. For Beveridge the labour market could be taken for granted. Those in employment were secure and it was necessary to provide support only for those excluded from it, either temporarily or permanently. Since the 1980s, by contrast, it has frequently been argued that the labour market is a much less secure and more volatile environment (see, for example, Commission on Social Justice, 1994, pp.221–4). As a result, policy emphasis shifted towards enabling people to find employment in the new context; instead of 'welfare' for those out of work, it has been argued, the need is for 'workfare' so that income is generated from employment, even if the only jobs available are low paid. In the words of the Commission for Social Justice (1994, p.224), the emphasis of policy shifted towards providing people with a 'hand-up rather than a hand-out.'

This stress on the close relationship between social security and changing labour markets has been used to reinforce arguments for a shift to training as a means into employment and an indication of an individual's readiness to prepare her or himself for the rigours of the 'riskier' labour market.

The move towards workfare also implies a shift back towards the Poor Law's notion of 'less eligibility', since the assumption is that no-one should be better off out of work than would be the case if she or he had a job. But one sharp difference is that in contemporary debates providing forms of subsidy to those offering low-paid employment is increasingly seen as the way to tackle the problem. Family credit and the social fund illustrate this approach in that they provide extra support to ensure that people remain in work, even if their incomes are low. In other words, so far as workfare is concerned, the 'less eligibility principle' does *not* rely on forcing levels of income support below the lowest pay available locally.

ACTIVITY 8.5

Extract 8.5 comes from an official leaflet on the jobseeker's allowance. This benefit, first introduced in 1996, replaced both unemployment benefit and income support for unemployed people looking for work. In reading the extract, try to assess the main emphasis of the policy which lies behind the allowance. What are the main objectives of the jobseeker's allowance as implied by the leaflet?

Extract 8.5 'Jobseeker's allowance: helping you back to work'

What to do when you start looking for work

As soon as you are unemployed or know that you will be unemployed and looking for work, contact your local Jobcentre. You should do this straight away because, if you can get Jobseeker's Allowance, you may lose money by not claiming at once. When you first contact the Jobcentre you will be asked about your situation and requirements. You will be given information about what you have to do to claim Jobseeker's Allowance and advice about other courses of action you can take.

If you decide to claim Jobseeker's Allowance, you will get an appointment for a New Jobseeker Interview and you will be given a claim pack to complete before the interview. You can get help to complete the claim forms if you need it ...

New Jobseeker Interview

At the New Jobseeker Interview the Employment Service Adviser will

- make sure you understand the conditions for receiving Jobseeker's Allowance
- discuss the types of work you are looking for and the best ways of finding it
- give you information about jobs, training and the other opportunities that are available
- discuss with you and draw up a Jobseeker's Agreement

and

- check that you have completed the claim form fully and provided all the information needed to work out your Jobseeker's Allowance claim …

Jobseeker's Allowance

To get Jobseeker's Allowance you must

- be capable of, actively seeking and available for work, usually for at least 40 hours a week …
- have paid enough National Insurance contributions, or have income and savings below a certain level …
- be out of work or working on average less than 16 hours a week
- be, normally, 18 years old or over and under pension age …
- have a Jobseeker's Agreement which is signed by you and an Employment Service Adviser
- not be in relevant education

and

- be in Great Britain.

To receive Jobseeker's Allowance based on your **income**, you must also

- be habitually resident in the United Kingdom, the Channel Islands, the Isle of Man or the Republic of Ireland

or

- be treated as habitually resident in the United Kingdom.

If your partner is working, it may affect your entitlement to income-based Jobseeker's Allowance …

Availability for work

You should be willing and able to start a job **immediately**. However there are some exceptions from having to be able to take up work straight away. These are if you are

- providing a service such as an emergency service
- undertaking voluntary work

or

- have caring responsibilities.

You should be available for work for at least 40 hours a week, but you may agree with an Employment Service Adviser the times in the week when you are prepared to be available. You may be able to restrict your availability if, for example, you have

- a physical or mental condition which affects the work you do
- caring responsibilities

or

- a conscientious or religious objection.

If you are looking for work **in your usual occupation**, you may be allowed a period of between one and 13 weeks at the beginning of your claim (this is know as the **permitted period**), during which you are able to restrict your availability to that occupation and your normal rate of pay. After the permitted period jobseekers are expected to be available for a wider range of jobs. You cannot normally refuse a job on the basis of pay after six months.

Actively seeking work

In order to meet the *actively seeking work* condition you must actively seek work in each week you are receiving Jobseeker's Allowance. To do this you need to take appropriate steps to improve your employability and to help you find work. Taking one step each week is not usually sufficient. As well as contacting possible employers, you could, for example, also be improving your employment prospects by putting together a Curriculum Vitae (CV). Taking more than one step will count towards meeting the *actively seeking work* condition.

Your Jobseeker's Agreement

To get Jobseeker's Allowance you must have a Jobseeker's Agreement which is signed jointly by you and your Employment Service Adviser. At your New Jobseeker Interview, your adviser will help you draw up an Agreement which takes account of your skills and experience. The agreement will be in writing and will set out

- your availability for work and any agreed restrictions
- the type of work you are looking for
- what you will do to look for work and improve your chances of finding work
- what you must do to remain entitled to Jobseeker's Allowance

and

- the services which are provided by the Employment Service to help you back into work.

(*Jobseeker's Allowance*, n.d., pp.3–8)

COMMENT

The main emphasis in Extract 8.5 is on the link between the jobseeker's allowance (JSA) and the need for claimants to be available for and actively looking for work (or seeking training to help them find work). A core condition of receiving the benefit is that 'You should be willing and able to start a job **immediately**', and the section headed 'Actively seeking work' spells out what this means. Anyone receiving the allowance has to sign a personalized written agreement with the employment service, which specifies a range of conditions about availability for work, type of work sought and the obligation to look for work or appropriate training. The emphasis, therefore, is on the position of the individual and her/his commitment to find work, rather than on the provision of benefits because of any perceived imperfection in the labour market (or lack of employment opportunities because of economic recession).

Two further points are worth noting, although they are not clear from the extract. First, only the first six months of JSA payment is at a standard rate based on the payment of national insurance contributions. After six months, or if there have been insufficient national insurance payments in the relevant period, claimants seeking work may be eligible for income-related JSA. That means that their allowance will be means tested, that is influenced by other sources of household income (including that of children and partners in the same household) along the same lines as income support. In some cases, of course, this may mean that there is little point in claiming the allowance, since claimants effectively become defined as dependants on the income of others. Second, 16 and 17 year olds are generally excluded from receiving JSA, because if they are not employed or in full-time education it is assumed that they are on training courses. Their fall-back position is likely to be income support, or dependence on parental income (including benefits).

The key defining principle of the JSA is that employment should be the main source of income for those who are economically active – that is, able to work – and it operates to define this more sharply than was the case with unemployment benefit. Others are assumed to have left the labour force, perhaps receiving benefit on another basis (for example, because they have caring responsibilities, or through incapacity benefit), or are redefined as dependent on parents, partners and sometimes children. The purpose of the JSA is to get people back into paid employment of some sort, and welfare generally has increasingly been defined in terms which stress this.

In a highly critical commentary on the JSA, Novak (1997) emphasizes the 'toughness' of the regime, pointing to the way in which it now generates 'pointless tasks' for claimants which are 'experienced more often as punishment than an aid to finding work' (Novak, 1997, p.105). In other words, he suggests, the key aspects of the jobseeker's allowance are to be found in the scope for using it to police and control those who are likely to rely on it. One of its aims, he argues, is to force the unemployed to take whatever work is available, and to 'punish' those who are either unprepared or unable to do so.

■ ■ ■

Whether one accepts the more positive language of 'enabling' people to move from 'welfare to work', or the more negative interpretation which sees the JSA as being about 'punishment', it is important to acknowledge the extent to which there has been a shift towards the regulation of the labour market and away from the state provision of benefits. This could simply be dismissed as a change in emphasis, since the Beveridgean settlements also implied that employment was the key to welfare. However, the shift was nevertheless significant enough to suggest that a new settlement may be emerging. The balance is increasingly directed more at individual responsibility and less at forms of universal entitlement. This has also been reflected in the nature of political debates, which focus on different ways of introducing responsibility and of regulating and shaping the labour market. It is for this reason that the introduction of a minimum wage has been a matter of contention, alongside claims from each political party that it offers ways of ensuring higher levels of individual welfare and prosperity through its labour market policies. Although the debate about a minimum wage in the UK has frequently been associated with the policies of the European Union (and specifically the Social Chapter of the Single European Act), it is also a feature of the US labour market, which is otherwise acknowledged to be highly flexible.

ACTIVITY 8.6

This chapter has not tried to summarize all the different benefits available at the time of writing, although it has briefly referred to many of them. One reason for not outlining each in detail is simply that policy-makers introduce changes on a regular basis. More important, however, we have been concerned to identify and explore the direction of change in the period up to end of the 1930s, and between the 1950s and 1990s, particularly in terms of what it tells us about the way in which the 'problem' of income maintenance and welfare recipients has been constructed.

Extracts 8.6 and 8.7 are taken from statements made by leading 1990s' politicians of different political parties. The first comes from a lecture given by Gordon Brown in 1996 when he was in opposition as Labour's Shadow Chancellor, while the second comes from a book by David Willetts, a Conservative MP centrally involved in the Conservative Party campaign during the 1997 General Election.

You should first try to identify the main arguments in each extract. They emphasize differences in approach, but there are also clear similarities. In reading these extracts you should:

- identify the differences;
- identify the similarities;
- note the continuities and differences with the income maintenance policies associated with Beveridge.

You may find it helpful to use a table such as this to make your notes:

	Brown/Willetts	Beveridge/Brown	Beveridge/Willetts
Differences			
Similarities/ continuities			

Extract 8.6 Gordon Brown: 'A chance to start again'

The 1945 welfare state meant a shift from charity to rights, from discretion to legal entitlement, from eligibility to meeting need, from local patchwork to national provision, from conditionality to universal opportunities. The underlying belief was that no one should be denied chances in life because of accidents of birth and temporary misfortunes.

Since 1979 each principle has been subverted …

The market is replacing need as a guiding principle – even in the NHS – and in many services we are seeing the emergence of a two-tier system of provision: new opportunities available to only some but not all. In its treatment of the poor the government is returning to the punitive principles of the 1834 Poor Law. The underlying philosophy is that the poor are somehow to blame for their poverty … It is assumed that the unemployed are unemployed because they do not want to work and that they can be made to by cutting their benefits. And one symptom of the profound change is the aura the term social security has acquired.

Social security: the very words chosen in 1945 to signify a fresh start. Once a dignifying concept that replaced the Poor Law, the words social security have now acquired, for millions, the stigma that the old Poor Law possessed. It is time to rebuild the welfare state from the original underlying principles of 1945, a universal system for all citizens, treating all citizens equally.

But we must face up to the fact that the challenges of the 1990s are not the same as those of 1945.

The 1945 welfare state assumed that its beneficiaries were passive recipients. When you became unemployed your responsibility was simply to wait until another job came along. Job changes were infrequent, unemployment was principally caused by fluctuations in demand, and the duty of the unemployed was clear: wait for the recession to become a recovery.

Today all this has changed. Job changes are frequent, the need to upgrade skills is constant and universal, and the unemployed can remain unemployed even when demand is high. They can be and are, of course, victims of low demand but they are more likely to be the victims of technological change, lacking the skills for the jobs that are available.

The answer lies in neither the post-1979 punitive welfare state nor a return to the post-1945 passive welfare state. The post-1996 welfare state must be one which actively tackles the causes of poverty and creates new opportunities for employment, providing the skills to take advantage of these opportunities. It means a welfare state where the unemployed person is encouraged to take steps to become employable and the welfare state gives active help …

We do not substitute state responsibility for individual responsibility; opportunities and personal responsibility go hand in hand …

My vision is of a welfare state which helps everyone realize their potential and where the task of government is to help people bridge the gap between what they are and what they have in themselves to become. We need policies that create work, create the skills for work, ensure that work pays and in particular give women new opportunities: work-creating employment practices, work-enabling education policies, work-friendly tax and benefit policies and work-permitting child care policies …

We will give young people two high-quality routes to qualifications: college- and school-based apprenticeship and training route. And where young people are in work we will place a statutory obligation on employers to provide unqualified young workers with training opportunities.

Even so, all our efforts will be of limited benefit if we do not break the cycle of disadvantage. We want more and more teenagers from lower income families staying on at school and going to university and college. That is why we have said we will replace the Child Benefit after 16 with a new National Education Attendance Allowance available at a higher level for those who need it most …

Educational opportunity for all will not work unless there is a second pillar: employment opportunity for all. What we call our new deal for the under-25s involves jobs, not schemes, wages not benefits, and opportunities and choice. To narrow the time between redundancy and re-employment we should create a modern jobs information highway that any unemployed or working person can access, backed up by an up-to-date careers service …

[T]o make sure money from Family Credit and other tax and benefit reforms goes to the employee instead of subsidizing bad employers we need to underpin benefit reform with a wages floor, and that requires a properly implemented minimum wage. Unless we have a minimum wage which underpins the benefits system, we are condemned to using the Family Credit system or any wage supplement, not as a way of helping those genuinely in need, but as a way of subsidizing exploitative employers who deliberately keep their wages low.

(Brown, 1996, pp.24–5)

Extract 8.7 David Willetts: 'Why vote Conservative'

Low pay: Family Credit versus minimum wage

Imagine a group of people serving behind the bar at your local pub and earning say £3 an hour. One might be a student boosting his grant. Perhaps another is a young woman with a husband who has got a good job at the factory but she is earning some extra money to pay for a good holiday. Then there is a single parent struggling to raise two children on her own. Finally, perhaps there is a forty-year-old man who has been made redundant and is earning some money to keep his non-earning wife and two children before he can get back into a well-paid job again. They are all doing the same work and so they are all receiving the same wage. But whether or not that is a living wage depends on their circumstances. That is why the single parent and the forty-year-old father would both be entitled to claim Family Credit to help keep their families. A man with a young family working full time at £3 an hour could receive over £55 a week in Family Credit. Family Credit now goes to over 660,000 low-income families and helps the vast majority of families on low incomes to be better off in work than out of work.

Some of our critics say that Family Credit just subsidizes employers who pay low wages. But a recent study showed that very few employers knew whether their staff were eligible for Family Credit or not, and so could not have pushed wages down to account for it. Family Credit costs almost £2 billion a year, it is true. But it is cheaper to pay someone Family Credit than for them to remain on income support – which would be the alternative if a minimum wage destroyed their jobs. And for many people, a low-paid job is a first step towards a better one. Only 12 per cent of people on Family Credit receive it for more than twelve months. And Sir Stanley Kalms of Dixons is fond of pointing out that many of his key managers started out in part-time jobs.

Labour do not like Family Credit. Instead they wish to force employers to pay the minimum wage. It is a striking reminder of the basic difference between the two parties when it comes to the free market. It would become a criminal offence to pay an employee less than the rate fixed as the minimum wage. This is a very clumsy way of dealing with poverty because a high proportion of those on low pay live in households with a higher earner. The Institute for Fiscal Studies calculate that a minimum wage would actually help households in the top third of the income distribution by more than those in the bottom third. So it is much worse targeted than Family Credit. Of the 10 per cent of people with the lowest wages, 95 per cent of them are not in the poorest 10 per cent of households. It does badly therefore at helping poverty and it does even worse when it comes to maintaining jobs ...

Many of the people affected by the minimum wage work in the public services ... Back in 1992 Robin Cook estimated that a minimum wage would cost the NHS £500 million. Local authorities would be hit too and schools would have to pay more for their ancillary staff ... Either Labour will end up increasing their public spending or they will have to cut back services in order to pay public sector unions more.

From dole to dignity

Even though British unemployment is significantly below the European average we obviously want to see it lower still. That is why we introduced the new Jobseeker's Allowance in October 1996 which requires unemployed people to be available for and actively seeking work. It makes clear their obligations as jobseekers and gives the Employment Service the power to apply sanctions if they do not fulfil their obligations: it is a powerful set of tools to prevent people languishing on benefit ...

We are also dealing with the notorious 'why work' problem to ensure that people are better off in work than out of work. For example, the new Back-to-Work bonus helps people working part time and in receipt of the Jobseeker's Allowance or Income Support to accumulate a tax-free bonus of up to £1,000 payable when they get back into full-time work. Any employer who takes on someone previously unemployed for two years now receives a one-year holiday from their National Insurance contributions. If people take a job after six months out of work they can keep their Housing Benefit at their existing rate for four weeks regardless of their earnings. Partners of JSA claimants can now work for up to twenty-four hours per week without the claimant losing entitlement to benefit, so dealing with the serious problem that if someone is unemployed it may become worth while for their partner to give up work. This is just a small selection of a range of imaginative measures and there are more to come ...

We are now developing the most ambitious range of measures aimed at encouraging people into work that any British Government has ever introduced.

(Willetts, 1997, pp.37–41)

COMMENT

In Extract 8.6 Gordon Brown explicitly takes on the Beveridgean settlements, claiming that substantial change is necessary, but he also questions the strategy of the then Conservative government, which he accuses of going back to the Poor Law. The main emphasis of his argument is on the need to create new opportunities for employment through a strategy of skills development: 'a welfare state where the unemployed person is encouraged to take steps to become employable and the welfare state gives active help.' At the heart of this model is a notion of individual responsibility, underpinned by opportunities for self development guaranteed (if not always provided) by the state. In other words, Brown's vision of welfare is one which highlights education and training and defines income maintenance in relation to access to employment and education (for example, through proposals for a new education allowance to replace child benefit for young people aged between 16 and 18). A corollary of this is that in many cases benefit payment will depend on the individual's readiness to take up the 'opportunities' which are offered. Introducing a minimum wage (sometimes reinforced by a commitment to lower the starting point of income tax) is seen as a means of ensuring that individuals do not lose out by moving from benefit to employment.

In Extract 8.7 David Willetts also focuses on the labour market, but his approach is rather different, particularly in the nature of the political rhetoric employed. Brown uses the language of the welfare state, suggesting that the state has a role in shaping the labour market. Willetts makes the opposite assumption his starting-point. Unlike Brown, he favours the use of a family credit approach instead of the introduction of a minimum wage. He presents two main reasons for this. First, the positions of those in low-paid jobs varies, and family credit makes it possible to adjust household income according to household needs instead of providing everybody with the same overall income just because of the job they occupy. In other words, Willetts argues that family credit allows better targeting of need than a minimum wage. Second, he argues that by forcing pay levels up, the introduction of a minimum wage will discourage employers from creating jobs. A third, subsidiary reason given is that, since many low-paid people work in the public sector (generally in health and social care), meeting the costs of introducing a minimum wage will either mean a significant increase in taxes, or a reduction in public services. Willetts goes on to stress the need for policies to encourage people back to work, and outlines a range of policies associated with the jobseeker's allowance.

■ ■ ■

In Willetts' discussion of the jobseeker's allowance, the similarities between his and Brown's approach are clear. Brown and Willetts share an emphasis on work, training and assistance with getting back into work as the solution to welfare problems. Even Brown's use of the term 'allowance' for the new benefits he wishes to introduce indicates that the debate is taking place within a shared set of understandings. The move away from the Beveridgean settlements involved a period in which the term 'assistance' seemed to dominate, through one in which everything was described as a 'benefit', to one in which the language of 'allowances' has taken over. Unlike the payment of 'assistance', which suggests an almost charitable approach, and the payment of 'benefits', which reflects a more universal approach based on rights, the notion of 'allowances' implies that those who receive them are supposed to be doing something in return.

assistance
benefits
allowances

The debate around the minimum wage highlights important differences between the approach of Brown and that of Willetts. But here, too, the debate is taking place on ground that is shared. The shared implicit assumption is that direct state provision is not the way forward; instead, it is in the labour market and its workings that solutions are to be found.

The arguments developed in these extracts suggest that there has been a move away from Beveridge. One casualty has been the principle that income maintenance policies existed to ensure that income from the good years (of full employment, of individual employment) would be used to cover costs in the lean years. Instead, by the late 1990s, the dominant principle was that individuals

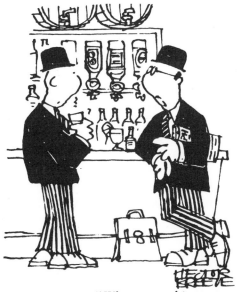

"What we need is a strong, authoritarian government with the courage to bring in compulsory laissez-faire."

needed to take advantage of opportunities to ensure that they were able to find work in an ever-changing labour market. The language of equality used in Extracts 8.6 and 8.7, as well as more generally in political discourse in this period, is a language of equal opportunity rather than equalization through a welfare system. The emphasis of policy has shifted substantially away from the achievement of 'equity objectives relating to living standards and the reduction of inequality to efficiency goals concerned with incentives' (Barr and Coulter, 1990, p.274).

Paradoxically, perhaps, these new frameworks also suggest more active state intervention in the operation of the labour market, something which Beveridge explicitly sought to avoid by emphasizing policies based on taxation and social insurance.

3.4 Moving beyond Beveridge

Until the mid 1970s, income maintenance policies in the UK were developed to incorporate increasingly wider sections of society. The introduction and development of various earnings-related schemes (particularly for pensions) and forms of financial assistance to those in low-paid employment meant that most people were directly involved in one way or another.

In the mid 1970s, however, this process came under challenge as the UK economy was perceived to be in crisis and a great deal of the blame was placed on what were said to be high levels of public spending. Tighter rules on rights to benefit were introduced and benefit levels were restricted. Moves towards privatized and occupational welfare arrangements were encouraged. The rules appeared to become more and more complex, made up of a range of specific allowances each with its own set of regulations.

Overall, there has been a move towards an income maintenance system which combines an increased emphasis on individual moral responsibility with the aim of reducing state expenditure. The most obvious examples include the Child Support Agency (which highlights the responsibility of the 'absent' parent and offers the prospect of reducing the costs of income support) and the jobseeker's allowance (which highlights the responsibility of the unemployed to get jobs, and regulates the number of people entitled to receive the allowance itself).

There has also been a move away from the notion that individuals might somehow have a right to levels of income support (above some very low minimum). On the contrary, in order to receive certain allowances, the requirement now is that a person must be prepared to undertake certain forms of activity (looking for work, undertaking appropriate training, preparing for a return to the world of work). Access to employment is defined as the means of escaping from welfare dependency and developing economic solvency and independence.

New approaches to income maintenance appear to be structured around the possibility of regulated markets rather than state provision. Some forms of welfare previously provided by the state (such as pensions or sick pay) are increasingly provided through employers or private insurance, while access to employment itself is now seen as a core aspect of welfare. The state's role, according to one expression of this, should be to move people from 'welfare to work'

welfare to work

These developments seem to confirm the emergence of an interrelated set of post-Beveridge welfare settlements in the area of income maintenance. Some aspects of this process can be summarized briefly as follows, although it is important to stress that these are projections of change which may be taking place, rather than a description of the completed process.

- The political settlement seems to mix a commitment to intervention on the supply side of the labour market (that is, improving the employability of people through skills training and education) with a reluctance to interfere with the operations of economic markets in other ways.

- The economy has been interpreted by successive governments as one dominated by global market forces in which there are no longer 'jobs for life' and labour flexibility is highly valued. This suggests that there is little scope for nationally based Keynesian strategies, but that the role of the state is to prepare its citizens for survival in the context of continuing rapid economic change.

- The social settlement is one which emphasises the importance of individual responsibility (for example, to train, to seek employment, to work, to contribute to occupational and other pension schemes), alongside rights to specified benefits, and reinforces the responsibility of those in employment to provide support for those defined as their dependants (for example, fathers for children, husbands for wives, etc.).

- The new organizational arrangements have involved the setting up of quasi-autonomous government agencies which are also charged with the development of individualized packages of income support intended to encourage different behaviour (for example, undertaking training, finding paid work, providing for children), and not just the distribution of social security budgets according to nationally determined rules.

4 Conclusion: the changing same?

It is possible to argue that we have come full circle – towards a 'late twentieth century high technology Poor Law' (Clarke *et al.*, 1992, p.196). Certainly, Brown (1996) accuses the Conservative governments of the 1980s and 1990s of moving in this direction. And some features of the new arrangements (including those espoused by Brown) are highly redolent of the old arguments. The emergent framework is dominated by growing concern about individual moral responsibility for the maintenance of household income, and it is accompanied by forms of intervention which are likely to discourage benefit take-up. There remains a fundamental – and increasingly explicit – concern that the availability of benefits should not undermine incentives to work. Various allowances are made available to those who follow the approved channels and accept their responsibilities to look for work. The implicit assumption remains that households are headed by male breadwinners, although this is no longer stated explicitly. Motherhood (or more accurately 'parenthood', which often amounts to the same thing in practice) is seen as a possible route to income support, as long as one parent (usually the father) is absent. There has been little change in many of the tensions and debates.

ACTIVITY 8.7

Think back over the arguments of this chapter – and of earlier chapters, particularly Chapter 2 – and try to make your own judgement about the changes in income maintenance policy over time.

1   Do you think we are seeing a return to the principles of the nineteenth-century Poor Law?

2   Or has the death of the welfare state been much exaggerated, to the extent that really nothing much has changed since Beveridge?

3   Or are we seeing the emergence of substantially new arrangements, which may borrow from the past, but are being put together in different ways?

COMMENT

I think it would be a mistake to conclude that we have simply gone back in time, to rediscover Victorian values. Although it is important to set contemporary debates in a longer-term context, it is also important that we use that context to inform those debates. It should not substitute for them, through the drawing of inappropriate historical analogies. We need to be ready to explore developments over the longer term, but we also need to assess the situation in which we find ourselves, exploring how the arguments and debates fit together today.

Whatever the pressures, in the late 1990s there were, for example, still entitlements to certain basic benefits which were not means tested (such as child benefit and state pensions). The role of the state has also changed significantly. Whatever the political rhetoric, state regulation is much more extensive in the contemporary period than it was at the beginning of the twentieth century. The rise of the insurance principle has changed the income maintenance landscape for those who are in long-term employment, although the predicted rise of a more flexible labour force has introduced new forms of insecurity for those whose jobs may be redefined or disappear. The emphasis of the Poor Law system on encouraging (or forcing) the able bodied back to work is reflected in some of the emergent arrangements, but the biggest growth in the need for income support is post-retirement, because the proportion of the population living to that age is much greater than before.

■ ■ ■

Income maintenance both reflects and helps to construct forms of differentiation. The jobseeker's allowance is based on individualized 'contracts'; the operation of the child support system depends on individualized deals arranged through the Child Support Agency (according to predetermined formulae); pensions increasingly depend on individualized packages – generally arranged through employers. The vast range of specific benefits helps to construct a complex and overlapping system, in which each person's individualized package may be rather different from those of other people. It is, of course, still recognized that some people will fall through the 'net', but the net itself increasingly looks more like a spider's web within which those involved are in danger of becoming trapped. As a last resort, means-tested income support is still available, but it is tightly controlled, and benefit levels have failed to keep pace with inflation. Moreover, it opens up households to extensive forms of social intervention and 'counselling'. A very high proportion of those reliant on means-tested benefit are women. Lone motherhood has in the past been one of the few officially uncontested routes to income support, and even the introduction of the Child Support Agency has not managed to undermine this fully.

As far as possible, the aim seems to be either to identify someone on whom those needing support might be defined as being dependent, or to ensure that they enter some form of employment. In the case of young people, for example, it is assumed that they are dependent on their parents for shelter until the age of 18 (they are not entitled to housing benefit until then); until the age of 25 they are entitled to housing benefit for shared (rather than self-contained) accommodation only. Following the Child Support Act, lone parents with children are assumed to be dependent on the absent (biological) parent, and the Child Support Agency is charged with the task of ensuring that child maintenance is collected from the absent parent. In part this is intended to ensure that the continued individual (moral and financial) responsibility of the absent parent is acknowledged, and in part to ensure that benefit costs are reduced. The responsibility for caring for those who cannot care for themselves has also increasingly been transferred back into the family, and new benefits (in the form of carers' allowances) were introduced to reflect this, alongside increased requirements to pay for other forms of care.

Some issues that were more or less taken for granted within the Poor Law and, even, the Beveridge Report, are under much greater contention. Although, for example, the male breadwinner model has survived (against the odds) in the field of income maintenance, it is also clear that its assumptions fit uneasily with the ways in which households, families and individuals live their lives. However much the rules are changed to reflect political ideology, the practice of survival often seems to reflect different understandings. So, for example, in contrast to Orwell (Extract 8.1), research by Graham (1987) suggests that women reliant on income support often find it easier to survive financially without a male partner than with one. Placing them under pressure to identify the 'absent' parent may therefore be counterproductive if the implicit assumption is that it would be better if he remained a member of the household. Similarly, despite the apparently dominant view that the gaps in state provision for pensions will need to be met by private insurance, it is also increasingly clear that private insurance can be expected to cover only a relatively small proportion of the risk. At best it will be able to top up state and quasi-state (occupational) provision.

The emergent system is characterized by four main features. The first is an increased emphasis on the importance of the labour market, which associates income maintenance overwhelmingly with involvement in the workforce; the second is a stress on individual responsibility (to seek work, to provide support for those 'dependent' on you); the third is a belief in the growth of a mixed economy of income maintenance, and specifically in the need for extended private sector (and possibly not-for-profit) provision in pensions, but also, in principle, a wider role for privately provided social insurance; and the fourth is an acceptance of the continued need to provide a welfare safety-net for a small group of people (who might be labelled the 'deserving' poor, or the residual population).

In terms of the three elements of income maintenance identified in section 1, the relief of poverty remains a concern, but the group eligible for support is more narrowly defined. The protection of living standards is largely to be achieved through mechanisms which prepare individuals to operate better within the labour market, but some short-term benefits remain, and other aspects are to be covered by non-statutory means. Smoothing income out over the life cycle remains an issue, and some benefits, such as child benefit and basic state pensions, remain, but the main ways in which this is to be achieved are through forms of dependency on others (parents for the young, spouses for the parents, and children for the retired), or through involvement in various insurance schemes. In other words, the 'subjects' of income maintenance are less and less defined by their direct relationship to the state and more by their relationship to other individuals and families or households.

Further reading

John Hills' report on the *Future of Welfare* for the Joseph Rowntree Foundation, whose second edition was published in 1997, is a very helpful and well-supported review of debates and issues. The mobilization of evidence is particularly well done, leaving readers to make up their own minds. Like Hills' report, the Commission on Social Justice's report *Social Justice: Strategies for National Renewal*, published in 1994, considers much more than income maintenance, reviewing the whole of the UK welfare system and proposing its own programme of renewal. Its arguments are interesting and often challenging; you may not always agree with its conclusions, but it is certainly worth reading.

One valuable source of information about the UK income maintenance system is readily available in most Post Offices: leaflets and forms produced by the various agencies responsible for benefits, allowances and social security. Since these change a lot over time, it is worth picking them up every so often. The Child Poverty Action Group regularly produces a book on poverty within the UK, which reviews the impact of the benefits system for those who are most reliant on it. It is always worth reading, even if you are not able to get hold of the most up-to-date one. At the time of writing, the third edition, published in 1996, is the latest. It is called *Poverty: The Facts* and is written by Carey Oppenheim and Lisa Harper.

References

Bacon, R. and Eltis, W. (1976) *Britain's Economic Problem: Too Few Producers*, London, Macmillan.

Barr, N. and Coulter, F. (1990) 'Social security: solution or problem?', in Hills, J. (ed.) *The State of Welfare: The Welfare State in Britain since 1974*, Oxford, Clarendon Press.

Benefits Agency (1996) *Which Benefit? A Guide to Social Security and NHS Benefits*, Leaflet FB2, Oldham, HMSO.

Beveridge, W. (1942) *Social Insurance and Allied Services* (The Beveridge Report), Cmnd 6404, London, HMSO.

Branson, N. (1979) *Poplarism, 1919–1925*, London, Lawrence and Wishart.

Brown, G. (1996) 'A chance to start again', *Community Care*, 28 November–4 December, pp.24–5.

Clarke, J., Cochrane, A. and Smart, C. (1992) *Ideologies of Welfare: From Dreams to Disillusion*, London, Routledge.

Cochrane, A. and Clarke, J. (eds) (1993) *Comparing Welfare States: Britain in International Context*, London, Sage.

Cohen, M. (1945) *I Was One of the Unemployed*, London, Gollancz.

Commission on Social Justice (1994) *Social Justice: Strategies for National Renewal. The Report of the Commission on Social Justice*, London, Vintage.

Ditch, J. (1993) 'Next steps: restructuring the Department of Social Security', in Page, R. and Deakin, N. (eds) *The Costs of Welfare*, Aldershot, Avebury.

Gazeley, I. and Thane, P. (1998) 'Patterns of visibility: unemployment in Britain during the nineteenth and twentieth centuries', in Lewis (ed.) (1998).

Ginsburg, N. (1992) *Divisions of Welfare: A Critical Introduction to Comparative Social Policy*, London, Sage.

Graham, H. (1987) 'Being poor: perceptions and coping strategies of lone mothers', in Brannen, J. and Wilson, G. (eds) *Give and Take in Families: Studies in Resource Distribution*, London, Allen and Unwin.

Hall, C. (1998) 'A family for nation and empire', in Lewis (ed.) (1998).

Hills, J. with Gardiner, K. and the LSE Welfare State Programme (1997) *The Future of Welfare: A Guide to the Debate* (2nd edn), York, Joseph Rowntree Foundation.

Jobseeker's Allowance: Helping You Back to Work (n.d.) Crown Copyright.

Lewis, G. (ed.) (1998) *Forming Nation, Framing Welfare*, London, Routledge in association with The Open University.

Macintyre, S. (1980) *Little Moscows: Communism and Working-class Militancy in Inter-war Britain*, London, Croom Helm.

Mooney, G. (1998) '"Remoralizing" the poor?: gender, class and philanthropy in Victorian Britain', in Lewis (ed.) (1998).

Morris, L. (1998) 'Legitimate membership of the welfare community', in Langan. M. (ed.) *Welfare: Needs, Rights and Risks*, London, Routledge in association with The Open University.

Novak, T. (1997) 'Hounding delinquents. The introduction of the Jobseeker's Allowance', *Critical Social Policy*, vol.17, no.50, pp.99–109.

Oppenhiem, C. and Harper, L. (1996) *Poverty: The Facts*, London, Child Poverty Action Group.

Orwell, G. (1937) *The Road to Wigan Pier*, reprinted 1962, Harmondsworth, Penguin.

Peck, J. (1997) *Work-Place: The Social Regulation of Labor Markets*, New York, Guilford.

Willetts, D. (1997) *Why Vote Conservative?*, Harmondsworth, Penguin.

CHAPTER 9

Managerialism and Social Welfare

by Janet Newman

Contents

1   Introduction

There is nothing new about the idea of managing welfare services. There is always a need for activities to be co-ordinated, budgets allocated, staff supervised, control exercised. The focus of this chapter, however, is the change in the organization and delivery of social welfare that took place in the UK through the 1980s and 1990s. That is, the chapter is primarily about changes to the

organizational settlement

organizational settlement that was discussed in Chapters 1 and 2 of this book. The aims of the chapter are to:

- Identify themes in the unravelling of the organizational settlement of the post-war years (section 2).

- Unpack the languages and practices of managerialism by studying different managerial *discourses* (section 3).

- Explore the interaction of managerial, professional and bureaucratic *power* (section 4).

- Suggest some of the *paradoxes and tensions* within managerial regimes (section 5).

- Suggest different standpoints from which managerialism might be *evaluated* (section 6).

- Raise questions about the interaction between social policy and management in the new institutions of social welfare, and ask how far managerialism can be said to form the basis of a new organizational settlement (section 7).

- Enable you to trace the languages and practices of managerialism through your own experience of welfare organizations as a manager, practitioner or service user.

The chapter outlines the ways in which managerialism affects our experience in a number of ways. First, managerialism is more than the actions of specific individuals who have job titles that include the word 'manager'. One of the achievements of the reform process was to install and disperse a 'managerial consciousness' throughout organizations involved in the delivery of welfare. Many kinds of staff at different organizational levels came to take on managerial responsibilities, roles and functions. The service-contracting mechanisms also served to disperse this managerial mode to voluntary and community-based organizations by requiring that they behave in a 'business-like' fashion.

Second, managerialism has to be understood as not just a set of knowledges (**Clarke and Cochrane, 1998**) and skills. It forms the nexus of a changing field of relationships within and beyond social welfare. This changing field of relationships includes those between the state and the business world; between employers and employees; between organizations in the public, private and voluntary sectors; and between organizations and their users, customers or clients. To explore the ways in which these relationships have become transformed, the chapter begins by reviewing the role of managerialism in unlocking the old 'organizational settlement' of the post-war welfare state.

2   Bashing bureaucracy

2.1   Dismantling the old organizational settlement

Think back to how the term 'organizational settlement' was defined in Chapter 1, and make a brief note identifying the main points.

As Gordon Hughes outlined in Chapter 1, the organizational settlement was one of four settlements on which the old welfare state was built. It was based on the rather different principles of bureaucratic administration on the one hand, and professional expertise on the other. As was the case with other settlements, it was characterized by compromise and accommodation rather than complete harmony and consensus. Bureaucratic administration was a rational, rule-bound and hierarchical approach to co-ordinating complex systems of people and resource processing. Bureaucratic administration provided the organizational context in which welfare professionals – doctors, teachers, social workers, etc. – exercised their professional judgement. This combination of administrative rationality and professional expertise guaranteed the 'neutrality' of the welfare state and protected the exercise of professional judgement in the delivery of social welfare. Despite recurrent tensions between 'bureaucrats' and 'professionals', this form of organizational regime provided a stable institutional base for the growth of the welfare state in the post-war years.

The regime was not without its critics. A variety of critiques from socialist, feminist and anti-racist perspectives were directed at professional and bureaucratic power through the 1970s and 1980s. Challenges emerged from the growing number of user movements among recipients of social welfare, notably among people with disabilities (Taylor, 1993; Williams, 1996). Challenges had also been emerging throughout the period from the political Right. For example, the Black papers on education, produced between 1969 and 1975, criticized the post-war education reforms for their attempts at 'social engineering' (Centre for Contemporary Cultural Studies, 1981). Despite the orthodoxy that the post-war period can be characterized as a period of consensus between the major political parties, tensions about the role and nature of the welfare state were evident throughout the 1960s and 1970s. However, as Gail Lewis outlined in Chapter 2, a new set of critiques began to emerge in economic and political theory which were picked up by the government during the Conservative administrations of the 1980s and 1990s. Rather than repeating Lewis's arguments here, I want to review three themes in these 'challenges from above': those of economic, social and political critiques of the established ways of delivering social welfare.

The economic critiques were rooted in neo-liberal theories of the proper relationship between the state and the economy. Within this broad set of ideas, public choice theory articulated a set of concerns about the inherent waste and inefficiency involved in the provision of services through the public sector rather than the market (for example Niskanen, 1971). Walsh (1995) neatly summarizes the main elements of public choice theory:

economic critiques

> There are three basic sources of failure in government organizations identified by public choice theorists. First, it cannot be assumed that politicians will demand the pattern of public sector outputs that reflects the best interests of society as whole.

They will have their own interests to pursue and they will be subject to conflicting demands and pressures from special interests. Second, the bureaucracy will not necessarily carry out the wishes of the politicians, even if the latter do express the public good, since it is likely not to be in the bureaucrats' interests to do so. Third, it is unlikely that bureaucrats will act efficiently in producing whatever it is decided should be produced, since it may be in their interests to be inefficient. These criticisms of politicians and bureaucracy lead to the conclusion that the public service will be characterized both by allocative inefficiency, the production of the wrong mix of services, and by X inefficiency ... that is the production of less than it is possible to produce with the given inputs.

(Walsh, 1995, p.17)

These views shaped the critiques of bureaucracy and informed the development of market mechanisms for the delivery of welfare services through the 1980s and 1990s. However, these neo-liberal economic critiques articulated powerfully with a second strand of New Right thinking: neo-conservatism. Here the focus was on the social consequences of welfare provision rather than its economic

social critiques inefficiencies. The social critiques focused on the paternalism of the old regime and the effects of what came to be called the 'nanny state', which supposedly encouraged a 'dependency culture'. The focus on needs and entitlements was seen to undermine self-reliance and, ultimately, the moral welfare of society. For example, the provision of housing and benefits to lone parents was seen by many commentators to offer 'perverse incentives' which encouraged unmarried women to have children in order to secure welfare provision, and disadvantaged 'normal' families (Parker, 1982; see also **Lentell, 1998**).

political critiques The third set of critiques were political: bureau-professional power was seen to threaten the project of political and cultural change. Professionals – especially the more powerful medical professionals – represented important power blocks in their own right, and were thus able to gain concessions in the process of reform. The institutional forms of welfare also created and sustained attachments between citizens and the organizational forms of social democracy, with, for example, local government acting as a focus of resistance to many central government agendas, and with citizens expressing continued loyalties to the National Health Service as a symbolic institution.

The different forms of critique served to legitimate the introduction of managerial techniques and the strengthening of managerial power. The critiques of the past and assumptions about what management could offer in its place are summarized in Table 9.1.

managerialism Managerialism played a central role in the programme of reform and restructuring through the 1980s and beyond. It offered a set of prescriptions for producing economies in what was seen as a rising spiral of welfare expenditure. It was also highly compatible with the idea of a more self-reliant welfare consumer. The strengthening of managerialism was central to the general political project of unravelling the complex of bureau-professional power and diminishing the power of local government. Government reforms of the 1980s and 1990s can be seen in terms of a series of attempts to destabilize these regimes through direct intervention, or through the introduction of market mechanisms. Each area of social welfare underwent a profound process of transformation in which the dominance of professional and administrative modes of organization was challenged, and partially or substantially displaced by a new managerial mode.

These shifts were both underpinned by, and legitimated through, managerialism as the basis of a new organizational settlement. In this sense,

Table 9.1

Bureaucracy is:	Management is:
rule-bound	innovative
inward-looking	externally oriented
compliance-centred	performance-centred
ossified	dynamic
Professionalism is:	**Management is:**
paternalist	customer-centred
mystique-ridden	transparent
standard-oriented	results-oriented
self-regulating	market-tested
Politicians are:	**Managers are:**
dogmatic	pragmatic
interfering	enabling
unstable	strategic

Source: Clarke and Newman, 1997, p.65

managerialism can be understood as an *ideology*, not as a set of neutral techniques. It was not just a means of doing things – it formed a new set of principles which shaped the process of change itself by presenting answers to economic and social problems. Take, for example, *Reinventing Government*, one of the key texts of the early 1990s, which was closely associated both with the first Clinton administration in the USA, and with John Major and the Citizens' Charter in the UK (Osborne and Gaebler, 1992). The preface states:

> Our governments are in deep trouble today. This book is for those who are disturbed by that reality. It is for those who care about government – because they work in government, or simply want their governments to be more effective. It is for those who know something is wrong, but who are not sure just what that is; for those who have launched successful experiments, but have watched those in power ignore them; for those who have a sense of where government needs to go, but are not quite sure how to get there. It is for the seekers.
>
> If ever there was a time for seekers, this is it. The millennium approaches, and change is all around us. Eastern Europe is free; the Soviet Empire is dissolving; the cold war is over. Western Europe is moving towards economic union. Asia is the new centre of economic power. From Poland to South Africa, democracy is on the march ... The emergence of a post-industrial, knowledge based, global economy has undermined old realities throughout the world, creating wonderful opportunities and frightening problems. Governments large and small, American and foreign, federal, state and local, have begun to respond.
>
> (Osborne and Gaebler, 1992, pp.xv–xvi)

The idea of the need for 'reinvention' and 'transformation' is established by convincing the reader that there is a problem which it is important to address. Like all good ideologies, a logical sequence of ideas is established which together point to a seemingly unchallengeable conclusion – dramatic change. Different ideas (globalization, democracy, technological change) are juxtaposed to provide an overarching narrative which creates the necessity of dramatic changes to the forms and institutions of government. The reader is addressed directly, and offered a range of positive identifications: 'problem solver', 'radical thinker', frustrated 'change agent' and, above all, 'seeker'.

The promise of managerialism's ability to deliver radical change was a recurring theme. If you look at the business management section of any major library or bookshop, you are likely to find a series of titles on particular activities and techniques: strategic management, marketing, 'human resource' management, managing quality, managing change, managing for competitive success. The topics change to reflect the very rapidly shifting fads and fashions coming from an ever-changing cast of management 'gurus'. But there is something about the tone that remains constant. The books are not just outlining a set of techniques: they are extolling the virtues of change. New forms of competition, the new 'global' market-place, the new demands from consumers, the new need for flexibility and quality to respond to these demands – all, it is argued, require a fundamental change of approach, new attitudes and new ideas.

In the 1980s there was an enormous growth in the rate of publication of management books. Some (for example Peters and Waterman's *In Search of Excellence*, published in 1982) reached a level of world-wide sales unprecedented for management books. Management 'gurus' proliferated, and many leaders of business, from John Harvey Jones to Richard Branson, attained the status of national heroes (though rather fewer heroines gained this sort of public profile). Clarke and Newman locate this phenomenon in the context of deep-rooted economic problems, especially in the US economy:

> Managerialism was being revived, if not re-invented, by the emergence of new 'schools', of excellence, culture management, Human Resource Management, Total Quality Management, and re-engineering (to name but a few). Each of these promised a more or less coherent philosophy of and approach to managing and all testified to the potency and rewards of doing management. They changed the face of managers away from their previous image as dull organisational time-servers to those of entrepreneurial and inspirational change agents. Like all good discourses, the new managerialism announced the conditions of its own necessity – elaborating a tale of the failings of the old management and their dire consequences. The new manager was born out of a climate of crisis and disillusionment – located in the start of a long drawn out crisis of US capitalism in the late 1970s and more specifically in its competitive failure in the face of the industrialising Pacific Rim. This climate of American failure was the precondition for the new managerial literature's promise of salvation. It announced the possibility of a way forward which linked the fortunes of the individual manager, the corporation and the nation. The born-again manager could rescue the situation brought about by the old corporate mentality: the 'playing safe' organisation man; the ossified corporation; and the over-regulatory state produced by the politics of 'corporate liberalism'.
>
> (Clarke and Newman, 1997, p.35)

The success of this new managerialism was based on its vision of the power of management to transform rule-bound, inert and bureaucratic corporations into dynamic and competitive enterprises. This notion of managerial knowledge as the driver of change had close affinities with the New Right agenda of social and economic transformation. Both stood against excessive state regulation; both required individuals to be 'liberated' from bureaucracy in order to play their part as the dynamic agents of change. In addition, the neo-liberal agenda of the New Right explicitly looked to the business world – and to the techniques of business management in the private sector – to solve the problems of what was considered to be an over-large, bureaucratic and self-seeking state sector: 'Efficient management is the key to the [national] revival ... And the management ethos must run right through our national life – private and public companies, civil service, nationalized industries, local government, the National Health Service' (Michael Heseltine, then Secretary of State for the Environment, 1980, quoted in Pollitt, 1993, p.vi).

The 1980s and 1990s saw a shift in the dominant ethos and style of public management – indeed, many have talked of the emergence of a 'new public management' (Hood, 1991). This offered a powerful set of ideas and techniques which have helped to establish the need to reform the institutions of social welfare. To understand the principles of this new regime, the following sections explore managerialism from a number of perspectives. Section 3 views managerialism as a *set of discourses* which offer individuals particular points of identification and which prioritize certain forms of knowledge and expertise. Section 4 explores managerialism as a *field of relationships* through which activities are co-ordinated – relationships which are shaped around a particular set of priorities, strategies and judgements.

new public management

3   Managerialism as discourse

Managerialism does not form a unified body of knowledge, but can be understood as a set of discourses, each of which draws on a different knowledge base, legitimates particular goals, and underpins a particular ordering of relationships. Each discourse is a structured set of ideas which has an internal coherence. The different discourses can be see as a number of different languages of management. However, a discourse is more than just a language. As du Gay comments,

> Throughout the twentieth century a range of discourses have appeared, each of which has offered a certain way of drawing the map of the organizational world. These discourses … have all offered novel ways of 'imagining organization' and have played an active role in 'making up' new ways for people to conduct themselves at work.
>
> (du Gay, 1994, p.130)

What do you think du Gay means when he talks of a discourse as 'making up new ways for people to conduct themselves'?

What du Gay is suggesting is that a discourse offers a particular set of identifications for those who speak it or are spoken by it. For example, the identification of being a 'leader' is rather different from that of being a 'senior social worker': it implies different relationships and priorities, and requires different skills and a new focus of expertise. Discourses, then, imply actions as well as identities. Of course, calling someone a leader rather than a social worker does not necessarily change their loyalties and identifications. However, studying the different discourses of managerialism can help us to unlock some of the changes in role, practices and purposes that accompanied the process of state restructuring discussed in this book. We begin with one which is rather confusingly titled 'neo-Taylorism'.

3.1   Neo-Taylorism

Pollitt (1993) viewed the initial period of change in the UK, characterized by cost control and decentralization, as a 'neo-Taylorist' form of managerialism. This referred to the scientific management principles set out by Frederick William Taylor in the early years of the twentieth century. Taylor argued that previously unmeasured aspects of the work process could and should be measured in order to fix and control the effort levels of workers. Neo-Taylorism was based on an assumption that workers were individual units responding directly to fairly simple incentives and punishments, and that managerial control of the workforce could be enhanced by the application of scientific principles of work design and organizational structure. As applied to public management, neo-Taylorism referred to a strengthening of the control and measurement of work through mechanisms such as target-setting, performance indicators, and monitoring and control of the work process (through time recording and the use of information technology in a way which records the performance of individual workers). It was functional and mechanistic in its orientation:

> The central theme, endlessly reiterated in official documents, is to set clear targets, to develop performance indicators to measure the achievements of those targets, and to single out, by means of merit awards, those individuals who get 'results'. The strengthening and incentivizing of line management is a constant theme ... In official terms, what seems to be required is a culture shift of a kind that will facilitate a more thorough-going functional/Taylorist management process.
>
> (Pollitt, 1993, p.56)

This strengthening of control was linked to the drive for economy and efficiency in public management. Metcalfe and Richards (1990, p.17) suggest that this emphasis in the early stages of civil service reform had led to an 'impoverished' concept of management whose implementation would 'drag British government kicking and screaming back into the 1950s'. Nevertheless, neo-Taylorism remained firmly in place. There were continual pressures to control costs, to increase productivity, to manage performance and above all to demonstrate 'value for money' through a focus on the three Es of economy, efficiency and effectiveness. This was encouraged by external bodies such as the Audit Commission which, through a series of reports, set out appropriate management arrangements for local government, the health service, the probation service and other bodies.

The discourse of neo-Taylorism offered roles based on the elimination of waste, cost control and performance management. The dominant language was based on calculation: counting, measuring, assessing. The focus was on inputs (the acquisition and deployment of resources) rather than outputs: that is, there was much greater focus on the first two of the three Es (economy and efficiency) rather than effectiveness. The setting of objectives and the close monitoring of performance strengthened central control within organizations. Rather than getting rid of bureaucracy, neo-Taylorism sometimes reproduced it, albeit in the rather different guise of formalized systems of planning and monitoring.

3.2   The excellence approach

Pollitt contrasted neo-Taylorism with the 'excellence' approach, so labelled because of the importance of Peters and Waterman's *In Search of Excellence*, first published in 1982. Peters and Waterman studied a group of successful US companies and identified the ingredients of their success, focusing particularly on the role of organizational culture: 'Without exception, the dominance and coherence of culture proved to be an essential quality of the excellent companies. Moreover, the stronger the culture and the more it was directed towards the marketplace, the less need there was for policy manuals, organization charts, or detailed procedures and rules' (Peters and Waterman, 1982, p.75). The role of top managers was to build a strong, unified culture and to encourage workforce commitment rather than exert detailed control over the work process. The mode of control was *affective* rather than *directive*: that is, it was concerned with creating motivation through meaning and with sustaining attachments between managers-as-leaders and the workforce. As such, it has strong links with a set of related discourses: those of human resource management, leadership and staff 'empowerment'.

The ideas of the excellence school were of great significance in the process of transforming the organizations of social welfare. This significance stemmed from its critique of bureaucracy. As du Gay comments,

> The norms and values characterizing the conduct of 'excellent' organizations … were articulated in explicit opposition to those constituting the identity of 'bureaucratic' enterprises. Whereas bureaucratic organization encouraged the development of particular capacities and predispositions among its subjects – strict adherence to procedure, the abnegation of personal moral enthusiasms, etc. – the new discourses of work reform stressed the importance of individuals acquiring and exhibiting more 'market oriented', 'proactive' and 'entrepreneurial' attitudes and behaviours. 'Bureaucratic culture', it was argued, had to give way to 'new approaches that require people to exercise discretion, take initiative, and assume a much greater responsibility for their own organization and management' (Morgan, 1991, p.56 [see end references]). In other words, governing organizational life to ensure 'excellence' was deemed to necessitate the production of certain types of work based subject: 'enterprising', autonomous, productive, self regulating, responsible individuals.
>
> (du Gay, 1994, pp.130–1)

This antipathy to bureaucracy resonated with a range of existing critiques of the public sector, from those which saw bureaucracy as a source of waste and inefficiency to those who saw it as the source of unresponsive paternalism. Its paternalism was challenged by the emphasis in the excellence school on customer centredness and service quality, ideas which were picked up widely both by government and by service providers.

ACTIVITY 9.1

What are the main differences between the discourses of excellence and of neo-Taylorism? You might like to summarize these by making notes using the following chart:

	Neo-Taylorism	Excellence school
Focus (what is held to be important)		
Mode of control (how managers control the activities of staff)		

COMMENT

The different modes of control meant that these discourses gave rise to very different sets of injunctions for staff. For example, neo-Taylorism might hold 'meeting your financial targets' as the top priority, while the excellence approach might stress 'achieving service improvements' and 'satisfying customers'. Charts like this can help to identify contrasts between different managerial discourses. What they do not do, however, is look at how both may be present in a single organization, giving rise to 'mixed messages' for staff. We return to this point in section 5.

■ ■ ■

3.3   Consumerism and quality

The idea of the recipient of welfare and other public services being a 'consumer' or 'customer', rather than a client or citizen, was a central reference point in the reform of welfare services from the mid 1980s onwards (see **Hughes, 1998**). It underpinned a range of market reforms in which the language of consumerism was used to legitimate the breaking up of the old welfare state monopolies and the introduction of competition as a means of increasing customer choice and improving service quality. The consumerist emphasis was welcomed by many modernizers within the welfare organizations because of its challenge to the paternalism of the 'old' systems of welfare delivery. Consumerism viewed the service user not as a passive recipient of bureau-professional decisions but as an active participant in the process of defining needs and wants. Thus although it was connected to the new managerial regime, the emphasis on customers was welcomed by many professionals seeking to 'empower' service users.

In Chapter 2, Gail Lewis talked of the creation of customers and consumers as being among a series of 'new welfare subjects'. What did she mean by this term? And what were the problems she raised about the shift of emphasis from 'citizens' to 'consumers'?

The language of the customer presents some difficulties in many areas of social welfare. Nevertheless, the ideas of customer centredness, quality and customer choice provided a new logic of legitimation for government reform. That is, changes were driven through in the name of the customer, and legitimated in terms of greater choice or increased consumer power. This can be contrasted with the efficiency-driven 'logic of legitimation' of neo-Taylorism, which is based on the presumed interests of the taxpayer rather than the welfare consumer.

logic of legitimation

The discourse of consumerism implied shifts in the roles, relationships and identities of welfare providers. They were to be 'responsive', 'enabling' and 'empowering' in their interaction with users; they were to measure levels of customer satisfaction; they were to be judged in league tables which ranked providers according to their performance; and they were to compete in the 'market-place' of public services (real or imaginary) for customers in order to survive. They were, in short, to model themselves more on the entrepreneurial images drawn from the business world than on the 'public servant' images of the old welfare state.

3.4 Business entrepreneurship

The fourth key discourse that informed welfare reform was the language of business, based on the notion that welfare services could be improved by modelling them on ideas and practices drawn from the private sector. This flowed across and interacted with both neo-Taylorism and the excellence discourse: sometimes it meant that organizations should be more efficient, with a firmer managerial grip on performance; sometimes it meant that managers should have more freedom to respond to the demands of customers. Underpinning both, however, was a more general valorization of the business world, and the search for solutions to the perceived problems of social welfare from the private sector. Key figures were imported from industry and commerce to help transform the institutions of government. For example, Sir Derek Rayner's move from Marks and Spencer to set up an 'efficiency strategy' for the civil service received wide press coverage:

> With a few honourable exceptions, the newspapers presented a picture of the Prime Minister's champion, bringing with him the good news from the private sector, carrying her colours into the heartland of the enemy, the Civil Service, and there single handedly belabouring the inefficient and the wasteful ... It says something about the lack of public understanding of top management styles in the private sector that the myth took hold.
>
> (Metcalfe and Richards, 1990, p.6)

Models of management drawn from the business world (albeit often based on inaccurate understandings of how the business world actually operated) informed the practices of reform and restructuring. The training of public sector managers placed more emphasis on business management techniques. Competition was introduced as a stimulus to change, requiring managers to develop entrepreneurial skills and styles and challenging the professional paternalism of many providers, as Michael Pryke noted in Chapter 4.

These various discourses offer different kinds of subject positions and identifications for managers, with neo-Taylorism emphasizing managers as controllers, the excellence discourse emphasizing the role of managers as organizational innovators and transformers, and the business discourse locating managers as entrepreneurial actors. Some of the discourses represent managerial roles and practices as fundamentally rational (neo-Taylorism); others imply affective modes of engagement (leadership, culture and the excellence school). But together the new managerial discourses imply a fundamental shift in the institutions of social welfare, involving a reordering of relationships, shifts in power, and changes in the basis of decision-making.

4 Power, decision-making and the reordering of relationships

While the previous section explored differences *within* managerialism, the focus here is on the interaction *between* managerialism and bureau-professionalism. Each is the source of a different form of power; each orders relationships (internal and external) in a particular way; and each gives rise to different forms of judgement in the process of decision-making. The three different forms of power – bureaucratic power, managerial power and professional power – are likely to be present in most welfare organizations, interacting in complex ways. To help understand the way in which these forms of power work, we want to look at each as an 'ideal type', abstracted from reality, before exploring ways in which they interact.

4.1 Power and decision-making: managerialism as a 'logic of decision-making'

As we have seen, managerial discourse partly redefined relationships with users, subordinating notions of clients and citizens to those of consumers and customers. This helped to dismantle the much criticized paternalistic effects of professional power by emphasizing customer choice, customer care and customer power, however shallow these turned out to be in practice. Professional power was largely based on the acquisition of specialist knowledge and the claim to expertise in making judgements within a defined field of decision-making. The forms of knowledge varied widely, but it typically enabled professionals to diagnose 'problems', identify and formulate 'needs', and categorize and treat 'clients'. These processes were allied to those of rational bureaucratic administration, in which formalized sets of rules underpinned the allocation of resources, including the resource of professional expertise itself. The knowledge basis of the professional bureaucracy therefore legitimated particular goals ('solving problems' and 'treating clients'). Professional power was derived from outside the organization (the professional body) and was organized through distinct sets of relationships within it (hierarchy and bureaucracy).

In professionally dominated organizations, such as health, decision-making was based on the exercise of professional judgement, and the basis of calculation was that of need (see **Langan, 1998**). For example, in the case of doctors in the NHS, decisions about treatment were made primarily on the basis of clinical need. Resources were allocated on this basis, though there was some prioritizing or targeting where particular groups were deemed to be 'at risk' (as in the case of flu inoculations for the elderly). Professional regimes accorded a great deal of discretion to the individual worker to define need and make judgements about the best allocation of resources.

In bureaucracies, such as those organizations concerned with the payment of welfare benefits, decision-making was based on the exercise of rules, and the basis of calculation was that of whether an applicant was entitled to the provision (see Chapter 8). The much maligned bureaucratic structures and processes of many welfare services could be viewed as a means to ensure that decisions were made fairly on the basis of the equitable application of universal rules of entitlement. Unlike professional organizations, bureaucracies allowed little discretion to the individual worker.

Neither professional nor bureaucratic organizations were particularly resource sensitive, in that decisions about the allocation of resources tended to be made separately from the control and management of budgets. Indeed, this was one of the criticisms levelled against the 'waste' and 'inefficiency' of public bureaucracies. The pursuit of economy and efficiency was a recurrent theme in social welfare as successive governments sought to manage the tensions between rising welfare demand and the drive to reduce public expenditure. 'Good management' lay at the heart of resolving this tension. It did so partly by the introduction of *economic* forms of knowledge and expertise as the basis for decision-making alongside the professionally derived and rule-based forms of knowledge enshrined in welfare bureaucracies. The 'logic of decision-making' of managerialism was based on predominantly economic criteria, with the bottom line of financial viability becoming of much greater significance.

This focus on financial criteria of success worked by instilling greater cost consciousness among both managers and front-line staff, leading to what Mackintosh (1995) calls the rise of economic culture in both purchaser and provider organizations. Mackintosh (1995, p.8) defines economic culture as a particular 'thought world' which is 'not just a set of ideas; it is also a way of making decisions, and hence a self-reinforcing way of individuals interpreting their own working worlds and making decisions in them'. For example, the devolution of care budgets to front-line staff in the social service departments she studied had the effect of sharpening competitive cost pressures on provider organizations as purchasers 'shopped around' for care provision. The effectiveness of managerialism in partly displacing professional bureaucracy as a mode of co-ordination can be traced in how far those who are not themselves 'managers' become subject to this new logic of decision-making. That is, how far professional decisions about 'needs' or administrative requirements of access and equity become subjected to the logics of resource management and to organizational goals and priorities. A key feature of managerial regimes is the partial assimilation of new logics of decision-making among all staff through, for example, the devolution of decisions about how to balance needs against available resources. Indeed, Mackintosh's study of the growth of 'economic culture' among staff in social services departments found that cost consciousness was higher among front-line staff (care assessors purchasing services) than among their managers.

economic culture

Financial pressures also underpinned decisions about which groups services were targeted towards. Providers in a competitive field of relationships strove to control the conditions that affected their costs and performance. This produced two different, but related, strategies. The first, 'cream skimming', involved targeting a service towards particular groups of users (for example, schools seeking to exclude 'difficult' pupils and to attract pupils likely to achieve good exam performance to increase their success in the league tables of school performance). The second, 'boundary management', was concerned with shifting costs between organizations (for example, health and social services departments seeking to transfer the costs of 'expensive' patients to the budgets of other organizations). Both of these strategies helped define what or who should constitute a legitimate demand on an organization's resources. As such, they formed part of the managerial logic of decision-making.

4.2   Multiple and interacting regimes

Section 4.1 outlined three different forms of decision-making – professional, bureaucratic and managerial – and the logics that underpin each. Some of the key words reflecting the logics of the different regimes are highlighted in Table 9.2 (the 'Accountability' row has been left blank deliberately for the time being).

Table 9.2 Modes of relationship

	Bureaucratic	*Professional*	*Managerial*
Who has access	Citizens	Clients defined as having 'needs'	Customers or consumers
Gatekeeping mechanism	Legally defined entitlements	Professional needs assessment	Rationing or priority setting
Access shaped by	Extent of citizen knowledge of what is available	Gatekeeping by professional groups	'Cream skimming' and 'boundary management'
Basis of decisions	Application of universal rules (little workforce discretion)	Application of professional knowledge and expertise	Most efficient use of limited resources
Types of risk taken into account	Political	Clinical or social	Financial, organizational
Accountability			

Reality is, of course, more complex than charts like this suggest. Most organizations – and most managers – have to work within all of these frameworks and deal with the tensions and ambiguities that arise as different regimes interact. For example, let's take the case of a residential care establishment for the elderly seeking to minimize costs because of a squeeze on its financial resources. In doing so, it has made compromises on what, from a professional perspective, might be the best way of avoiding clinical or social risk. It has thus exposed itself to political risk (local scandals, headlines in the press, questions in the local council chamber, and so on). Such events may impact on the organization's reputation and therefore its capacity to attract new customers or win new contracts, thus reducing its competitive position. This takes us full circle back to the idea of managerial risk. In effect, the organization has to 'manage' multiple goals and success criteria. This is indeed a characteristic of most welfare and public service organizations, which have to respond to the requirements and interests of multiple groups and interests.

ACTIVITY 9.2

Look at the newspaper article from *The Guardian* reproduced opposite. What are the different goals and success criteria that are operating here?

NHS chiefs criticised over deaths

David Brindle

Health authorities must take important decisions in public if they affect patients and their families, the National Health Service ombudsman rules today.

In a damning judgement against the former Winchester authority, Sir William Reid says it acted in a totally undemocratic manner by deciding in secret to bring forward by 21 months the discharge of 24 elderly dementia patients from hospital to private nursing homes.

Four patients were moved the same day. Five died within 22 days of discharge, including one aged 95.

Sir William says the way in which the authority acted 'fell far short of the standards of accountability which a public body should display'.

His criticism was echoed yesterday by Alan Langlands, NHS chief executive, who told health authority and trust leaders that the principles of accountability and openness were non-negotiable in a publicly-funded service.

Addressing the annual conference in Harrogate of the National Association of Health Authorities and Trusts, Mr Langlands said: 'It is unacceptable for any board or any individual working in the NHS to ignore these public service values in the pursuit of results.'

The ombudsman has upheld a complaint made by the son-in-law of the 95-year-old man discharged from Park Prewett hospital, Basingstoke, to a nursing home. He died 17 days after the move.

Sir William's investigators discovered that the decision to bring forward the patients' discharge, in order to close two wards by March 31, 1994 instead of December 31, 1995, was taken at what was described as an 'informal' meeting of the authority.

The successor authority, North and Mid-Hampshire, has acknowledged that 'the only sense in which it was informal was that it was not held in public.'

Sir William criticises strongly all those involved in the affair, including the London community trust responsible for the hospital, and says the episode should serve as a 'grim warning' to any authority or trust planning to transfer long-term patients.

Expressing 'considerable doubt' that the authority had the necessary medical consent for the transfer of the 95-year-old, the ombudsman notes that the record of the decisive meeting referred to pleasure at bringing forward the discharge despite what he calls unresolved risks.

Sir William concludes: 'I find it totally undemocratic that a public body should have considered it justifiable to discuss a policy matter of such importance at a meeting closed to the general public.'

Mr Langlands told the Nahat conference ... that probity, as well as openness and accountability, was one of the crucial public service values underpinning the work of the NHS.

(The Guardian, 20 June 1996)

COMMENT

The different goals and success criteria underpin different forms of accountability – the means by which welfare organizations are held to account for their actions and decisions. In the article the health authority was viewed as having acted 'undemocratically' – that is, to have compromised on its accountability to the public at large.

accountability

You may want to try to fill in a few key words in the 'Accountability' row of Table 9.2. If you can't do this at present don't worry – we return to the idea of different forms of accountability in section 5.5.

■ ■ ■

Despite the importance of understanding the ways in which different regimes interact, it was the knowledges and forms of expertise that managerialism laid claim to that shaped the restructuring of social welfare. In doing so it fundamentally changed relationships both within welfare organizations and within the field of social welfare as a whole.

4.3 Reordering relationships

right to
manage

Managerialism is based on the idea that managers must be given the right to manage – the freedom to make decisions about the use of organizational resources, unrestricted by over-burdening state regulation on the one hand, or trade union power on the other. The 1970s and 1980s saw significant changes in the forms and relations of management in the private sector; these were accompanied by changes in the social composition of the labour force, which entailed greater labour 'flexibility' and a reduction in labour costs. The place of managerialism in state restructuring was therefore more than simply a transfer of private sector practices into welfare services; managerialism as a field of relationships was itself undergoing significant transformations.

4.3.1 Management/workforce relations

Enlarging the 'right to manage' meant displacing old forms of personnel management linked to bureaucratic regimes by a more strategic approach to human resource management. This focused on the development of direct relationships between managers and workforce in place of collective bargaining. The building of these relationships was based on a range of techniques from 'inspirational leadership' and culture change programmes to individual performance appraisals. New forms of employment contract were introduced in pursuit of greater workforce flexibility, and attempts were made to reduce labour costs by reorganizing work patterns (so that, for example, more of the work in some services was done by lower grade staff through a process of 'deskilling'). The activities of departments, groups and individuals became more closely tied to organizational goals through the mechanisms of funding, target setting and performance review.

ACTIVITY 9.3

The human resource management strategies combined a number of different elements: some were designed to reduce workforce costs, some to build employee commitment, and others to develop forms of control over working practices where direct supervision was not appropriate (for example where there are high levels of devolution or decentralization).

Recall (or if necessary re-read) the discussion of different managerial discourses in section 3.

1 Which of the changes in management/workforce relations outlined above do you think might be described as neo-Taylorist in its orientation?

2 Which do you think belongs more to the excellence approach?

3 How do you think the balance between 'control-oriented' and 'commitment-based' managerial strategies is changing in your organization (or an organization you know)?

4.3.2 Organizational and inter-organizational relationships

The processes of decentralization and the introduction of market mechanisms produced an increasingly fragmented array of welfare services. This had the effect of diffusing decision-making responsibility for defining and meeting needs.

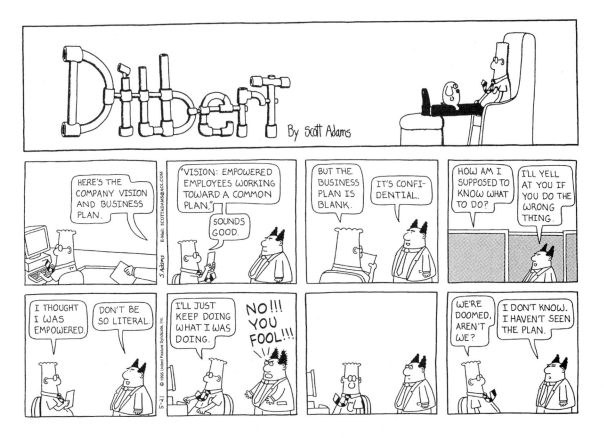

While central government kept a tight hold on expenditure and set national frameworks and standards, it also devolved and decentralized the management of implementation in complex ways. In some instances managerial responsibility was devolved from central government departments to executive agencies (for example the Benefits Agency); in others it passed to non-governmental organizations (such as training and enterprise councils and housing action trusts). Others involved passing responsibility to even more localized points of decision-making (headteachers and school governors, GP fundholders). In many cases the delivery of services passed to organizations in the private or voluntary sectors, controlled through an increasingly complex network of contractual relationships.

This fragmentation and localization of decision-making resulted in the problem of how welfare and other services were to be co-ordinated. Rather than hierarchical co-ordination, in which a line of direct control could be traced from ministerial policy to the point of service delivery, control mechanisms became obscured in a myriad array of contracts, framework documents, service level agreements, local business plans and devolved decision-making. Neither the complex rules of the bureaucratic regime nor the professional ethics and training of the professional regime could provide a coherent integrative framework. It is in this sense that managerialism might be said to form the 'glue' which co-ordinates the increasingly fragmented field of social welfare.

The processes of reform and restructuring, however, have had to address a number of tensions and paradoxes arising from the application of managerialism to welfare services. These are explored in the next section.

5 The paradoxes of managerialism

The idea that there has been a wholesale shift from 'old' public administration, characterized by bureaucracy and hierarchy, to a 'new' public management, characterized by efficiency, responsiveness and flexibility, has been challenged as an oversimplified view of change (Lowndes, 1996; Clarke and Newman, 1997). Narratives of change structured around clear oppositions between 'past' and 'present', or 'old and new', raise two important difficulties. First, there may be gaps between rhetoric and reality: that is, between what is described in textbooks or reports and what happens on the ground. When we talk about wholesale institutional change, we need to remind ourselves that we are talking about people who often have rather complex and ambiguous feelings about what is taking place. Sometimes change is welcomed because it is seen to bring benefits, perhaps to service users or groups of staff. Sometimes change is actively resisted. If the resistance is strong enough, a particular initiative may be modified (as happened when the introduction of general management met resistance from clinicians in the NHS). Another common response is for people to change the language they use and to adapt some of their practices to fit in with the new requirements, but to retain at least some of their old commitments and loyalties – for example to professional views of social work practice. This means that we can 'overread' the extent and embeddedness of change, and underestimate the important points of continuity with the old welfare regime.

continuity

The second reason why we should be suspicious of simple narratives of a wholesale shift from the 'old' to the 'new' is that they tend to tidy away some of the complexity and messiness of change. What is rather more interesting, but more difficult to describe, is how different elements of new and old are packaged and repackaged in ways which produce internal tensions, contradictions and paradoxes. For example, section 3 pointed to a number of different managerial discourses. These may not easily fit together since they require different management styles. They invoke different kinds of subject positions for managers (controller, leader, entrepreneur) and are based on different models of the subjects to be managed (neo-Taylorism assuming that workers require surveillance to perform effectively, the excellence school invoking the principle that workers want to use their creativity in the workplace, and market-based models of business entrepreneurship assuming that people work best when they are given incentives). In most organizations these different discourses are overlaid on each other in rather uncomfortable ways, giving rise to 'mixed messages'. There may be some tension between an approach based on winning commitment and giving staff responsibility for their own performance on the one hand, and the constant monitoring and checking by the centre on the other. This may be perceived in terms of hypocrisy on the part of senior managers, or a perverse desire to hang on to power. While each of these may contain glimmers of truth, there is something going on which is rather more structural: that is, a contradictory pull to centralize some forms of power and decentralize others.

The tensions between different discourses are not the only tensions we are concerned with. In section 4.2 we suggested that, rather than managerialism having displaced bureau-professionalism, it has operated alongside it in 'multiple and interacting regimes'. Managerial power may have become more dominant, but, as we have seen in the case of the NHS, it has not displaced professional power. Political accountability (achieved through the rules and decision-making hierarchies of bureaucracy) has continued to operate alongside managerial accountability (which emphasizes greater transparency in decision-making and a shift towards power to the consumer). Organizations have to respond to multiple sets of pressures from the different stakeholders who have some influence over their goals and objectives. For example, they have to satisfy the requirements of central government, and attempt to meet the performance targets that are set by government bodies and agencies such as the Audit Commission. They have to pursue business goals in order to secure organizational survival in an increasingly uncertain environment. They have to meet the needs of different sets of customers and users. They have to work in partnership with other agencies in the increasingly dispersed field of welfare service. At the same time, they have to demonstrate their accountability and to ensure probity in their use of public resources.

The combined effect of these multiple pressures is to produce a field of tensions which operate at different levels and in different ways. Some of the key tensions that arise are those between centralization and decentralization; between flexibility and standardization; between empowerment and control; between managerial and political forms of accountability; between management and politics. In the rest of this section I revisit some of the earlier chapters of Book 4 to identify ways in which these tensions are expressed in the delivery of social welfare.

5.1 Centralization and decentralization

Devolution and decentralization have been key themes in the new public management. Both involve a dispersal of power away from the centre to the managers of particular business units or service providers. This has multiplied the number of points at which financial decisions are made and has sharpened accountability for performance within organizations. Although devolution and decentralization are potent sources of efficiency, they bring some dilemmas for the centre: for instance, how is it possible to retain control while at the same time giving power away? The answer to this tricky question lies in the way in which the dispersal of power contains a double movement of centralization and decentralization.

dispersal of power

In Chapter 6 on education, for example, Ross Fergusson lists a range of decentralizing measures (such as devolved budgets for schools, enhanced powers for local governing bodies, schools being permitted to opt out of local authority control, the removal of FE colleges from local authority control) and balances this with a list of centralizing measures (the introduction of the national curriculum, the setting up of funding councils, new powers for the Secretary of State, greater control over teacher education, etc.). In this example it is possible to suggest that many of the professional decisions (for instance decisions about the curriculum) which had previously been made locally became centralized; on the other hand, resource decisions and decisions about service users (pupils) which had previously been made at the level of the LEA were decentralized.

The key issues are the distribution of powers between centre and periphery (what decisions the centre wishes to retain) and the nature of the control systems put in place by the centre. In terms of the former, it is important to look at the kinds of decision-making power held at different levels: professional decisions, resource decisions, staffing decisions, decisions about what services should be provided, decisions about which service users are to be targeted, decisions about where and how to involve service users or citizens in decision-making, and so on.

ACTIVITY 9.4

Consider a service with which you are familiar.

1   What kinds of power do you think have been decentralized?
2   What kinds of power do you think have been centralized?
3   How has this balance changed over time?

5.2   Flexibility and standardization

The pull towards centralization means that organizations need to structure and manage themselves in a way that will enable them to meet centrally determined goals. This in turn often results in a standardization of management styles and practices, and reduced flexibility of the system as a whole. However, there is still considerable discretion for many organizations to set their own goals and organize their work in the way they think best. One expression of the potential tension between these imperatives lies in the relationship between central government or national agencies on the one hand, and local government on the other. Chapter 7 described how local authority social services departments enjoy considerable discretionary powers in how to define local needs and organize services to meet them. At the same time bodies such as the Social Services Inspectorate and the Audit Commission have considerable influence through the establishment of national standards or targets and the publication of reports on 'best practice', both of which have a standardizing effect on social services departments. Similarly, Chapter 4 noted a continuing tension in housing policy between central government's desire to set a national framework for housing policy and the capacity of local authorities to determine local policies to reflect local circumstances.

Tensions between flexibility and standardization can also be seen in the changing role which voluntary, community-based and other 'not-for-profit' organizations play in the delivery of social welfare. Voluntary organizations have always had an important role in filling gaps in state provision, and in acting as advisers or advocates for individuals seeking to gain access to welfare services provided by statutory bodies. Their relative autonomy and high degree of flexibility meant that they were well placed to innovate by experimenting with new forms of provision, many of which were later incorporated into state agencies. However, the flexibility of voluntary organizations was threatened as cash-strapped local authorities became less able to provide funding to voluntary organizations to use as they wished, but instead began to set up contracts with them to provide core services (such as the transfer of housing management to housing associations, discussed in Chapter 4). Voluntary organizations found themselves having to sacrifice some of their autonomy and responsiveness in order to win and manage contracts. This required very different management arrangements in which the work of individual members of staff became more tightly controlled, supervised and standardized. Many voluntary organizations found that these 'neo-Taylorist' management arrangements sat rather uncomfortably with their ethos and purpose, and reduced their ability to attract volunteers.

5.3 Empowerment and control

Neo-Taylorism, as we know, is only one strand of managerialism. Others focus on diffusing responsibility and fostering self-control (through, for example, the 'discipline of the market' combined with the discipline of centrally set performance targets) rather than enforcing external controls. However, this rationale works rather imperfectly in the political context in which welfare services operate, where probity in the spending of public money is an important political requirement which may conflict with the entrepreneurial imperative of managerialism. The requirement that welfare organizations become more 'businesslike' implies a shift in culture: away from the values of stewardship and conservation to the more entrepreneurial and dynamic culture of the business world; from a culture which emphasizes the importance of the probity of process (accounting for the way we do things) to one which focuses on the achievement of results (being held to account for our success or failure).

The boundary between these is slippery, as is illustrated by a case reported by the news media in February 1997. This concerned a civil servant who worked for the special 'ghostbusters' division of the Inland Revenue. The civil servant had achieved spectacular outcomes in securing tax revenue from foreign nationals resident in the UK, but his downfall was caused when certain infringements in the process by which these were secured came to light. He was successful in terms of the new, business-oriented culture, acting with flair and ingenuity, but fell short of some of the values of probity embedded in the 'old' culture.

This is a rather stark example which became a high-profile media event, but tensions between multiple cultures, and the potentially conflicting values and practices which they embody, have to be negotiated every day. Many of them stem from the interaction of the worlds of politics and management. While managerialism requires 'hands off' control in order to allow managers to use their delegated powers to maximum advantage, politicians seeking to win popular support, or to respond to sudden crises or scandals in the media, continue to intervene in what the managers might view as day-to-day operational decisions. This tension between the 'right to manage' and political control was highlighted in the Prison Service in 1996, when Derek Lewis, the Chief Executive of the Prison Service Agency, engaged in open conflict with the Home Secretary, Michael Howard, about the level of political intervention into what Lewis regarded as managerial decisions. This leads us to consider the tensions that occur on the rather unstable boundaries between management, policy and politics.

5.4 Management, policy and politics

The relationship between politics and management has always been clouded with ambiguities. While in formal terms a clear distinction has been drawn between 'policy' (the realm of politics) and 'administration', in practice it has been difficult to sustain a clear boundary between them. Administrators have a role in advising on policy as well as delivering it, and the process of delivery involves a multiplicity of decisions about how policy is to be interpreted.

Many of the reforms attempted to create a stronger separation between policy and delivery by devolving responsibility for operations to agencies and other bodies working within some form of contract or framework document. Such a separation brought many potential benefits: it encouraged policy-makers to clarify their goals and to identify the outcomes they wanted, and to specify them in performance standards or targets. Managers could then be left to get on with the job, finding the best and most efficient ways of meeting their targets without undue interference, while being held to account for what they delivered. Such a separation addressed many of the presumed failings of bureaucracy identified by public choice theorists. There were also less explicit benefits. Decentralization provided a response to the potential political problems arising from the containment of welfare expenditure by distancing resource allocation and rationing decisions from the political realm. For example, the Minister for Prisons, Anne Widdecomb, announced on 11 March 1997 that the solution to the growing crisis of overpopulation in prisons was simply proper resource management by managers and governors. Decentralization enabled the problem of matching resources and needs to be de-politicized by defining them as a matter for local management.

However, the struggle to shift issues and problems from one domain to another (and indeed from one organization to another) provided a point of instability in the new order: what we might term an unsettled aspect of the struggle to create a new organizational settlement. Many issues stubbornly refused to be de-politicized in this way, and became the ready stuff of parliamentary question times and political campaigns. Thus the 1996 crisis in accident and emergency services was deemed by the minister concerned to be 'a matter for local managers', but this did not prevent him having to deal with difficult questions in the House of Commons. As I write this chapter a scandal is emerging about hospital records falling open to misuse as private agencies are contracted to process them for new computer record systems. What probably seemed to be a relatively straightforward management decision ('let's contract this out to someone who can do it more efficiently than we can') was to result in a question tabled by the Shadow Health Secretary. Decentralization, even with rigorous central controls and stringent performance targets, has remained inherently unstable in the politicized context of social policy. This is because however much power is decentralized, political accountability means that the exercise of that power, even at low levels of decision-making, remains open to public scrutiny and political debate. This takes us to our next set of tensions: those between political and managerial forms of accountability.

5.5   Managerial and political accountability

Issues of probity, ethics and accountability surfaced clearly in debates about the proper conduct of public business in the 1980s and 1990s. A number of high-profile failures of public sector bodies (most notably the West Midlands and Wessex Regional Health Authorities in the 1980s) drew attention to the need for probity and 'good governance' in the use of public resources. Such failures have been blamed on the rise of more entrepreneurial forms of management and the demise of public service values. Concern has also been expressed about the removal of public functions from the control of democratically elected bodies, with the stripping of powers from local authorities, the rise of 'quangos' (such as training and enterprise councils) which are appointed rather than elected bodies, and the development of new systems of governance in the NHS and elsewhere (see Ferlie *et al.*, 1996). Indeed, it has been suggested that we are now faced with a 'democratic deficit' resulting from the weakening of direct forms of political forms of political accountability (Stewart, 1993).

Others have argued that the structural reforms of public services have enhanced accountability by making decision-making more transparent: that is, by clarifying who is responsible for what, setting clearer goals and targets, and holding managers to account for their performance in achieving them. William Waldegrave, then Chancellor of the Duchy of Lancaster, contested the idea of democratic deficit, arguing that the reforms not only clarified responsibilities, but they also significantly enhanced a different form of accountability: not upwards to politicians, but downwards to consumers (Waldegrave, 1993). The research conducted by Ferlie *et al.* showed that a number of the members of NHS Trust boards (who are appointed by the Secretary of State) saw their accountability as being to patients, to communities and to staff, rather than to government. As one put it,

> I could not care a hang about the Secretary of State. I am accountable to the people who actually work within the institution, and to the patients. If I fail, I fail the people who work here and I fail the people who are our customers. That to me is far more important than failing the Secretary of State.
> (quoted in Ferlie *et al.*, 1996, p.209)

It has also been argued that accountability to consumers had been strengthened through new forms of representation (such as league tables on performance, which enable consumers to make more informed choices) and through the development of charters which set out service entitlements and provide certain forms of redress for consumers.

The debate about whether or not there is a 'democratic deficit' or whether managerialism has actually enhanced accountability by making service providers more responsive to consumers lives on. What is more important in the context of this section is the interaction between different forms of accountability. Managers have to be accountable to politicians *and* to consumers; to staff *and* to the wider community. This requires them to balance the tensions between different forms of legitimation. That is, actions which may be legitimated by the idea of 'good management' (for instance greater efficiency) may be seen as less legitimate from the framework of 'good governance' (perhaps, in seeking greater efficiency, undue risks were taken with public resources). Similarly, actions which might be taken to be successful in the market-place (by, say, targeting customers with high incomes) may not be seen as legitimate from a public interest perspective.

ACTIVITY 9.5

This might be a good point to look again at your answers to Activity 9.2 and to reconsider what you put in the 'Accountability' row of Table 9.2.

COMMENT

Accountability in bureaucratic regimes is upwards through line managers and eventually to elected politicians (at least in theory). Professional accountability is usually to professional colleagues and to a professional body (such as the accountability of doctors to the British Medical Association for their professional conduct). Managerial accountability places emphasis on the accountability of staff to the organization for which they work (for example being held to account for the achievement of individual targets which contribute to corporate goals) and to the customers it serves. As the newspaper article reproduced in section 4.2 illustrates, these different forms of accountability exist alongside each other in particular organizations. Doing well in one area appears to be no compensation for being weak in others.

■ ■ ■

This section has placed particular stress on the difficulty of identifying clearly the boundaries between politics, policy and management for a number of reasons. First, this is a key site of tensions and instabilities. Despite the injunctions of managerialism, managers in the public domain do not have an unfettered 'right to manage', free from political interference, because of the nature of political accountability. Second, we are not just concerned with tensions between management and politics; many of the dilemmas which organizations have to work with stem from oscillations between different government departments. Given the paradoxes and tensions outlined in this section, how well does managerialism deliver on its promises? Furthermore, are there other criteria that should be used in evaluating its impact? These issues are examined in the next section.

6 Evaluating the new public management

The shift towards managerialism in social welfare has not gone uncontested. Professional associations and trade unions have formed powerful centres of resistance to change. Conflict over health reforms has been particularly intense, with doctors and other health workers sometimes entering into direct conflict with government. Many workers in service organizations have resisted changes in the content of their jobs (for example social workers finding the balance of their work shifting towards assessment rather than the provision of care). Others, however, have welcomed the 'modernizing' thrust of managerialism, seeing it as a source of innovation and a potential challenge to the paternalism, protectionism and parochialism that characterized the 'old' welfare state. User and consumer groups have challenged specific outcomes of change, but have also used the new spaces which restructuring has provided to pursue particular agendas and interests. Politicians and policy groups reflecting different political traditions have come to view managerialism and markets as necessary (though perhaps uncomfortable) means of finding resolutions to the perceived gap between rising needs and declining resources.

Given this range of views and opinions, how can we set about the task of evaluation? This section begins by discussing what kind of evidence might be used in evaluating the new public management (section 6.1) and then explores different types of criteria or judgements which might be used in the process of evaluation (section 6.2). Section 6.3 goes on to develop an assessment of managerialism from the point of view of 'the public' as taxpayer, customer and citizen.

6.1 Weighing the evidence

An obvious starting-point is to look at the claims made about the benefits of managerialism and to consider how to assess their validity. Pollitt (1995) suggests that the claims of the 'new public management' can be summarized as follows:

- greater economy
- greater efficiency
- rising standards of public service
- keener 'ownership' and enhanced autonomy for service managers and service providers
- greater responsiveness by staff to the users of services.

ACTIVITY 9.6

Before reading on, ask 'how would we know if this were true' of each of the above claims. It might help to consider the following questions:

1   What kinds of evidence might be needed to assess this claim?
2   What difficulties might arise in collecting and evaluating the evidence?

Pollitt (1995) summarizes a number of difficulties in assessing the evidence relating to the impact of the new public management. We shall look at each of these in turn.

Attribution problems

The new public management is multifaceted, with different kinds of initiatives interacting with each other. For example, budgetary reform may be accompanied by the decentralization of authority, the setting of quality standards and perhaps the installation of new IT systems. How, then, can particular effects be attributed to a single cause? Furthermore, might not outcomes such as increased productivity simply be a response of old-style bureaucrats to severe budget cuts rather than to the introduction of new-style management?

Benchmarks

A second set of difficulties arises from the absence of clear benchmarks against which to measure the impact of change. For example, how might we decide when exactly the changes began, or establish the baseline against which the impact of change might be assessed? How might we establish how a particular organization might have changed over time, irrespective of any managerial impetus or government reform agenda?

Estimating financial effects

The claim that the new public management has led to greater economy in the delivery of welfare services obviously needs evidence about the comparative costs of delivering specific services before and after a particular change (for example purchaser–provider splits) was introduced. However, any assessment and comparison of costs may encounter difficulties such as deciding what to include in the costs; judging how competition interacted with other changes going on at the time, which may have an influence on the cost of services;

weighing short-term costs against possible long-term savings (or short-term savings against long-term costs); and deciding how to measure the 'transaction costs' involved in paying for the setting up and monitoring of contracts.

Theorizing contexts

Pollitt argues that there is a need to theorize the political and organizational contexts into which reforms are being introduced, as well as the characteristics of the reforms themselves. Different sorts of management and co-ordination may be appropriate in different fields of social policy. For example, the management of health services, housing, criminal justice and so on each raises rather different sets of problems which may need to be resolved in different ways. The evaluation process requires that account be taken of the appropriateness of the new public management in different contexts: no single set of criteria can be arrived at against which all organizations can be assessed.

Choice of criteria for evaluation

The most common basis for evaluation is that of measuring the identifiable effects of a particular reform against its stated objectives. Pollitt suggests that there are at least two drawbacks to this approach. First, such an evaluation may miss any unintended effects of that reform since it may not be looking for them. Second, the goals of a reform may themselves be ambiguous. Evaluating reforms only in terms of how far they deliver their stated goals 'omits or backgrounds consideration of other criteria or values which are normally deemed highly relevant for public sector reforms … These include equity and equality, honesty and public accountability' (Pollitt, 1995, p.149).

6.2   Assessing the arguments

A second approach to 'weighing the evidence' is to identify the standpoint and value base which underpin different assessments of the new public management. This section contains three extracts, each of which explores the new public management from a different standpoint.

ACTIVITY 9.7

Read Extracts 9.1–9.3 and consider what kinds of evaluation criteria are being used in the development of the arguments. Try to identify the *assumptions* each is making about the conditions that prevailed in the past (the 'benchmarks' against which the impact of change is assessed). For example, what assumptions about how accountability worked in the past may underpin the critique of the democratic deficits of the new public management?

Extract 9.1 by Jervis and Richards (both UK academics) is based on a series of workshops held for senior managers from the public sector in the UK. In tracing the 'three deficits', try to think about what difference it makes that their analysis is based on the views of managers themselves. Also, consider which of the 'paradoxes' of managerialism outlined in section 5 are illustrated in the experiences of these practitioners.

Extract 9.1 Jervis and Richards: 'Public management: raising our game'

The analysis contained in this article follows from our work with groups of public managers and the accounts they provide of what works, and what does not work, in the system as they experience it. ... These accounts paint a picture of a system where recent reforms have produced dramatic increases in two of the Audit Commission's three Es – economy and efficiency – but where the ability to achieve effectiveness, both in policy formulation and implementation and service delivery, is being frustrated. The paradox is that the 'recipe' which has produced substantial gains in economy and efficiency is being revealed as increasingly unsuitable for the pursuit of effectiveness.

An effective public policy and management system is one that functions equally well at both the collective level and the level of single organizations. In this article we explore what might be involved in developing an improved system. In particular we focus on what this might mean for public managers with whom, we argue, a major responsibility for ensuring effectiveness of the system must rest. It is clear that the old governance formulation – that political leaders decide and public managers implement – no longer provides an adequate foundation for collective action. We suggest that public managers need to raise their game to meet the challenges now facing all of us.

The UK public policy and management system – the public managers' view

A unique insight into the operation of the public policy and management system comes from those working within it. In seminars with groups of senior public managers we have sought to take stock of the state of public management and identify the issues of greatest current concern. Public managers tell us, first, of the new structures, skills and cultures which have improved their capacity, and that of the organizations they lead, to deliver efficient services. The bad news is that these same people report increasing frustration at their inability to tackle effectively the major, complex, deep-rooted, intractable and multi-faceted problems that face communities and society, those issues that have been termed 'wicked problems' (Rittel and Weber, 1973, Stewart, 1995). Effectiveness is being inhibited among other things by continued centralization, on the constraints of a functionally-organized core executive in central government, and the increasing burden of audit and monitoring which has in the past been instrumental in promoting efficiency. All these militate against the effective tackling of complex problems requiring co-ordinated multi-disciplinary, multi-organizational responses.

Having listened to these accounts, we deduce that the UK public policy and management system suffers from three serious, separate, yet inter-related deficiencies. We have referred to these as *three deficits of public management* (Jervis and Richards, 1996):

- Public management as practised in the UK today suffers from a *democratic deficit*. This has developed as, one by one, a succession of public services have been removed from the framework of local democratic accountability. Public managers cite many examples of ways in which this lack of local democratic accountability inhibits their ability to operate effectively.

- Public managers report a second class of problem, related to the difficulty public service providers face in developing the business of their organizations, and exploiting the freedoms open to organizations operating in markets. We have termed this constraint the *development deficit*. It manifests itself in public service providers which improve significantly their operational performance but which cannot evolve and develop their organizations at the strategic level, and thus find their longer-term viability threatened.

- A further series of problems stems from the failure to design an effective overall system of policy formulation and implementation. By 'effective' in this context we mean a system of policy formulation and implementation which will enable society to tackle the 'wicked problems' it faces. We attribute these issues to a *design deficit* in the public policy process.

The democratic deficit has had several significant impacts. It has devalued electoral mechanisms as a principle in the process of making collective choices, and thus led to a decline in the capacity for democratic expression. In removing some but not all local services from the control of local government, it has placed structural obstacles in the way of effective service integration across organizational boundaries at the local level. Additionally, lack of democratic legitimacy in policy-making at the local level has forced contested issues up into central government, as local losers in policy decisions raised the stakes, believing they have not had a fair hearing. This overloads the centre.

The development deficit arises because public organizations acting as service providers have found limitations placed on their capacity to develop further their capacity and their services, unlike private sector providers. Competitive success for private sector organizations comes from being able continually to 're-invent themselves' (Hamel and Prahalad, 1994; Normann and Ramirez, 1993). This freedom is denied to many public service providers as the 'system' imposes restrictions on development which may be expressed in the phrase 'thus far and no further' (Jervis and Richards, 1995).

Sometimes these limitations may occur in the form of centrally imposed rules and regulations such as those preventing effective public service units from competing with the private sector, curbing their desire to expand into new markets, and forcing them to privatize or atrophy. There are examples of both local government and central government services which fall into this category. 'Market management' in the NHS provides another example, as in the ruling when NHS trusts were established that providers of acute and community services should be separate, thus preventing, for example, acute hospitals developing their service by providing primary care on an out-reach basis. Because of these 'strategic strait-jackets' the successes in service development which have accompanied the early stages of public management reform, and which have largely been based on improved operational efficiency, increasingly appear to have run their course. In fact there are signs that the constraints on strategic development will also threaten to erode the efficiency gains that have been achieved ...

The design deficit refers to those features of the architecture of public policy which consign key issues to the margin. Stewart (1993) has attributed the existence of 'wicked issues' in the public sector partly to the gaps which occur between different jurisdictions. Changes put in place since 1979 have increased the capacity of local public service managers to do an efficient job. Often they enjoy increased powers which enable them to take hold of the managerial reins, particularly in professional service organizations where previously power and authority have been dispersed. However, while being more powerful on management of service issues, centralization of the system of policy-making has reduced the ability of local service managers to contribute to policy development and to shape the policy agenda in the light of service experience ... While the idea that Ministers make policy and public officials implement it may conform to the old constitution's impoverished concept of governance, it is much too simplistic a formulation to support effective policy-making, which requires that experiential knowledge be brought to bear in the process.

Instead, particularly in the last few years as performance measurement has increased, local managers find themselves responding on ever tighter feedback loops into the centre, either through formal performance requirements, or through the back-door centralization which often seems to result from increased monitoring and audit ... This seems to be happening despite the formal intention to decentralize, evident in such changes as the NHS and Community Care Act 1990 and the establishment of training and enterprise councils. The level of monitoring and audit in a service system which purports to be decentralized seems to reflect some entrenched centralist aspect of the British state, the governance in the old constitution, which leads to the reassertion of central control despite the overt intention to decentralize.

All of this is compounded by the fact that policy decisions are being focused in a central government structured around functional specialism, which exacerbates the problem of integration across service boundaries. If the problems we need to solve fell neatly into functional boundaries, there would be no difficulty in working with this design. Wicked problems do not and centralization into a functionalist setting makes things worse. ...

The three deficits are inter-related and inter-dependent. They interact to produce a system of public policy and management that is underperforming ... Addressing the problem of underperformance requires a focus on the operation of the system, not just attention to any of its parts – policy changes aimed at only one or other of the deficits will not work.

References

Hamel, G. and Prahalad, C. (1994) 'Competing for the future', *Harvard Business Review*, July-August.

Jervis, P. and Richards, S. (1995) 'Strategic management in a re-invented government: rowing 1, steering 0', paper presented to the 15th International Conference of the Strategic Management Society.

Jervis, P. and Richards, S. (1996) *Three Deficits of Public Management*, School of Public Policy, University of Birmingham.

Normann, R. and Ramirez, R. (1993) 'From value chain to value constellation: designing interactive strategy', *Harvard Business Review*, July-August.

Rittel, H. and Weber, M. (1973) 'Dilemmas in a general theory of planning', *Policy Science*, vol.4, pp.155–69.

Stewart, J. (1993) *Local Government Today: An Observer's View*, Luton, Local Government Management Board.

Stewart, J. (1995) *The Rebuilding of Public Accountability*, London, European Policy Forum.

(Jervis and Richards, 1997, pp.1–3)

The focus in Extract 9.2 is rather different from that of Jervis and Richards. Lane, based in the University of Oslo, contrasts the 'administrative state', which has grown up across Europe, with the managerial state. As well as evaluating managerialism in terms of its capacity to accommodate the 'justice' principles enshrined in public administration, Lane identifies criteria against which the claims that managerialism produces more efficiency might be assessed. He suggests some 'optimality conditions' for managerialism as the source of efficiency – that is, the conditions in which efficiency gains are most likely to be delivered.

Extract 9.2 Lane: 'The management state vs the administrative state'

Over time, the management approach has driven out the public administration framework when it comes to modelling public sector reform in the advanced economic countries. The new phrase public management reflects the insertion of the management perspective into the public sector. Efficiency is considered more important than rule obedience, effectiveness comes before legality, flexibility and adaptation are more vital than predictability and responsibility. If public operations can give a profit, then profitability is a highly relevant objective besides the public interests that are served.

The managerial revolution has slowly crept into the public sector, increasing the role of managers, on the one hand, and reorienting governance towards the management philosophy, on the other hand. The managerial revolution … implies that public organizations such as hospitals, schools and infrastructure departments be run as firms and that state enterprises be made into joint-stock companies, operated as a private firm. What are the pros and cons of the management state? …

Pros and cons of the management state

Pros	Cons
Clear goals	Neglect of means
Measurement of outputs and outcomes	Insensitivity towards intangible values
Cost consciousness	Unresponsiveness to demand
Discretion	Transaction costs
Manpower manoeuvrability	Loss of tenure
Separation between purchaser and producer	Small numbers problem
Competition in supply	Lack of demand-revelation mechanisms
Motivation transparency: self-interests	Lack of institutions and a democratic deficit

Creating internal markets within the public sector increases the scope for managers to direct the provision of goods and services in accordance with clear goals that may be monitored by measuring outputs and outcomes. Managers may raise efficiency – effectiveness as well as productivity – because their discretion provides them with a scope for cost-cutting strategies. …

The establishment of internal markets within the public sector is a rejection of the administrative state. Proper procedures count for less than efficiency in outputs and outcomes and intangible values connected with the public sector will receive less attention. Due process values underlining the means employed in the public sector figure less prominently, because they cannot be quantified or measured in terms of value: equal treatment, openness of procedures, legality and predictability. …

Internal markets enlarge the discretion of managers in the process of supplying goods and services. They will not be bound by earlier commitments but may make contracts with the lowest bidder. However, the internal market model will not resolve basic problems on the demand side. Consumer demand will still be channelled by means of the political election mechanisms, as the internal market model does not include any extensive employment of user charges as a demand-revelation mechanism.

The strong emphasis on bidding by means of short-term contracting raises the question of transaction costs within the new management framework. Traditional budget-making in an incremental model lowered transaction costs by means of so-called standard operating procedures. Internal markets must raise transaction costs, as there will be no long-term contracts or any fixed assignment of task to bureaux. In internal markets competition will take place all over the budget, as there will be no base that remains protected from one year to another.

A rise in transaction costs will also raise the possibility of opportunistic behaviour within the bidding process that takes place in short-term contracting. Persons or organizations with transaction-specific assets may engage in strategic behaviour in order to raise the price for their products – the small numbers problem. The management approach promises increased efficiency in the public sector, but will it achieve the conditions for optimality in resource allocation?

Optimality conditions
… Optimality in the public provision of goods and services requires that the marginal willingness to pay of the consumer/citizen is equal to the marginal cost of producing the good or the services and that marginal costs are minimized. Will internal markets (1) reveal the marginal willingness to pay and (2) result in cost minimization? Is it altogether improbable that there may occur X-inefficiencies and Y-inefficiencies in the internal market regime?

The answer to these optimality problems depends upon how the management state scores in relation to (a) information, (b) motivation and (c) opportunistic behaviour. The management approach appears to be weak with regard to information about citizen preferences, since it does not employ user charges. It is an open question whether managers may be hired in such a manner that they have the motivation to promote the conditions that lead to efficiency in allocation. There is a risk that high transaction costs reduce the efficiency gains from increased competition. There is also a danger of opportunistic behaviour when short-term contracts are drawn up, as persons with transaction-specific assets will have a strategic advantage in such budgetary biddings. The role of politicians will have to change, because they have to ensure that the managers themselves do not engage in opportunistic behaviour.

Conclusion
There are several signs to the effect that public administration is about to be driven out by public management as the paradigm for interpreting the public sector, in particular in relation to problems of organization and leadership. The trend away from the public administration framework towards the public management approach is no doubt part of the general process of public sector reform, searching for greater efficiency in the delivery of goods and services by the state and local governments.

However, there are drawbacks in the transformation process. The public administration framework cannot easily be replaced by the new management approach, as the former has qualities not covered by the latter. In its most radical version, the management approach calls for the introduction of internal markets in the public sector, replacing hierarchy and long-term contracts with bidding and short-term contracts. If implemented on a large scale, internal markets will drive up transaction and switching costs, which could erase the efficiency gains from increased competition.

In addition, internal markets will not be able to meet the non-pecuniary goals connected with the public sector, in particular the strong emphasis upon legality and its various values. There is more to the public sector than efficiency. How can procedural values be taken care of in the management approach, not to speak of the rights to voice, remedy and legal control? The notion of justice looms large in the public sector, but where does it fit into the internal markets framework?

(Lane, 1995, pp.197–200)

In Extract 9.3 Kooiman and van Vliet (two academics from the Erasmus University in Rotterdam) are concerned with the relationship between governance and management. They argue that modern societies are characterized by increasing complexity, dynamics and diversity, and that this has led to new social needs that can only be answered by new forms of governance. This places particular requirements on public management. As you read this extract, try to identify what the authors mean by 'governance' and its relationship with 'management'. This is a hard extract – don't worry if all is not clear. However, do think about the key terms they use to describe modern society – complexity, dynamics and diversity – and think about how well placed conventional public management is to deal with these.

Extract 9.3 Kooiman and van Vliet: 'Dilemmas of and responsibilities for public management'

The aim of this chapter has been to develop criteria for the performance of 'modern' public management, that is public management that copes with the central features of contemporary advanced (western) society: increasing complexity, dynamics and diversity. We conclude that high quality public management in '(post)-modern times' is public management that contributes to 'good governance'. Good governance refers not only [to] the quality of the government's own actions alone but also to the quality of the politico-social order as a whole and the process of governance that is resulting from that order. The importance ... is not so much within the quantitative extension of the performance criteria for public management but in the manifestation of the dilemmas that face modern public management today. These dilemmas confront contemporary public management with the task to re-model its responsibilities towards societies and its citizens. In our opinion, it is the confrontation between a perspective 'from inside out' [and] a perspective 'from outside in' that makes the public management task a difficult one.

With regard to dynamics, the task of public management is to relate effectiveness and efficiency measures more to learning and learning capacities. Effectiveness cannot be measured on [the] basis of fixed *ex ante* objectives alone. In a dynamic context one must reckon with changing circumstances that can develop in changing problem definitions, better solution methods and fresh insights that can develop over time. Learning, the capacity to learn and the capacity to develop learning capacities must be part of new definitions and conceptions of effectiveness and efficiency. Management of problems which are dynamic in character, such as environmental problems, [has] to sail between two forms of failure. On the one hand there is the risk that new insights are continuously translated into new problem definitions and new targets so that governing and other social actors do not know where they stand and what they are supposed to do, with the result that developments stop and usual criteria of effectiveness and efficiency are not met. On the other hand the risk is that not incorporating new insights could mean that the achievement of *ex ante* determined objectives is less or not at all useful at the time of accomplishment.

Diversity seems to be the most difficult factor to deal with in contemporary society. Rules and regulations in a constitutional state are based on the principle of equality [before] the law. However, in a diversified society the equality principle is less applicable if everyone is 'different'. Implementation of social security regulations in the Netherlands shows us that, due to an increasing diversification in living situations, rule-implementation without interpretation is increasingly difficult and is often regarded as not justified. On the other hand more freedom of interpretation in the hands of implementing personal decisions could lead to a sense of arbitrariness. Governmental action in a diversified world seems to depend more and more, neither on 'impersonal' application of general rules on special cases, nor on the personal but arbitrary choice of implementing (executive) public officers but on the development of communication structures in which reasonable argumentation leads to acceptable and legitimate governmental intervention. 'Reasonable argumentation' means that there is an (ongoing) interaction between 'general rules' and 'special cases' within the government itself and between government and society. Within this interaction process governments and social actors have to consider governmental action and its intended and unintended consequences.

Public management must create time and room for 'self-reflection' but it must also support society and its citizens in its consideration of public action. In Reich's (1985, 1988) opinion the responsibility of public managers is not only taking decisions in the public interest but also in helping the population to deliberate about the collective decisions that should be taken: 'Thus the public manager's job is not only, or simply, to make policy choices and implement them. It is also to participate in a system of democratic governance in which public values are continuously rearticulated and recreated' (Reich, 1988, p.124).

In a society that is increasingly complex, dynamic and diverse, 'the' government is not capable of deciding alone in which direction society develops. Societal development is necessarily a result of interactive social forces. The fact that societal developments are dependent on the actions of a variety of social actors, however, does not mean that public management does not have a special responsibility. On the normative level it has the responsibility to stimulate public debate about public values, governmental tasks and collective decision-making through which government's role in society is being legitimized and a public 'purpose' is given to governmental action. On the level of the political-governmental process public management has to take care that all involved interests, also wide-spread and/or interests difficult to organize such as the interest of future generations, are represented to take part in public decision-making. On the level of implementation public management must innovate and experiment with new instruments of public management, such as public–private partnership for infrastructural investments and urban development, negotiated rule making in environmental issues, and forms of (semi-) autonomization of public services.

Conclusion

Within this chapter we have developed the idea that modern societal development described by means of increasing complexity, dynamics, and diversity, leads to new collective and social needs that only can be answered by newly developed forms of governance. These governance forms have to take into account the *Eigendynamik* of society in social subsystems directed in the development of processes of interaction [within] which political-governmental interventions and social self-organization are co-ordinated. The government has to take care of both the performance and quality of its own actions/interventions as the performance of the evolving governance structure. In the governance perspective public

> management ... is set ... to implement these governmental responsibilities by supporting and making possible 'responsible' decision-making within and between social organizations and citizens, by 'balancing' social forces ... and by making use of innovative public management instruments.
>
> ### *References*
>
> Reich, R. (1985) 'Public administration and public deliberation: an interpretative essay', *Yale Law Review*, vol.94, pp.1617–41.
>
> Reich, R. (1988) 'Policy making in a democracy', in Reich, R., *The Power of Public Ideas*, Cambridge, Mass., Harvard University Press.
>
> (Kooiman and van Vliet, 1993, pp.70–2)

COMMENT

This section has looked at a range of extracts which illustrate different standpoints against which managerialism might be assessed. Lane evaluates managerialism in its own terms, questioning whether it delivers the efficiency it promises. Others use criteria based on other sets of values and concerns. Jervis and Richards explore the effectiveness of the new public management system as a whole to deliver effective public policy, while Kooiman and van Vliet suggest that managerialism needs to be evaluated in terms of its capacity to meet the needs of a complex, dynamic and diverse society, and that the 'governance' needs of this society require a distinctive approach to public management.

■ ■ ■

The claims and counter claims about the outcomes of managerialism are often couched in the language of 'the public' or 'the public interest'. The next section develops this theme by exploring different conceptions of the public that these might refer to.

6.3   The public as stakeholder: complementary or competing assessments?

In discussions of managerialism, notions of the public are employed in statements such as the following:

1   'Better management leads to more effective use of public money.'

2   'The reforms of the last decade have made services more responsive to the public.'

3   'Competition has given the public more choice.'

4   'Organizations have become more transparent – it is clear who is responsible for what, and this makes services more accountable to the public.'

Such statements raise a number of difficulties. Who does the speaker assume is included or excluded? What parts of the public count most? Are all members of the public assumed to want the same things? These questions reflect the difficulties identified in Chapter 2 of assuming a common social settlement which ignores issues of diversity and power.

Individuals and groups stand in different kinds of relationship to welfare services, with different sorts of 'stakes' in the outcomes of change. They may be at the same time a taxpayer, with an interest in reducing or containing the costs of welfare; a user, with an interest in receiving high quality and responsive services; and a citizen, perturbed about, say, increased numbers of people sleeping on the streets, and anxious that the problem of homelessness be addressed. They may also be an informal, unpaid producer of welfare in the home and community.

Which of the statements at the beginning of this section do you think reflect the ideas of the public as (a) taxpayer; (b) service user; and (c) citizen?

Let's take each in turn. The idea of the public as taxpayer has been used **public as taxpayer** throughout the reform process to legitimate calls for curbs on public expenditure. As suggested in the first statement, managerialism is viewed as the driver of efficiency. How far it has been successful is difficult to assess because of the problems of attribution, benchmarking and cost assessment outlined in section 6.1. For example, managerial changes cannot be isolated from policy changes (in terms of how benefits are calculated, how health services are rationed, or how social needs are assessed). Second, claimed efficiency savings are usually based on the degree of cost reduction that is achieved from, say, contracting out services or introducing internal purchaser–provider splits. But the costs of writing, managing and monitoring contracts – the *transaction costs* that are incurred – are not easy to measure, and may outweigh some of the economy gains. These costs will be higher in some services than others, depending on the level of complexity and therefore the difficulty of writing specifications. This takes us back to Pollitt's point about the importance of theorizing context, and to Lane's list of 'optimality conditions'. Lane argues that, in any case, there is 'more to the public sector than efficiency'. However, it is important to note the critical importance of the emergence of the 'citizen-as-taxpayer' in political discourse through the 1980s and 1990s.

When we look at managerialism from the standpoint of the public as **public as consumer** consumer (as reflected in statements 2 and 3) the shift from bureaucratic paternalism to a greater focus on quality, responsiveness and choice holds considerable promise. There is a range of criteria that can be used to evaluate services from a consumer's perspective:

- Access: how do consumers get to know about, and gain access to, a service?
- Choice: is there a choice of providers, a choice of services, and/or a choice about how the service is to be provided?
- Voice: how much power do consumers have to influence or complain about the service?
- Exit: the ability to go to other providers if dissatisfied.

Some of these criteria have been seen as more legitimate than others, and consumerism in reality takes a very partial and limited form (Pollitt, 1988). Consumer surveys and questionnaires have proliferated, but actual participation by users in decisions about service design or service priorities has been limited since it challenges the managerial 'right to manage'. The criterion of choice is also limited in that it rests on an assumption that 'meaningful choices can only be made by individuals and only in the context of a market exchange relationship.

It fails to recognise the possibility of choice being exercised collectively by citizens with a common interest' (Prior *et al.*, 1995, p.131). It is this which leads Ranson and Stewart (1994, p.19) to argue that 'Consumerism provides an incomplete language for the public domain'.

public as citizen

This notion of the public domain, in which the public can express collective interests, takes us to yet another standpoint: the idea of the public as citizen. The collective interests of the citizen are usually assumed to be expressed through the formal channels of elections and representation through MPs, local councillors, and so on. However, this section has highlighted two other issues. The first is how effective managerialism is as a means of delivering collectively determined social policy. Jervis and Richards argue that fragmentation, linked to the imperative to focus on an organization's core business, leads to a design deficit. It follows that the system as a whole cannot deal with 'wicked issues' which do not fall neatly into the 'business' of a particular organization. While public managers do attempt to work across boundaries to deal with these problems of integration, their effectiveness in doing so is limited by the government performance targets which are based on organizational effectiveness rather than policy effectiveness. Managerialism, then, is limited in its ability to hold together an increasingly fragmented field of social welfare services.

The second issue relates to how well collective interests are addressed in the managerial order. Ranson and Stewart (1994) argue for a conception of the 'public domain' which can embody both individual and collective purposes. They suggest that a model of public management is needed which contributes to a 'learning society' by promoting public discourse which gives expression to notions of citizenship. They view the dominant language of consumerism as unable to promote such public discourse or express public purpose.

These ideas raise important questions about the nature of 'the public' which is addressed in the different extracts. Before reading on, you might like to review Chapters 1 and 2, where Gordon Hughes and Gail Lewis discuss the social settlement. How do you think the 'subjects' constituted through the discourses of public as taxpayer and public as consumer differ from the welfare subjects of the Beveridgean social settlement?

The notion of 'governance', which was introduced in Extract 9.3 by Kooiman and van Vliet, takes us into a rather different set of perspectives, though the vision offered is not dissimilar to that of Ranson and Stewart. Kooiman and van Vliet use the term governance to indicate the creation of social order through the interaction of a plurality of actors. These actors include government itself, but also organizations involved in purchasing, providing or commissioning services, or acting as advocates or representatives of service users or communities. In this sense, public management must be evaluated in terms of how well it steers, integrates and regulates social action in ways which respond to the needs of a complex and diverse society. This conception blurs the boundary between management and politics and offers a more expansive role for public management as both a part of and a catalyst for governance.

7   Conclusion: managerialism and the restructuring of social welfare – a new welfare settlement?

Chapters 1 and 2 argued that the 'old' welfare state was based on a number of settlements: economic, political, social and organizational. This final section asks the question: how far does managerialism provide the basis for a new set of settlements which together might form a 'new welfare order'? It does not provide answers – at the time of writing a new government has not long been in power and a number of issues remain unresolved – but it does seek to suggest some potential points of instability which may mean that the idea of a 'closure' based on a new set of settlements can be contested. Since this chapter has mainly dealt with the organizational settlement, this is where we begin.

It seems that managerialism has indeed become embedded as the basis for a new organizational settlement. The new public management has become a dominant set of ideas which are drawn on in the design and management of organizations across the UK and in other modern industrial societies. However, there are two cautionary points about variability that need to be made. The first concerns the idea that all such nations have adopted the same solutions to the 'problems' of welfare in the late twentieth century. Different nations have followed rather different reform processes, and there is no wholesale convergence around a common set of organizational solutions (Flynn and Strehl, 1996; Ferlie *et al.*, 1996). Flynn and Strehl comment:

> The pressures on the public sector do not produce a common set of responses from politicians and managers. There are many variables which affect how reforms are designed and implemented, including the constitutional arrangements in place, political opinions at national and sub national level, public attitudes towards the state and its employees, and the skills and knowledges of public sector managers.
>
> (Flynn and Strehl, 1996, p.4)

The second source of variability derives from the processes of accommodation between bureau-professionalism and managerialism in different sectors. The nature and extent of this accommodation depend on the degree of professional power, the extent of the introduction of market mechanisms, and the culture and ethos of specific organizations. So, for example, professional power has remained strong in the NHS, and managerialism has developed more strongly in the executive agencies of central government than in the policy-oriented departments.

These sources of variability mean that there is a need to question the idea of a common organizational settlement. It is clear, though, that managerialism has formed the basis of an emerging *political* and *economic* consensus about how best to run welfare organizations, whether in the private, public or voluntary sectors. Managerialism has shifted from its place at the heart of the ideological politics of the New Right in the 1980s towards forming the basis of a multi-party consensus on how best to solve the economic problems of the welfare state. It has become de-politicized – as Labour Party leader Tony Blair commented in the run-up to the 1997 General Election, 'what counts is what works'. Disagreements between the major parties remain, but the concerns that preoccupy them, and the language used to debate them, are remarkably similar.

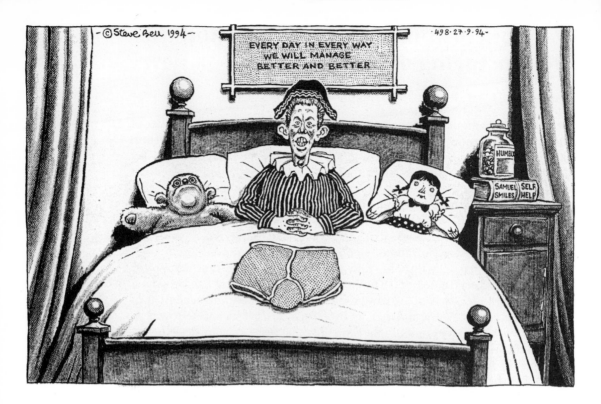

The 'glue' which appears to stick this emerging political consensus together is an agreement that managerialism plus markets will deliver answers to some of the economic problems linked to rising public expenditure. However, it is less clear that they can resolve some of the intractable social, environmental or community-based policy agendas – the 'wicked issues' – which flow from an increasingly complex and differentiated society. Many of these do not fit neatly into linear goals that can be translated into clearly defined organizational objectives, but are concerned with interaction between different policy agendas – for example those concerned with social, environmental, economic, health and education issues. Managerialism tends to produce a concentration by single organizations on narrow agendas defined around their core business. This reduces its capacity to address complex social policy issues.

More fundamentally, the problems which managerialism seeks to resolve do not lie in the old organizational settlement alone. That is, the problems of the welfare state were not just about the perceived waste and inefficiency of bureaucracies: they stemmed from contradictions and conflicts in the relationship between the state and its citizens (and other residents). The old welfare state was based on a notion of social citizenship and the construction of a new social order. It had built into it a number of contradictions based on the narrow (racialized and gendered) view of citizenship it embodied, but installed a notion of a socially democratic public which was the basis of the social settlement of the post-war years. The new public management has helped dismantle this settlement in two important ways: first, by reconstituting the 'social citizen' into a series of fragmentary relationships as the customer of welfare services (see **Hughes, 1998**); and, second, by dismantling the institutions of welfare into a dispersed set of agencies and organizations. In a society characterized by sharpening social tensions and increasing mistrust between citizens and political institutions, and by the 'complexity, dynamics and diversity' highlighted by Kooiman and van Vliet, managerialism may do little to help resolve the instabilities in the social settlement.

The question, then, is not just about whether managerialism forms the basis of a new organizational settlement. It is about the impact of managerialism on the political and social settlements. In each there are important points of instability which may militate against the formation of a new series of settlements and a new (marketized and privatized) welfare order. In the social domain, there are tensions between the notion of citizens as political subjects, as consumers and as self-reliant providers of social welfare within the family and community. The organizational domain, as we have seen, contains a number of internal contradictions and tensions. Finally, the slippery boundary between management and politics produces points of instability in the new order which managerialism cannot resolve and which politicians may be reluctant to address.

7.1 Review

Managerialism is likely to continue to be seen as a solution to economic problems of high welfare expenditure. It helps to deliver economies by bringing decisions about how to meet welfare needs closer to decisions about resource availability and the best use of scarce resources. Section 4 of this chapter described how managerialism prioritizes particular sets of goals which are concerned with organizational survival and success alongside the professional goals of meeting needs or solving problems. It invokes particular ways of thinking about how activities should be carried out, based on notions of efficiency. It lays claim to particular types of expertise which underpin the exercise of discretion and judgement. As such, managerialism serves as the 'glue' which integrates and co-ordinates an increasingly fragmented field of social welfare delivery across the public, private and voluntary sectors. However, as section 3 outlined, there is no single managerialism, but a number of different discourses and practices. These have different sorts of consequences for decision-making, and reshape relationships in different ways. As a consequence, managerialism embodies a number of internal tensions and paradoxes, some of which were explored in section 5. These mean that change has been complex and uneven. Social actors have tried to find ways of resolving contradictions on the ground, working with multiple goals and success criteria, or reshaping the managerial agenda around other sets of values and goals – for example around professional goals or in the interests of staff, users or communities.

All of this means that evaluating managerialism is not an easy task. Section 6 highlighted some of the problems of providing evidence, and looked at some of the different standpoints and arguments in the debate. The aim has not been to come up with a single conclusion, but to enable you to assess the arguments of others or develop arguments of your own. This is important because of the central role that managerialism seems to have played in the shaping of a new political settlement between 'neo-liberalism' and 'New Labour'. While the post-war project of building the welfare state looked to a mix of professional expertise and bureaucratic rationality, the project of containing welfare growth and reshaping the welfare order was seen to require a new form of co-ordination and control. The logic of efficiency has become the dominant ethos in this new managerial regime. However, efficiency may not be sufficient as either a single tool for evaluation or as a single imperative to be pursued in developing new policy agendas to meet the requirements of a complex and diverse society. The unravelling of the old social settlement raises critical questions about the effectiveness of managerialized and fragmented organizations in creating effective relationships between policy-makers and service users, and ultimately between state and citizen.

Further reading

Many of the arguments in this chapter are more fully developed in Clarke and Newman (1997). An earlier but nevertheless valuable collection which traces the development of managerialism in different areas of social policy is Clarke *et al.* (1994). This also has a chapter on the gender and equality implications of the new public management (Newman, 1994). A different but complementary perspective is provided in Ferlie *et al.* (1997), which is particularly strong on the interaction between professionalism and managerialism, especially in the NHS, and on issues of accountability. Flynn (1997) provides a good guide to management practice in the public sector, while a more comparative perspective is presented in Flynn and Strehl (1996).

References

Centre for Contemporary Cultural Studies (Education Group) (1981) *Unpopular Education: Schooling and Social Democracy in England Since 1944*, London, Hutchinson.

Clarke, J., Cochrane, A. and McLaughlin, E. (1994) *Managing Social Policy*, London, Sage.

Clarke, J. and Cochrane, A. (1998) 'The social construction of social problems', in Saraga, E. (ed.) *Embodying the Social: Constructions of Difference,* London, Routledge in association with The Open University.

Clarke, J. and Newman, J. (1997) *The Managerial State: Power, Politics and Ideology in the Remaking of Social Welfare*, London, Sage.

du Gay, P. (1994) 'Colossal immodesties and hopeful monsters: pluralism and organizational conduct', *Organization*, vol.1, no.1, pp.125–48.

Ferlie, E., Pettigrew, A., Ashburner, L. and Fitzgerald, L. (1996) *The New Public Management in Action*, Oxford, Oxford University Press.

Flynn, N. (1997) *Public Sector Management*, 3rd edn, London, Prentice-Hall/ Harvester Wheatsheaf.

Flynn, N. and Strehl, F. (eds) (1996) *Public Sector Management in Europe*, London, Harvester Wheatsheaf.

Hood, C. (1991) 'A public management for all seasons?', *Public Administration*, vol.69, spring, pp.5–19.

Hughes, G. (ed.) (1998) *Imagining Welfare Futures*, London, Routledge in association with The Open University.

Jervis, P. and Richards, S. (1997) 'Public management: raising our game', *Public Money & Management*, April–June, pp.1–3.

Kooiman, J. and van Vliet, M. (1993) 'Governance and public management', in Eliassen, K. and Kooiman, J. (eds) *Managing Public Organizations: Lessons from Contemporary European Experience*, 2nd edn, London, Sage.

Lane, J. (1995) *The Public Sector: Concepts, Models and Approaches*, 2nd edn, London, Sage.

Langan, M. (1998) 'The contested concept of need', in Langan, M. (ed.) *Welfare: Needs, Rights and Risks*, London, Routledge in association with The Open University.

Lentell, H. (1998) 'Families of meaning: contemporary discourses of the family', in Lewis, G. (ed.) *Forming Nation, Framing Welfare*, London, Routledge in association with The Open University.

Lowndes, V. (1996) 'Change in public service management: new institutions and management regimes', *La Journée d'Etude Local Governance*, February, Paris..

Mackintosh, M. (1995) *Putting Words into People's Mouths? Economic Culture and Its Implications for Local Governance*, Open Discussion Papers in Economics, no.9, Faculty of Social Sciences, The Open University.

Metcalfe, L. and Richards, S. (1990) *Improving Public Management*, 2nd edn, London, Sage.

Morgan, G. (1991) *Images of Organisation*, London, Sage

Newman, J. (1994) 'The limits of management: gender and the politics of change', in Clarke *et al.* (eds) (1994).

Niskanen, W.A. (1971) *Bureaucracy and Representative Government*, New York, Aldine-Atherton.

Osborne, D. and Gaebler, T. (1992) *Reinventing Government: How the Entrepreneurial Spirit is Transforming the Public Sector*, Wokingham, Addison-Wesley.

Parker, H. (1982) *The Moral Hazard of Social Insurance*, London, Institute of Economic Affairs.

Peters, J. and Waterman, R.H. (1982) *In Search of Excellence: Lessons from America's Best Run Companies*, New York, Harper and Row.

Pollitt, C. (1988) 'Editorial: consumerism and beyond', *Public Administration*, vol.66, summer, pp.121–4.

Pollitt, C. (1993) *Managerialism and the Public Services*, 2nd edn, Oxford, Blackwell.

Pollitt, C. (1995) 'Justification by works or by faith? Evaluating the new public management', *Evaluation*, vol.1, no.2, pp.133–54.

Prior, D., Stewart, J. and Walsh, K. (1995) *Citizenship: Rights, Community and Participation*, London, Pitman.

Ranson, S. and Stewart, J. (1994) *Management for the Public Domain: Enabling the Learning Society*, Basingstoke, Macmillan.

Stewart, J. (1993) *Accountability to the Public*, London, European Policy Forum.

Taylor, G. (1993) 'Challenges from the margins', in Clarke, J. (ed.) *A Crisis in Care? Challenges to Social Work*, London, Sage.

Waldegrave, W. (1993) *The Reality of Reform and Accountability in Today's Public Services*, London, Public Finance Foundation.

Walsh, K. (1995) *Public Services and Market Mechanisms: Competition, Contracting and the New Public Management*, Basingstoke, Macmillan.

Williams, F. (1996) 'Post-modernism, feminism and the question of difference', in Parton, N. (ed.) *Social Theory, Social Change and Social Work*, London, Routledge.

CHAPTER 10

Review

by John Clarke, Gordon Hughes and Gail Lewis

Contents

1   Introduction

This book has concentrated on the reconstruction of the purpose, place and provision of social welfare in the UK in the late twentieth century. At one time the focus of the book would have been described as that of 'the welfare state', but the changes made to the organization and delivery of welfare over the last two decades of the twentieth century have meant that this phrase no longer provides a simple and easy point of reference. In the preceding chapters we have explored not only the reconstructions that have occurred in the shape and organization of social welfare, but also the changing role of the state during the 1980s and 1990s, which have called both the idea and the practice of 'the welfare state' into question. In this book you have encountered a large amount of rich, and at times very detailed, material relating to the reconstruction of social welfare in the UK since the Second World War. The main aim of this review chapter, therefore, is to offer you:

- an overview of the principal themes and concepts employed in the previous nine chapters; and

- a review of where these processes of change have left social welfare and the role of the state at the end of the twentieth century, with a particular emphasis on the extent to which new 'welfare settlements' and 'welfare subjects' have been constructed.

Chapters 1 and 2 offered an overview of the major features of the welfare settlements in the UK during the post-war era. In particular, Chapter 1 'plotted a story' of the Beveridgean welfare state during the decades from the 1940s through to the 1970s.

ACTIVITY 10.1

Look back quickly at Chapter 1. Why was the term 'story' used there, with all its connotations of fiction, narrative and imaginary elements?

As you may recall, it was argued in Chapter 1 that the post-war welfare state in the UK was a complex institutional entity, involving policies, processes and practices of welfare provision which embodied a rich ideological and representational dimension. This dimension included the way in which our understandings of 'the welfare state' were enmeshed in myths and symbols of 'Britishness' and 'citizenship' and about the relationship between 'the people' and the state. Chapter 1 went on to question the image of a monolithic and homogeneous welfare state and, central to our purposes in this book, emphasized the importance of the four settlements that underpinned the Beveridgean welfare state. This 'de-mythologizing' of the welfare state is not intended to undermine or underestimate its social significance. On the contrary, paying attention to both its institutional and its ideological role in UK society is important as a way of grasping its *full* significance. Indeed, we would argue that any study of social welfare in the UK has to address the intensive period of reform and innovation which surrounded the end of the Second World War. These processes of post-war reform and reconstruction produced what we have variously referred to as the 'Beveridgean welfare state', the 'Keynesian welfare state', the 'social democratic welfare state' or the 'old welfare state' and established the broad shape of social welfare that persisted into the 1980s. This period of reform was also crucial in establishing the frameworks from which we can assess and evaluate the changes, 'unsettlements' and 'reconstructions' in welfare institutions, policies and discourses that occurred in the 1980s and 1990s. Furthermore, this book has emphasized that we need to understand welfare as the object of both political and theoretical controversies.

Chapter 2 provided an overview of the major processes of welfare reconstruction in the UK since the 1970s. In particular, the chapter focused on the major criticisms of the Beveridgean welfare state and the subsequent welfare reforms and reconstitution of the public sphere during the last decades of the twentieth century. Although note was made of the resilience of the levels of welfare spending (due largely to the high levels of demand for social security payments both for unemployment and retirement pensions) throughout the latter part of the twentieth century, it was also noted that the 'ground rules' of welfare provision changed. 'The welfare state' was thus restructured in ways that changed both the character of social welfare and the role of the state in providing it. The shift to more 'mixed' economies of welfare, the introduction of markets or market-mimicking processes (such as 'quasi-markets') and the creation of new organizational structures, all within commitments to contain public spending and reduce 'welfare dependency', were features of these changes.

As well as providing this overview of the changing fortunes of the welfare state in the UK, Chapters 1 and 2 were also intended to set the context, for the subsequent chapters, of the specific forms of welfare restructuring in relation to health services, housing, probation, education, social care and income maintenance. Finally, Chapter 9 focused on the emergence of a new 'organizational settlement' constructed around the discourse of managerialism. Chapter 9 provided one way of drawing connections between some of the wider processes of welfare restructuring discussed in Chapters 1 and 2 and the specific manifestations of change in social welfare policy and practice explored in Chapters 3 to 8. In the following sections we review both the general themes and concepts employed in this book and their relationship to the specific forms of welfare reconstruction in the different areas of welfare provision. We begin by revisiting the core themes and concepts of the book as a whole.

2 The welfare state: from the cradle to the grave

The first two chapters of this book traced the rise and fall of the Beveridgean welfare state through the 50 years following the Second World War. They did so by focusing on the 'settlements' that underpinned the construction and development of this 'old' welfare state – the economic, political, social and organizational conditions that enabled and shaped its role in UK society. Chapter 2 traced both the unravelling of those settlements and the attempts to construct new ones, as well as the restructuring of the welfare state. As a result of these processes of unravelling and restructuring, the last two decades of the twentieth century saw significant changes in both the social character of social welfare and the role of the state in providing or promoting welfare. This section reviews the main dimensions of the post-war settlements and the principal directions of change.

2.1   The settlements

Throughout this book great emphasis has been placed on the idea of settlement as a conceptual means of understanding the complex nature of the thing we call 'the welfare state'. We have emphasized that the settlements, past and present, around social welfare should not be viewed as a case of complete unity or consensus, but rather as the outcome of compromise and accommodation between different social interests. They not only reflect but also result in both privileged and subordinated/marginalized inclusions as well as systematic exclusions of specific categories of people. Let us begin with the political and economic settlements – which in combination produced what is often referred to as the 'social democratic consensus'.

2.1.1   The political and economic settlements

What were the key components of the social democratic consensus identified by Kavanagh and Morris (1994) in Chapter 1, section 5.1?

According to Kavanagh and Morris, the key components of this cross-party political consensus included a commitment to:

- the 'mixed economy', including both public and private enterprise;
- a role for government in economic planning and in identifying and promoting the conditions for national economic goals;
- government action to promote full (male) employment;
- the provision of a structure of welfare benefits and services for citizens of the UK.

The foundation stone of this consensus was the assumption of – and policies directed towards – the creation of continued economic growth. The consensus emerged in what might be called cross-class and cross-party forms. It was carried through 'corporatist' arrangements between the representatives of 'big capital' and 'organized labour' (typically the Confederation of British Industry and the Trades Union Congress at national level). It was also sustained by a relatively high degree of agreement between the main political parties about the management of the economy by government. This economic 'settlement' (see Chapter 1, section 5.2) combined a number of elements:

- the view that a 'reformed', 'managed' or 'moderated' capitalism could provide economic growth without economic crises;
- the commitment to state economic management through macro-economic Keynesian policies;
- the acceptance of corporatist bargaining arrangements between capital and labour (which were seen as the major contending social interests), with government as the 'neutral arbiter' of conflicts of interest.

We noted in Chapter 1 that there were party political differences within this consensus, regarding both economic and social policies, but that these were framed by the common, overarching assumptions about the relationship between the state, the market and welfare. As a consequence, the broad framework of welfare provision became a relatively taken-for-granted element of the post-war consensus. The state provision of welfare thus emerged as one of the apparently unchangeable commitments of post-war UK government policy. Welfare provision appeared to be the inevitable duty of the state even though there might be party disagreements about the *levels* of benefits and services provided. There was a shared assumption that there would be public welfare programmes funded from public expenditure raised through general taxation and national insurance.

2.1.2   The social settlement

The welfare state was embedded in a set of assumptions about the social order of society in the UK – or 'pictures of the nation' – in which the expected or desired relationships between 'the Family', 'Work' and 'the Nation' were delineated. These relationships can be seen as mutually reinforcing or sustaining. Full male employment (to be maintained by state action) enabled men to earn a 'family wage'. The 'family wage' was supposed to 'keep' or sustain a family – including a housewife/mother – which in turn would be a self-sufficient social unit. Occasionally, there would be welfare needs that could not be met through the market or the family for which the state would be required to make collective provision so as to enable all citizens to lead full and useful lives (or to be cared for, if they were deemed unable to care for themselves). We have seen that these assumptions also articulated conceptions of class, gender, 'race', able-bodiedness and age in structures of both privileged and subordinated/marginalized inclusion as well as patterns of structured exclusion. To the extent that the Beveridgean welfare state addressed issues of social inequality and social redistribution, these were largely understood in terms of 'socio-economic groups' (sometimes called classes). Other axes of division, 'difference' or inequality were conceived of as belonging to 'nature' – that is, the perceived biology of 'race', gender, age and disability tended to make them invisible as *social* divisions (see **Saraga, 1998**).

2.1.3   The organizational settlement

Despite the diversity and complexity of the institutional arrangements of the welfare state – combining central and local government bodies as well as creating new services such as the National Health Service (NHS) – these institutions shared common elements. In particular, Chapter 1, section 5.4 suggested that the organizing principles of bureau-professionalism formed a common thread in the development of the old welfare state. Welfare services and benefits were produced and delivered through large-scale professional bureaucracies in which specific forms of knowledge and expertise provided the means of ensuring 'public service'. Although the balance between professionalism and bureaucracy differed between welfare services – for example, with medical professionalism predominating in the NHS, but with bureaucracy providing the dominant principle in social security – the welfare state was ordered around the combination of these organizational principles.

What were the social implications of professionalism and bureaucracy for conceptions of public service?

3   Towards new settlements?

Chapter 2 plotted the growth of criticisms of the welfare state from the late 1970s, especially both from the New Right and from critical voices 'from below' challenging the social inequalities and injustices of welfare provision. It was also argued that the New Right appropriated some of the criticisms made by the voices 'from below' and that it became the dominant critic of the 'old' welfare settlement. We saw that there were three main themes to the New Right's arguments about state welfare:

1   the proper role of the state (and the need for selectively 'rolling back' the state);

2   the costs of state welfare (in apparently excessive spending and the stifling of initiative and enterprise);

3   the effects of state welfare (particularly the assumed creation of dependency).

Both Chapter 2 and Chapter 9 also pointed out that these themes about the state and welfare were linked to four major imperatives of reform and restructuring after the mid 1970s in the UK. These were:

1   the economic imperative based on financial reform, cost containment and the search for 'value for money';

2   the drive to break up established organizational hierarchies through processes of devolution, decentralization and, in some cases, centralization;

3   the introduction of quasi-markets and competition within social welfare provision;

4   the imperative of creating 'more and better' management as the condition of a more efficient, effective and economic provision of social welfare.

Again, it is vital to remember that these imperatives were not just neutral, improved 'technologies' of governance. Rather, as Chapter 9 pointed out, they were aimed at transforming the underlying organizational and political principles of the social democratic welfare state in the UK.

3.1   A new political settlement?

The New Right put radical reforms of social welfare and the state into the centre of political debate in the UK. By the late 1990s, it was clear that their efforts had been successful, at least to the extent that there were very few arguments that the country could – or should – return to the 'old' welfare state. The extensive restructuring of social welfare undertaken by the Conservative governments of the 1980s and 1990s established the basis for a new political settlement with regard to social welfare and the state. By the late 1990s the Labour party, and the Blair government elected in 1997, appeared to have accepted the main framework of assumptions developed by the preceding Thatcher and Major Conservative governments. It is also crucial to note that this new political settlement was also part of a wider agenda regarding the UK economy, its defects and the 'solution' to these problems.

Chapter 2 outlined how the critique of the 'nanny state' opened up a series of opportunities for critics of the 'old' welfare state. The chapter usefully summarized the critique in terms of the models of the 'old' and 'restructured' welfare regimes, shown here in Table 10.1.

Look at Table 10.1 and think about how these notions resurfaced in the particular areas of welfare examined in Chapters 3 to 8. You might find it helpful to refer back, and perhaps add to, your notes on those chapters concerning this issue.

Table 10.1 Contrasting the 'old' and 'restructured' welfare regimes

'Old'	'Restructured'
Disincentive	Incentive
Dependence	Independence
Irresponsibility	Responsibility
Constraint	Opportunity

The New Right self-consciously attacked and unlocked the old institutional arrangements of the 'corporatist' settlement and the negotiating spaces and rights of organized labour. This was part of a concerted attack on what were described as 'special' or 'vested' interests, whose activities were seen as antithetical to the workings of either free markets or efficient public services. Such vested interests included trade unions, local government officials and councillors, and, especially, the 'liberal welfare professions', such as teachers, social workers and doctors. But, in addition to remaking the institutional arrangements of the old welfare state, the New Right also changed the conception of the 'proper role of the state' – redefining what government could and should be expected to do. In relation to social welfare, this meant shifting 'responsibility' from government to the market, individuals and families as a way of breaking the 'culture of dependency' and promoting initiative and choice. Increasingly, this meant government 'at a distance', acting 'at arm's length' through agencies, contracts or devolved powers. Chapter 2 described these changes as 'realigned statecraft' – the creation of new relations, processes and practices of governing.

To what extent do *you* think it is reasonable to suggest that a new political settlement has been established?

3.2 A new economic settlement?

We saw throughout Chapters 2 to 9 that the market came to occupy the centre stage in discourses on welfare and in social policy in the last two decades of the twentieth century. The virtues of the market as a self-regulating system were attributed an almost magical status. It was argued by many on the Right that markets, freed from government interference, would produce what customers wanted at the keenest prices through the co-ordination of the market's 'invisible hand'. In reshaping the role of government, these arguments were influential both in reducing the role of the state in macroeconomic management (setting markets free both nationally and internationally) and in supporting government action to remove 'blockages' to free markets (such as government 'regulation' or 'red tape' and trade union bargaining rights). Setting 'enterprise' free came to be defined as the first – if not the only – obligation of government.

It was argued that these advantages of markets could be applied to the provision of welfare services just as much as to conventional goods and services: creating what we may term the 'shopping around' or 'consumerist' model of social welfare. However, in practice, the new welfare system was characterized not by markets in a pure form but by market-like relationships and processes that were effectively created, managed and regulated by the state. These are now generally termed 'quasi-markets' (Le Grand and Bartlett, 1993). Distinctions between purchasers and providers became established in a range of public services – including health care and social care – as ways of promoting market-like behaviour. Such distinctions operated both between organizations (for example, district health authorities purchasing health services from hospital trusts) and within organizations (with service units selling their services to central planning and purchasing departments).

As with the political settlement, many of these elements had become institutionalized as the new, taken-for-granted arrangements of the relationships between the economy and the state by the end of the 1990s. This applied to the general pattern of relationships between the state and the national economy, such that 'free markets' remained the symbolic reference point for economic growth and social well being. But the development of market-like relationships in social welfare and the move away from direct provision by public bodies towards 'welfare pluralism' also became part of the new political landscape (Rao, 1996).

3.3   A new social settlement?

Critics on the Right and Left in the 1970s and 1980s were increasingly sceptical about the Beveridgean image of the British way of life (namely nuclear families comprising husband, wife and children, with the husband as breadwinner). This image was viewed as increasingly disconnected from the more complex reality of lifestyles and households. For those on the Right, this pointed to the failure of the state to support and enforce the 'normal' way of life and the role of the 'traditional' family within it. In contrast, those on the Left argued that the state still favoured such traditional arrangements and thus disadvantaged alternative forms of domestic living. We saw in Chapter 2 that there were also social and demographic factors at work in challenging the old welfare regime beyond these particular ideological onslaughts, such as the changing patterns of need associated with the steady increase in numbers of people over retirement age, the changing patterns of employment and unemployment, and changes in household structure, all taking place in a context of limited economic growth and rising social inequalities.

Out of this crisis of the social settlement emerged a new discourse based on the idea of the 'active citizen' and the virtues of self-reliance and voluntarism. In the last two decades of the twentieth century there was an explicit reassertion of voluntarism, particularly in terms of the role of 'the family' and 'the community' in social welfare. At this point we should note that welfare outcomes have always been the product of complex processes of interaction between public-, voluntary-

and private-sector provision, built around highly gendered assumptions about informal care in households and communities. However, with the new settlement, such voluntarism was explicitly developed around the notion of 'the mixed economy' of welfare rather than around a unified welfare state. It has been argued that we are currently witnessing the rise of what has been termed 'privatized prudentialism' (O'Malley, 1992) as the emergent rationale for 'governance' of welfare subjects. According to this new rationale, it is expected that individuals will privately calculate their own risks and opportunities in the realm of social welfare in contrast to previous, collective forms of risk management.

To some extent, this new set of assumptions addressed the more visible patterns of social diversity in terms of individualized differences – understanding them as the different wants or needs of individual consumers. This conception of differences thus fed the more 'market-like' restructurings of welfare. However, this left other issues about the composition of the contemporary social settlement – or at least the dominant set of assumptions about the desired social order – unresolved. Differences as structured divisions and inequalities remained a contested issue – whether around class, 'race', gender, 'ability' or age. Such problems gave rise to tensions between pressure for equalities of opportunity and citizenship rights on the one hand and the wish to restore 'traditional morality' on the other. There may therefore be doubts as to whether a new social settlement had emerged by the late 1990s.

3.4   A new organizational settlement?

In the remaking of the relationship between social welfare and the state, it was not just 'welfare' that changed but also the institutional arrangements and organizational processes through which social welfare was produced and distributed. As Chapter 9 demonstrated, new organizational forms were accompanied by a shift to 'managerialism' in the new form of the state. In these processes power relationships were reordered; most dramatically, bureau-professional power was challenged and increasingly subordinated to the 'decisional calculus' of managerial power. Here we saw the rise to dominance of a narrow 'economistic' view of how to evaluate social policies. This development involved the spread of modes of financial calculation and budgetary obligations to areas previously governed according to bureaucratic, professional and other norms (Rose, 1996, p.351). Rose has argued that the effects of this shift have been to give an accounting value to issues that were previously subject to the esoteric languages of the designated expert.

What might be the benefits of this new approach for the lay person using public services?

According to Rose, it is likely that this 'no-nonsense' accounting model may have punctured the enclosures within which many forms of expertise in the past were able to insulate themselves from 'political interference'. It also shifted power to other forms of expertise – accountants and managers – and changed the terms in which experts calculate and enact their expertise. The mechanism of the audit would seem to have replaced the 'trust' that government – and perhaps members of the public – invested in professional wisdom and the decisions of experts. The services to be delivered were defined in terms of measurable goals and targets (Rose, 1996, pp.351–2). Clarke and Newman (1997) have argued that this process of managerialization in social welfare has had 'perverse effects' on the policies, processes and practices of welfare provision. For example, the pressure on welfare providers to be 'business-like' encourages behaviour that tries to reduce costs rather than meet needs. So, the care needs of older people became a focus of disputes between health and social services, as neither wished to face the costs of meeting these needs. This move to managerialized co-ordination of social welfare may not have been wholly beneficial to service-users, since it subjected them to new forms of decision-making, new criteria and new evaluations of their worth or costs to the organization.

These processes were also part of the rise of what we earlier called government 'at a distance': the organizational co-ordination of services realized through 'arm's length' agencies, through contractual arrangements for the purchase of services and through new forms of 'partnership' between statutory and private or voluntary agencies and members of 'the public'. Notions of partnership became particularly evident in legislation on children, families and community care, in crime prevention strategies and in social housing policy. As a consequence of such developments, the delivery of services was increasingly organized through independent agencies and co-ordinated and regulated through formal agencies of the state (that is, the state acting as an 'enabler' rather than as a direct provider of services). Even where agencies were not directly independent of the state (such as most hospitals, the probation service and most schools), the mechanisms of state delivery were restructured to imitate the forms of such independent, business-like agencies. In these new structures and relationships the connecting thread was the recurrent claim that 'more and better management' would be the key to making them work effectively.

Chapter 9, section 5 focused on the way in which the new managerial discourse did not distinguish between the public realm and private enterprise. Four main paradoxes of managerialism are noted in Chapter 9, which were also visible throughout the discussions in Chapters 3 to 8. These relate to the tension between:

1   standardization and flexibility;

2   centralization and decentralization;

3   empowerment and control;

4   the different 'logics' of managerial versus political accountability.

You may wish to look back at Chapters 3 to 8 to see how these tensions were played out in particular sectors of social policy.

4   Subjects in welfare restructuring

Section 7.1 of Chapter 2 explained the meaning of 'subject' as we have employed it in this book. You will recall that the 'subject' was contrasted with 'naturalized' notions such as that of the 'individual' as used in common sense. It was also pointed out that the concept of subject is linked to the perspective of 'social constructionism' (see **Saraga, 1998**). The chapter emphasized six key points in connection with the idea of the 'subject'. These were that:

1   Subjects are constantly 'made up', constructed or constituted during their life-times (that is, 'what we are' is not fixed from birth or as a result of any essential characteristic).

2   Subjects are 'made up' within webs of intersecting relations and through processes of recognition.

3   Subjects are statuses or positions in a field of knowledge (or what we have termed 'discourses').

4   Subjects are constructed through the operation and contestation of power and are also the targets of the practical power of welfare practitioners.

5   Subjects are constituted psychically (that is, our 'self' of self-identity and psychological being derives in part from our subject status).

6   Subjects have identities (which are shared with others, associated with 'belonging' to a particular category of person).

These points should be borne in mind in any discussion of the changing subjects of welfare which follow.

4.1   'Old' welfare subjects

Chapter 1, section 5.3 suggested that the Beveridgean welfare state's social settlement enshrined a powerful representation of the welfare subject at its heart as the white, British, male, able-bodied, 'worker/father/husband' citizen. We also saw in Chapters 1 and 2 that the creation of this subject was the result of, and had the consequence of, the construction of forms of subordinated inclusion – or even the exclusion of whole categories of the population in the UK from the status of being a citizen. Chapter 1 showed us that, in the demographics of the immediate post-war period, the nation was also ideologically represented as a homogenous 'British race'. By the 1970s and 1980s this social settlement had been subject to a profound destabilization, not least due to challenges from women, black people, gay men, lesbians and disabled people aimed at overcoming their apparent 'invisibility' in the old social settlement of the Beveridgean welfare state. The myths of universalism and of a unified people embodied in this 'old' welfare state were thus exposed.

4.2   'New' welfare subjects

The dismantling of the old welfare state in the UK and elsewhere (Esping-Anderson, 1996) was coupled with the implementation of the principles of economic and political individualism. This was perhaps most succinctly summed up in the New Right's rhetorical conception of 'the enterprise culture'. Together with the subjects constituted by the formation of new social movements, these political changes inaugurated and brought to life 'new' welfare subjects as detailed in Chapter 2, section 7. Furthermore, Chapter 8 noted in the discussion of income maintenance that particular policies define who is 'poor' and who is or is not 'deserving', thus producing the 'subjects' of this field of welfare. The chapter went on to make the crucial point that policies also 'help to frame the way in which we interpret and understand the world and what is possible within it' (Chapter 8, section 1). This is an important point to bear in mind across all the sites of welfare which we have covered in this book. In a similar manner, Chapter 9 argued that new discourses, in this case the managerialist discourse, have the important effect of 'making up' new ways for people to conduct themselves – for example, in the shift from *social work professional* to *social care manager*.

ACTIVITY 10.3

Think back to Chapter 9, section 3 on the discourse of managerialism. Bearing in mind conceptions of the 'citizen' and the 'client' in the social democratic discourse of the Beveridgean welfare state, can you remember the key changes in terminology that occurred in the notion of the 'welfare subject' in the new discourse of managerialism?

COMMENT

In the new discourse of managerialism, the terms 'consumer' and 'customer' increasingly replaced those of 'client' and 'citizen'. This shift of emphasis was part of the break-up of what may be called the old welfare bureaucracy and paternalism and of their replacement by an emphasis on entrepreneurialism and individual initiative.

■ ■ ■

5 Trends and variations: the uneven impact of reconstruction

So far we have emphasized the general trends of welfare restructuring. However, it would be misleading to treat these processes as if they have had a uniform impact across the whole range of welfare services. It is clear from reading Chapters 3 to 8, which deal with specific forms of welfare, that, while all these forms of welfare have been subject to change, they have not all changed in the same way or at the same speed. The general trends of welfare restructuring have been played out in specific ways in the different areas of welfare, some giving greater emphasis to 'marketizing' reforms while others were dominated by strong cost-control pressures. There are a number of reasons for these processes of *uneven development* and it is worth taking a little time to think about why these general trends and tendencies might have worked out differently in the particular welfare services discussed in this book.

The first, and most obvious, point is that they have involved the restructuring of a welfare state which was not a single, simple and monolithic institution. As we have seen, 'the welfare state' was a convenient term for referring to a set of institutional arrangements, policies and practices and formed an important public and political symbol. Nevertheless, the policy, practice and organizational realities were much more complex. So the processes of restructuring have addressed different starting-points of policy and practice within the welfare state. For example, the reconstruction of the benefits system posed different problems of reform from those presented by the NHS.

In one sense, this issue of divergent starting-points is a policy and organizational matter. The organizational character of benefit administration was different in important respects from that of the NHS. But it is also worth thinking about these differences in terms of political and social symbolism. Distinct parts of the welfare state were used by and, to some extent, politically supported by different social groups or constituencies. So, Le Grand (1990) pointed to the relative protection that had been given to some policy areas (health and education spending, for example) because they were seen as important to the political support for the government among the middle classes. But there may also have been issues beyond this narrow conception of party support. There were also significant differences about which aspects of the welfare state commanded widespread public respect and loyalty. Those aspects most associated with universalism and mutual support and protection continued to command much more public enthusiasm and support than did more narrowly focused or targeted benefits and services. In this sense, the NHS in particular 'stood for' something more than just the provision of health care services and proved a difficult target for reform as a consequence.

Second, it is important to recognize that the institutional components of the welfare state were not just the passive recipients of reforming action by government. There were significant differences between parts of the welfare state in terms of policy, practice and power. As all the earlier chapters have indicated, the organizational processes of welfare provision were the focus of conflict in the restructuring. Some groups – the medical profession in particular – were better able than others to defend aspects of professional autonomy and control of work processes and resources. Such issues had consequences for the pace and scale of change and also shaped which trends and tendencies had most impact in particular welfare areas. This 'active' sense of institutional practices and power was not only important in the reformation of public-sector organizations, it also played a role in the way in which the voluntary and private sectors were looked to for a greater involvement in some areas of welfare provision. So, for example, plans to reform the benefits system in the mid 1980s stalled when it became clear that the private-sector financial institutions did not wish to take over the whole pensions process, preferring to concentrate on narrower, but more profitable, 'niche markets'.

Third, although the 1980s and 1990s saw extensive reconstruction of the welfare state, it is worth noting that the emphasis of reform changed during this period such that aspects of welfare varied according to when they were reformed. Although, as Chapter 9 pointed out, all agencies of welfare have been confronted by a centrally driven search for greater economy and efficiency aimed at the reduction of public spending costs, the means of achieving this changed, as did the other policy objectives being pursued alongside this overriding quest for economy. So we could point, for instance, to the processes affecting public housing (an early target for reform) where the model of 'privatization' or 'selling off' public assets dominated, in contrast to the introduction of market-like mechanisms into the public sector, such as internal markets in the NHS (a much later phase of reform).

Finally, we also need to bear in mind that processes of reform rarely work out exactly as the reformers claimed or intended (and, of course, what they 'claimed' might not be the same as what they 'intended'). Although there are many reasons for this, one which has been particularly important in the context of this book is how reforms are received in the institutions being reformed. This issue is of special significance for the reconstruction of the welfare state in the late twentieth century because so many of the reforms were addressed to the organizational processes and relationships of welfare provision and delivery. The 'organizational settlement' occupied a central role in these changes. So, despite the common tendency towards managerialized control, the way in which managerialism has affected forms of welfare organization has varied. As Chapter 9 suggested, 'the processes of accommodation between bureau-professionalism and managerialism' took different forms in different sectors. This relates to what Pollitt (1995) referred to as the important task of 'theorizing contexts' in studying the reform of public services. What we have tried to do in this book is to strike a balance between attending to the general trends and tendencies of reconstruction and recognizing the specific contexts of welfare services and sites that were the target of reform.

ACTIVITY 10.4

Before you leave this section, you may find it helpful to use Table 10.2, opposite, as a way of summarizing the impact of change in the different welfare areas discussed in Chapters 3 to 8. You could use it for making notes on the way in which any of the specific areas of social welfare that you have read about have been involved in the deconstruction and reconstruction of the political, economic, social and organizational settlements.

6   Conclusion: a new welfare order?

This book suggests that there has been no simple and uniform shift from the 'old' welfare state to a 'new' welfare order in the UK. Nevertheless, it is clear that there were some strong trends and tendencies that were visible across most of the forms of welfare restructuring. These are especially associated with the emergence of new political, economic and organizational settlements. Above all, the new political–economic consensus that had emerged by the late 1990s seemed to frame questions about the role, purpose and limits of state-provided welfare in very distinctive ways. The increasing subordination of social policy to the 'needs of the economy' – understood as combining low taxation, low regulation and high labour 'flexibility' – implied a structural move away from the Beveridgean model of a welfare state. The emphasis on controlling public spending, both as a means of ensuring low personal taxation and as a way of making the UK economy more 'competitive' in world markets, had shaped the approach of both Labour and Conservative governments to social welfare in this period. This had led some analysts to talk about a new political consensus – represented in terms such as 'Blaijorism' as a way of linking convergences between the Conservative Party after Thatcher and the Blair-inspired 'New Labour' Party. Some commentators dubbed this emergent new consensus the attempt to create 'Thatcherism with a human face'. Despite some party differences, this new settlement was framed by a common view of the economic problems and of the limited role of government in relation to markets (Hay, 1996). Hay's argument stressed the ways in which this new consensus inhabited a political terrain whose main parameters were inherited from the New Right (or Thatcherite) transformations of the economy, society and politics of the UK during the 1980s and early 1990s.

Table 10.2 Impact of change in the different areas of welfare

AREA/SERVICE	SETTLEMENTS			
	Political	Economic	Social	Organizational
Health				
Housing				
Probation				
Education				
Social care				
Income maintenance				

Hills (1993) argued that some aspects of the welfare state needed to be seen as a continuing 'success story' in their capacity for delivering provision for inescapable needs such as health care and education. However, he also noted that, with one in six of the population in the early 1990s dependent on the safety net of income support, this was hardly indicative of the triumph of the welfare state. Rather, it is a sign that the welfare state had been picking up the pieces of failure elsewhere in the economy. Indeed, it might be that the wider issues around national (social and economic) regeneration may be the most crucial factors for the future of welfare in the next century (Hills, 1993, p.84). The placing of social welfare in these terms, however, indicated its increasing subservience to objectives defined in terms of national economic performance. This result was reflected in calculations suggesting that forms of social inequality or social exclusion should be a matter of public concern because they are indicative of inefficiency rather than because they are 'unjust' (Mandelson, 1997).

These new political and economic settlements seemed to have guaranteed that there would be 'no going back' to the old model of the welfare state, in terms either of its cost, its social purposes or its organizational structures. Certainly, the reformed structures of welfare – towards more mixed economies, markets and managerialism – looked to be firmly established by the late 1990s. So, too, were the rationales for them: the claims for their ability to be effective, economic and efficient; to provide value for money; and to be flexible and responsive to users/customers in a more complex society. The discourses of managerialism and marketization formed the basis of the emerging, cross-party, political–economic consensus about how best to run welfare organizations. As Chapter 9 suggested, we might best see managerialism as the 'glue' which holds the new organizational forms of social welfare together in a fragile unity. In the face of pressures towards fragmentation and disintegration resulting from competition, contracting and new budgetary responsibilities, managerialism promised to make things work and provided a culture shared by many welfare organizations (no matter in which sector they might be based). At the same time, however, the chapters in this book have argued that managerialism and marketization were unable to resolve the continuing tensions and instabilities of the social settlement. Some of these involved the inability to establish new norms for the contemporary formations of 'Family', 'Work' and 'Nation'; some related to the links between social welfare and forms of social difference; while others manifested themselves particularly around the mistrust between citizens and political representatives and institutions in conditions of complexity, dynamics and diversity that characterized UK society at the end of the twentieth century. There were continuing tensions between the discourses of citizens as legitimate members of a political society, citizens as consumers and citizens as self-reliant providers within families and communities. Some of these issues are explored in **Hughes (1998)**.

In this book we have shown that the welfare state, in both its Beveridgean and restructured forms, has been a major site of continuing political and social conflict. The involvement of the state in social welfare has been constantly contested, particularly around the following questions:

■ What is the social purpose of welfare provision? (Should it redress inequalities and injustices? Should it maintain a 'way of life' and a social order? Should it promote economic efficiency?)

- What is the proper role of the state? (How should the state be involved: as an agency of political intervention or by adopting a 'hands-off' stance and allowing individuals and communities to meet their own needs through the market?)

- How is welfare to be provided? (Should it be universally, as of right; selectively, on the basis of tests of means and desert; as a broad social strategy through state welfare services; or as a residual/minimal safety net to back up market choices?)

- Who are the people/the public who are to be served by social welfare? (What 'pictures of the nation' are to be reproduced through welfare policies and provisions?)

During the last two decades of the twentieth century, we witnessed the transformation of the 'old' welfare state in the UK. The social and political struggles over its future resulted in the phrase 'the welfare state' becoming less and less meaningful as a way of conceptualizing the purpose, place and practices of social welfare. The restructuring of the welfare state involved changes in both of its words: welfare and state. Social welfare was reformed to make it more efficient, more 'targeted', more rationed, more selective, more productive of 'independence'. Similarly, the state itself was reformed to create new institutional structures and processes that promoted efficiency, economy and flexibility, together with new forms of control and accountability. In the process of reform, though, the relationship between the state and social welfare was itself changed. The state's role as the primary provider declined, although most welfare provision has remained publicly funded. Rather, the state's role became the engagement of a range of diverse organizations, families and individuals in the production and distribution of social welfare: what is conventionally termed the 'mixed economy of welfare' or 'welfare pluralism' (Rao, 1996). Although the state still directed these processes, they constituted something other than a 'welfare state'.

References

Clarke, J. and Newman, J. (1997) *The Managerial State*, London, Sage.

Esping-Anderson, G. (ed.) (1996) *Welfare States in Transition*, London, Sage.

Hay, A.C. (1996) *Re-stating Social and Political Change*, Buckingham, Open University Press.

Hills, J. (1993) *The Future of the Welfare State: A Guide to the Debate*, York, Joseph Rowntree Foundation.

Hughes, G. (ed.) (1998) *Imagining Welfare Futures*, London, Routledge in association with The Open University.

Kavanagh, D. and Morris, P. (1994) *Consensus Politics from Attlee to Major* (2nd edn), Oxford, Blackwell.

Le Grand, J. (1990) 'The state of welfare', in Hills, J. (ed.) *The State of Welfare: The Welfare State in Britain Since 1974*, Oxford, Clarendon.

Le Grand, J. and Bartlett, W. (eds) (1993) *Quasi-Markets and Social Policy*, Basingstoke, Macmillan.

Mandelson, P. (1997) Speech to the Fabian Society, 14 August.

O'Malley, P. (1992) 'Risk, power and crime prevention', *Economy and Society*, vol.21, no.3, pp.251–68.

Pollitt, C. (1995) 'Justification by works or by faith? Evaluating the new public management', *Evaluation*, vol.1, no.2, pp.133–54.

Rao, N. (1996) *Towards Welfare Pluralism: Public Services in a Time of Change*, Aldershot, Dartmouth Publishing Company.

Rose, N. (1996) 'The death of the social? Refiguring the territory of government', *Economy and Society*, vol.25, no.3, pp.321–56.

Saraga, E. (ed.) (1998) ***Embodying the Social: Constructions of Difference***, **London, Routledge in association with The Open University.**

Acknowledgements

Grateful acknowledgement is made to the following sources for permission to reproduce material in this book:

Text

Chapter 1: *Royal Commission On Population Report* (1949), Crown copyright is reproduced with the permission of the Controller of Her Majesty's Stationery Office; ***Chapter 2:*** *The Patient's Charter* (1991), Crown copyright is reproduced with the permission of the Controller of Her Majesty's Stationery Office; ***Chapter 3:*** Green, D.G. (1996) *The New Right: The Counter Revolution in Political, Economic and Social Thought,* Harvester Wheatsheaf; Lister, J. (1988) *Cutting the Lifeline: The Fight for the NHS,* Journeyman Press Ltd; Timmins, N. (1996) *The Five Giants: A Biography of the Welfare State,* HarperCollins Publishers Ltd; Owen, CH, Lord D. (1976) 'Patient, help thyself', *The Sunday Times,* 3 October 1976, courtesy of the Right Honourable Lord David Owen, CH; Calman, K. *The Chief Medical Officer's Challenge,* Department of Health, Crown copyright is reproduced with the permission of the Controller of Her Majesty's Stationery Office; Skrabanek, P. (1994) *The Death of Humane Medicine and the Rise of Coercive Healthism,* The Social Affairs Unit; ***Chapter 4:*** Page, D. (1993) *Building for Communities: A Study of New Housing Association Estates,* Joseph Rowntree Foundation; Burrows, L. and Walentowicz, P. (1992) *Homes Cost Less than Homelessness,* Shelter; Bulgin, S. (1994) 'The sinister arrangement for black homeless people', *Black Housing,* March–April 1994, Federation of Black Housing Organisations; ***Chapter 5:*** *Probation Services in England & Wales: Statement of National Objectives & Priorities* (1984), Crown copyright is reproduced with the permission of the Controller of Her Majesty's Stationery Office; Patten, J. (1992) 'The Criminal Justice Act 1991 – the underlying philosophy', *The Magistrate,* 48(2), March 1992, Magistrates' Association; Worthington, M. (1990) 'The responsibility of probation officers – letter to the editor', *The Independent,* 31 January 1990; *Home Office: Control and Management of Probation Services in England & Wales* (1989), Crown copyright is reproduced with the permission of the Controller of Her Majesty's Stationery Office; *National Standards for the Supervision of Offenders in the Community* (1992), Crown copyright is reproduced with the permission of the Controller of Her Majesty's Stationery Office; Blatch, Lady (1995) 'Quality recruitment', *The Guardian,* 18 October 1995; Henry, W. (1995) 'Criminal cuts that will increase crime', *The Guardian,* 22 November 1995; ***Chapter 6:*** Green, K.G. (1975) 'Why comprehensives fail', from Cox, C.B. and Boyson, R. (eds) *Black Paper 1975,* J.M. Dent, The Orion Publishing Group Limited; *The Omega File: Education Policy,* Adam Smith Institute; ***Chapter 7:*** *Making a Reality of Community Care: A Report by the Audit Commission* (1986), Crown copyright is reproduced with the permission of the Controller of Her Majesty's Stationery Office; *Working Together Under the Children Act 1989: A Guide to Arrangements for Inter-agency Co-operation for the Protection of Children from Abuse* (1991), Crown copyright is reproduced with the permission of the Controller of Her Majesty's Stationery Office; *Progress Through Change: The Fifth Annual Report of the Chief Inspector Social Services Inspectorate 1995/96* (1996), Crown copyright is reproduced with the permission of the Controller of Her Majesty's Stationery Office; ***Chapter 8:*** Cohen, M. (1945) *I Was One of the Unemployed,* Victor

Gollancz Limited; Beveridge, Sir W. (1942) *Social Insurance and Allied Services*, Crown copyright is reproduced with the permission of the Controller of Her Majesty's Stationery Office; *Jobseekers Allowance: Helping You Back to Work* (*c*.1996), Crown copyright is reproduced with the permission of the Controller of Her Majesty's Stationery Office; Brown, G. (1996) 'A chance to start again', *Community Care*, 28 November–4 December 1996, Reed Business Publishing Ltd; Willetts, D. (1997) *Why Vote Conservative?*, reproduced by permission of Penguin Books Ltd; **Chapter 9:** Brindle, D. (1996) 'NHS chiefs criticised over deaths', © *The Guardian*, 20 June 1995; Jervis, P. and Richards, S. (1997) 'Raising our game', *Public Money and Management*, 17 (1997) 1–3, CIPFA; Lane, J.E. (1995) *The Public Sector: Concepts, Models and Approaches* (second edition), reprinted by permission of Sage Publications Ltd: Eliassen, K.A and Kooiman, J. (1993) *Managing Public Organizations: Lessons from Contemporary European Experience*, reprinted by permission of Sage Publications Ltd.

Photographs/Illustrations

p.7: Getty Images; *pp.11, 12:* Solo Syndication. Cartoon supplied by The Centre for the Study of Cartoons and Caricature, University of Kent at Canterbury; *p.20 (left):* Getty Images; *p.20 (right):* Val Wilmer Photography; *p.28 (top):* The Advertising Archives; *p.28 (bottom):* Getty Images; *p.30:* Imperial War Museum, London; *p.31:* Getty Images; *p.51: Independent on Sunday*, 5 December 1993, © *The Independent*; *pp.56, 61:* Format Photographers; *p.66:* Brent Community Health Council; *p.76:* Mark Power/Network; *p.84:* Murray, M./Format Photographs; *p.85:* Kobal Collection; *p.87:* Isherwood, P./Format Photographs; *p.97:* P.A. News Photo Library; *p.103: Eight Guidelines for a Healthy Diet*, © 1996 Crown copyright is reproduced with the permission of the Controller of Her Majesty's Stationery Office; *p.113:* Press Association; *p.118:* Alan Wylie; *p.122: Socialism and Housing Action; p.125: The New Statesman*, 20 December 1996, © Tim Major; *p.128: Private Eye*, 18 July 1980, © Ken Pyne; *p.130:* reproduced by permission of *Punch*; *p.133: Architects' Journal; p.139:* © Paul Smith; *p.165:* Ronald Grant Archive; *p.173: The Times*, 14 October 1993, © Angus Mewse; *p.185:* © *The Guardian*; *p.186:* Lee Stannard; *p.192:* © Don McPhee/ *The Guardian; p.197 (top):* © Malcolm Croft/Press Association; *p.197 (bottom left and right):* © Dave Cheskin/PA News; *p.199:* photo supplied by City Press Services; *p.219 (top): Lancashire Evening Post; p.219 (bottom):* Getty Images; *p.222:* Getty Images; *p.229:* Guzelian; *p.235:* Jeremy Long/TES; *p.236:* Steve Bell; *p.246:* reproduced by permission of Bill Stott, *p.254:* Manchester City Libraries, Local History Collection; *p.263:* Steve Bell; *p.268:* Steve Bell; *p.269:* Harry Venning; *p.297:* Getty Images; *p.300:* Getty Images; *p.301 (top):* cartoon by Sidney 'George' Strube, © Express Features plc, supplied by the Centre for the Study of Cartoons and Caricature, University of Kent at Canterbury; *p.301 (bottom):* cartoon by David Low, © Solo Syndication/*Evening Standard*, supplied by the Centre for the Study of Cartoons and Caricature, University of Kent at Canterbury; *p.302:* Getty Images; *p.310 (left and right):* Photofusion; *p.325:* reproduced by permission of *Punch*; *p.349:* Knight Features; *p.370:* Steve Bell.

Figures

Figure 4.1: Greve, J. and Currie, E. (1990) *Homelessness in Britain*, Joseph Rowntree Foundation; *p.147 (top):* Burrows, L. and Walentowicz, P. (1992) *Homes Cost Less than Homelessness*, Shelter; *Figure 4.2:* Withers, P. and Randolph, B. (1994) *Access, Homelessness and Housing Associations*, National

Housing Federation; *Figures 5.3, 5.4 and 5.5: Criminal Justice: A Working Paper, Revised Edition 1986* (1986), Crown copyright is reproduced with the permission of the Controller of Her Majesty's Stationery Office; *Figure 5.6:* Barclay, G.C. (1995) *The Criminal Justice System in England & Wales*, Crown copyright is reproduced with the permission of the Controller of Her Majesty's Stationery Office; *Figure 5.7 (top):* Barclay, G.C. (1991) *A Digest of Information on the Criminal Justice System, Crime and Justice in England & Wales*, Crown copyright is reproduced with the permission of the Controller of Her Majesty's Stationery Office; *Figure 5.7 (bottom):* Barclay, G.C. (1993) *Information on the Criminal Justice System in England & Wales,* Crown copyright is reproduced with the permission of the Controller of Her Majesty's Stationery Office; *Figure 5.9: Going Straight: Developing Good Practice in the Probation Service,* 16 October 1991, p.3, Audit Commission; *p.260: Making a Reality of Community Care: A Report by the Audit Commission* (1986), Crown copyright is reproduced with the permission of the Controller of Her Majesty's Stationery Office; *Figure 8.1:* Hills, J. (1997) *The Future of Welfare: A Guide to the Debate*, Joseph Rowntree Foundation.

Tables

Table 1.1: Stevenson, J. (1984) *British Society 1914–45*, Penguin Books Ltd; *Table 2.2: Social Trends 27*, Office for National Statistics (1997), Crown copyright is reproduced with the permission of the Controller of Her Majesty's Stationery Office; *Table 4.1:* Hills, J. (1987) 'What happened to spending on the welfare state?', Walker, A. and Walker, C., *The Growing Divide: A Social Audit 1979– 1987*, Child Poverty Action Group; *p.152:* Bulgin, S. (1994) 'The sinister arrangement for black homeless people', *Black Housing*, March–April 1994, Federation of Black Housing Organisations; *Table 6.1:* Dearing, R. Sir (1997) *Higher Education in the Learning Society* (Dearing Report), Crown copyright is reproduced with the permission of the Controller of Her Majesty's Stationery Office; *Table 9.1:* Clarke, J. and Newman, J. (1997) *The Managerial State: Power, Politics and Ideology in the Remaking of Social Welfare*, Sage Publications.

Index

The Open University Course Team

The Open University

Sally Baker	*Liaison Librarian/Picture Researcher*
Melanie Bayley	*Editor*
David Calderwood	*Project Controller*
Hilary Canneaux	*Course Manager*
John Clarke	*Author/Course Team Chair*
Allan Cochrane	*Author*
Lene Connolly	*Print Buying Controller*
Troy Cooper	*Author*
Nigel Draper	*Editor*
Ross Fergusson	*Author*
Sharon Gewirtz	*Reading Member*
Fiona Harris	*Editor*
Rich Hoyle	*Graphic Designer*
Gordon Hughes	*Author and Editor, Books 4 and 5*
Jonathan Hunt	*Co-publishing Co-ordinator*
Kate Hunter	*Editor*
Maggie Hutchinson	*Reading Member*
Sue Lacey	*Secretary*
Mary Langan	*Author and Editor, Book 3*
Patti Langton	*Producer, BBC/OUPC*
Helen Lentell	*Author*
Gail Lewis	*Author and Editor, Books 2 and 4*
Vic Lockwood	*Producer, BBC/OUPC*
Lilian McCoy	*Author*
Eugene McLaughlin	*Author*
Tara Marshall	*Print Buying Co-ordinator*
John Muncie	*Author/Co-Course Team Chair*
Pam Owen	*Graphic Artist*
Doreen Pendlebury	*Secretary*
Sharon Pinkney	*Author*
Michael Pryke	*Author*
Esther Saraga	*Author and Editor, Book 1*
Paul Smith	*Liaison Librarian/Picture Researcher*
Pauline Turner	*Course and Discipline Secretary*

External Contributors

Marian Barnes	*Author, Department of Social Policy and Social Work, University of Birmingham*
Janet English	*Tutor Panel, Region 11, The Open University*
Ian Gazeley	*Author, School of Social Sciences, University of Sussex*
Catherine Hall	*Author, Department of Sociology, University of Essex*
Mary J. Hickman	*Author, Irish Studies Centre, University of North London*
Eluned Jeffries	*Tutor Panel, Region 02, The Open University*
Chris Jones	*External Assessor, Professor of Social Work, University of Liverpool*
Gerry Mooney	*Author, Department of Applied Social Studies, University of Paisley*
Lydia Morris	*Author, Department of Sociology, University of Essex*
Janet Newman	*Author, School of Public Policy, University of Birmingham*
Lynne Poole	*Tutor Panel, Region 11, The Open University*
Pat Thane	*Author, School of Social Sciences, University of Sussex*